THE EIGHT ROLES
OF THE **MEDICAL**
TEACHER

Dedication

We dedicate this book to all the passionate and enthusiastic teachers we have met around the world who strive to provide for their students and trainees the best possible education experience.

THE EIGHT ROLES OF THE **MEDICAL TEACHER**

The purpose and functions of a teacher in the healthcare professions

Ronald M. Harden OBE MD FRCP(Glas) FRCS(Ed) FRCPC

General Secretary, AMEE – An International Association for Medical Education

Editor, Medical Teacher

Professor Emeritus Medical Education, University of Dundee, UK.

Pat Lilley BA (Hons)

Operations Director, AMEE – An International Association for Medical Education

Managing Editor, Medical Teacher.

Foreword by

John Norcini PhD

President and Chief Executive Officer, Foundation for Advancement of International Medical Education and Research (FAIMER®), USA.

ELSEVIER   Edinburgh   London   New York   Oxford   Philadelphia   St Louis   Sydney   2018

ELSEVIER

ISBN: 978-0-7020-6895-9

Executive Content Strategist: Laurence Hunter
Content Development Specialist: Carole McMurray
Project Manager: Julie Taylor
Design: Christian Bilbow
Illustration Manager: Karen Giacomucci
Illustrator: Libby Wagner
Marketing Manager: Deborah Watkins

Printed in Poland

Last digit is the print number: 9   8   7   6   5   4   3   2

Contents

Foreword

No bubble is so iridescent or floats longer than that blown by the successful teacher.

William Osler

Teachers are agents of change and they are central to the health of communities and the reform of health professions education. However, individuals often assume these responsibilities are based on their professional competence, without preparation for the roles of the teacher and without the broad support of a community of practice. Systematic faculty development, along with active participation in networks and consortia, is central to addressing these challenges and this book provides a much needed resource to support such efforts.

In Chapters 1 and 2, the authors offer an important and comprehensive framework for the competencies of teachers built around the roles they are expected to fill. This approach is consistent with the wider movement toward competency-based education, and it serves as a basis for comprehensive programs of faculty development and teacher assessment.

In the remaining chapters the authors populate this framework with practical information that will support teachers on their journey to excellence. Historically, the primary role of the teacher has been to provide information to students. Chapters 3 and 4 address this traditional role while reflecting the fact that the focus of education has shifted away from teaching and towards learning. These chapters underscore the notion that the learner-centric teacher must be able to curate information, to act as a coach, to facilitate and identify learning opportunities, and to mentor students on the path to their learning goals.

Chapters 5 and 6 explore the roles of the teacher related to curriculum and assessment but with an eye towards the increasing prominence of the learner and changes this newer focus brings about. Chapter 5 highlights the fact that the teacher not only has control over the delivery of the curriculum but also has a strong voice in its reform. Chapter 6 underscores the increasing emphasis on formative assessment, which is aimed at supporting and creating learning.

As the authors note, much of what students learn is based on observing others, especially those with more experience in their chosen field of study. This form of instruction is often unconscious, both for those learning and those teaching, and its consideration in faculty development programs has been limited. The important aim of Chapter 7 is to raise awareness about role modelling as a teacher and its potential to affect change, for both good and bad. Although they are not contiguous, it was instructive for me to consider Chapter 10 simultaneously because it addresses the critical issues of standards of behaviour and responsibilities.

Chapter 8 recognises the fact that expectations of professionals today, regardless of the discipline, include the ability to manage projects and lead teams. Fortunately, this chapter also stresses the importance of collaboration and the significant role it can play in achieving shared goals and driving reform.

Chapter 9 stresses the potential for all teachers to make scholarly contributions and the advantages this brings to teaching. Important to teachers fulfilling this role will be the implementation of a broader definition of scholarship as well as recognition of the importance of teaching in the tenure and promotion process.

Finally, Chapter 11 looks at the changing roles of the teacher today and into the future. The capstone of the chapter is a series of case studies of the roles of the teacher in practice. Their wonderful contributions to the curriculum are both instructive and inspiring.

The Eight Roles of the Medical Teacher offers a rich and accessible resource for those who are new to the field and for those of us interested in "raising our game". It fills a critical role by helping to create teachers who touch the lives of patients through the excellence of their students.

John Norcini, PhD

Preface

In education, the choice of curriculum model, learning strategy or assessment approach is important, but the evidence is that the impact of the teacher is more important. More important than whether there is a problem-based or traditional curriculum model is the quality of the teacher or trainer. The good teacher will inspire, motivate and facilitate the learning by the student or trainee (Pullias and Lockhard, 1963). But can anyone become a good teacher? What makes a good teacher? Steiner (2003), in his text, *Lessons of the Masters*, asks, "What empowers a man or a woman to teach another human being?" (p. 1) These are questions we address in this text.

Competence in the teacher's professional practice as a surgeon, dentist or nurse is important and is learned. Competence in teaching, however, is also required and like other competencies, can be learned. In faculty development programmes, in printed texts on medical education such as *A Practical Guide for Medical Teachers* (Dent et al., 2017) and in evaluations of teaching, the emphasis is on the tasks performed by a teacher – giving a lecture, leading a small group, organising problem-based learning or designing an assessment. These are important but do not represent the whole story. This book explores teaching from a different and broader perspective. It describes how we can ensure quality in teaching and job satisfaction for the teacher through a better understanding of the range of functions and roles of a teacher.

As teachers, we are concerned with what our students know, the skills they have, how they behave and for what they strive. Will they be competent to work as members of the healthcare team, meeting the needs of the population they serve? Will they have the value judgements, creativity and critical thinking that are necessary? How can we assist our students or trainees to achieve these goals? To do so effectively, we need a clear understanding of the roles we can play as teachers in the complex and difficult job of facilitating a student's learning. These roles have changed over time. The teacher is more than a dispenser of information and is recognised now as having a range of different roles in the education programme.

We describe eight key roles for the teacher or trainer. A consideration of these roles illuminates what is expected of you as a teacher and illustrates how you can more easily achieve your potential. You should be aware of and have a measure of familiarity with all eight roles described. You cannot be expected, however, to be an expert in all of the roles: as a teacher you may wish to develop particular expertise in one or more of the roles. Teachers vary in their goals, styles, idiosyncrasies, values and in the context in which they work. You should establish what is for you the most appropriate function you can fulfil in the education programme given your interests and experience. Different levels of mastery are explored in relation to each role and what is expected of all teachers, of an expert teacher and of a master teacher. For maximum effectiveness and job satisfaction, it is important that you establish your role in the education programme and how you can contribute most effectively. This book is written to assist you to do just that.

An earlier version of the teacher role model described in this book, published in AMEE (An International Association for Medical Education) Guide 20, *The good teacher is more than a lecturer – the twelve roles of the teacher* (Harden and Crosby, 2000), has been widely cited and used as a model in schools around the world for understanding the work of a teacher. It highlighted that teachers are able to identify and develop their personal role in the curriculum and that this role may be redefined and evolve over time. This book provides an updated analysis and expanded description of the roles of the teacher in the 21st century, combining some of the roles in the AMEE Guide and adding other roles not previously addressed. An understanding of the eight roles provided in this book should help you to decide what kind of teacher you want to be.

In the first chapter, we highlight the importance of the teacher in the education programme and how the teacher or trainer is critical to the success of the learner. We describe the attributes or qualities of a good teacher, including how a teacher works, not in isolation but as part of the education team, using evidence-informed practice alongside personal judgement. The second chapter provides an overview of the eight roles and how they are interconnected. The subsequent chapters describe in turn each of the roles, highlighting what is expected of a teacher, what is required of an expert teacher who has perhaps been given particular responsibilities relating to the role, and what is expected of a master teacher who is an innovator in the field relating to a particular role. The final chapter reviews the eight roles in the context of the day-to-day work of the teacher or trainer and how these roles might change in the future.

Each chapter in the book starts with a summary of the chapter's content, a quotation capturing the spirit of the chapter and a short statement highlighting the chapter's key message. The chapters close with key take-home messages, a summary of the role responsibilities of all teachers, "expert" teachers and "master" teachers, and suggestions for consideration by the teacher as to their personal role. Also provided in the "Explore further" section at the end of each chapter is a list of references which can help you to explore further the topics addressed in the chapter.

This book should be an essential read for all new teachers or trainers in medicine and the healthcare professions. It also provides a review or update for more experienced teachers, particularly those who may have been assigned new educational responsibilities. The book recognises the diverse and at times conflicting demands made of a teacher as a clinician, a basic scientist, a researcher or an administrator. An understanding of the roles of a teacher as presented in this book is relevant to education researchers and to administrators and managers, in particular, those responsible for faculty recruitment and promotion. While we have used the term "teacher" in the text and many of the examples are taken from undergraduate education, the roles described may be applied equally in postgraduate and continuing education and "trainer" may be substituted for "teacher". While the book is aimed primarily at those working in the healthcare professions, the roles described are also applicable to other professions and to higher education more generally. In the book, we address the medical teacher but the description of the roles and responsibilities is relevant to all engaged in undergraduate or postgraduate healthcare professions education.

A teacher's commitment to teaching may vary from an occasional lecture, to regular weekly clinical sessions, to responsibility for a course or curriculum and to a full-time education position with a range of educational duties. Whatever the context, being a teacher in the healthcare professions is not easy. As a teacher, you are likely to face conflicting demands, with time for teaching competing with other responsibilities including patient care, research activities or administration. Thinking of these pressures, we had two emotions in writing this book. On the one hand, we were concerned that finding time to read the book may simply add to your already full workload and be a distraction from other important activities. On the other hand, we believe that by reflecting on the issues raised and the role options presented in the book, you will be able to make more effective use of your time and ultimately to be more fulfilled.

The teacher's role framework as described in this book, reflecting both the art and science of teaching, is of value not only to help teachers and trainers to reflect on their personal work. It also has important implications for a medical school. It makes explicit an institution's commitment to teaching and to the different roles expected of a teacher; it assists with identification of the teaching skills required within an institution and highlights gaps that need to be filled; it contributes to the job specification of staff and their contracts; and it identifies the needs for staff development programmes and relates these to the requirements of individual teachers. We argue in this book that, whilst it is unrealistic to expect a teacher to be an expert in all of the roles described, expertise in all the roles needs to be recognised and represented in the faculty for the delivery of an education programme.

Essential Skills for a Medical Teacher (Harden and Laidlaw, 2017) is a companion text to this book. It looks at teaching from the perspective of the various tasks that a teacher has to perform, such as giving a lecture. Because of this, a prescriptive style was chosen. This book is different. It looks at teaching from the perspective of the functions or roles of a teacher and, while aiming to maintain both brevity and clarity, we have adopted a more personal style and approach in order to provide a flavour of what it means to be a teacher. We have included short narratives from colleagues from around the world, highlighting for them what it means to be a teacher. We have also included in the text itself personal anecdotes to provide an additional insight into the roles a teacher fulfils.

Teaching, it has been said, can be the best job in the world or the worst, depending on how you approach it. Through an appreciation of your different roles as a teacher, the aim of this book is to help you see teaching as the best job in the world. We also hope that the book will help deans, directors of postgraduate programmes, managers and administrators to assist you to achieve it. We hope that the book will also be of interest to educational researchers and will encourage more research in the area.

References

Dent, J.A., Harden, R.M., Hunt, D. (Eds.), 2017. A Practical Guide for Medical Teachers, fifth ed. Elsevier, London.

Harden, R.M., Crosby, J., 2000. AMEE Education Guide No 20: The good teacher is more than a lecturer – the twelve roles of the teacher. Med. Teach. 22 (4), 334–347.

Harden, R.M., Laidlaw, J.M., 2017. Essential Skills for a Medical Teacher. Elsevier, London.

Pullias, E.V., Lockhard, A.S., 1963. Towards Excellence in College Teaching. W.C. Brown, Dubuque, IA.

Steiner, G., 2003. Lessons of the Masters. Harvard University Press, Cambridge, MA, USA.

About the authors

Ronald M Harden

Professor Ronald Harden graduated from medical school in Glasgow, Scotland, UK. He completed training and practised as an endocrinologist before moving full time to medical education. He is Professor of Medical Education (Emeritus), University of Dundee, Editor of *Medical Teacher* and General Secretary and Treasurer of AMEE – An International Association for Medical Education.

Professor Harden has pioneered ideas in medical education, including the Objective Structured Clinical Examination (OSCE) which he first described in 1975, and has published more than 400 papers in leading journals. He is co-editor of *A Practical Guide for Medical Teachers*, now in its 5th edition, and the *Routledge International Handbook of Medical Education*. He is co-author of *Essential Skills for a Medical Teacher: An introduction to Learning and Teaching in Education*, and *The Definitive Guide to the OSCE*.

Professor Harden's contributions to excellence in medical education have attracted numerous international awards, including an OBE by Her Majesty the Queen for services to medical education, UK; the Hubbard Award by the National Board of Medical Examiners, USA; the Karolinska Institute Prize for Research in Medical Education, which recognises high-quality research in medical education; the MILES Award by the National University of Singapore; the ASME Richard Farrow Gold Medal; the AMEE Lifetime Achievement Award; and a Cura Personalis Honour, the highest award given by Georgetown University, Washington, DC, USA.

Pat Lilley

Pat Lilley joined the University of Dundee in 1995 and worked on a range of projects in the Centre for Medical Education. In 1998 she joined AMEE – An International Association for Medical Education, and has been part of its development into a leading healthcare education association, with members in over 90 countries. Now AMEE Operations Director, Pat is closely involved in all of AMEE's projects and initiatives. Since 2006, she has assisted in the development and execution of the AMEE Essential Skills in Medical Education (ESME) face-to-face and online courses for teachers, the ASPIRE-to-Excellence initiative, and AMEE's new journal *MedEdPublish*. Pat is Managing Editor of *Medical Teacher* and co-author of *The Definitive Guide to the OSCE*.

Acknowledgements

While this book is based upon our personal experiences working in medical education, we have greatly benefitted from others whose work and contributions to the field we have acknowledged in the references at the end of each chapter. We commend Geoffrey Squires' book, *Teaching as a Professional Discipline*, which addresses the question we have used in our text – "How would students learn if we were not there as their teachers?"

We are grateful to our colleagues from around the world who have contributed their own narratives which emphasise the personal nature of teaching and the satisfaction and rewards it can bring.

We would like to thank everyone who supported us in the preparation of this book, including Jake McLaughlin for work on the preparation of the manuscript, Jim Glenn whose cartoons we hope will entertain the reader, and John Norcini who has written the Foreword. Finally, we would like to thank the team from Elsevier, including Laurence Hunter, Carole McMurray and Julie Taylor, without whose support and assistance this book would not have been possible.

Ronald M Harden
Pat Lilley

Chapter 1

The medical teacher

A teacher affects eternity; he can never tell where his influence stops.

Henry Brooks Adams (1838–1918)

The teacher is a key player in the education programme. Recognised attributes distinguish a good teacher.

- The teacher is important
- The doctor as a teacher
- Challenges facing the medical teacher
- Competing demands on the teacher
  - Lack of a supportive environment or climate
  - Changes in medical education
  - Teaching as a craft and a science
- What is a good teacher?
  - Technical abilities
  - Approach to teaching

- The teacher as a professional
- The attributes of the good teacher
- Outcome frameworks and the abilities required of a teacher
- Anyone can become a good teacher
- Take-home messages
- Consider
- Explore further

The teacher is important

In recent years, emphasis has been placed on student autonomy, on student engagement with the curriculum and on students taking more responsibility for their own learning. In the ASPIRE-to-Excellence initiative, student engagement is one of the areas in which excellence in a medical school is recognised (www.aspire-to-excellence.org). There may even be a perception among teachers and others responsible for delivering the education programme that the emphasis has moved away from the teacher and closer to the student. Indeed, it has become fashionable to talk about learning and learners rather than about teaching and the teacher.

The increased prominence given to the learner may be seen by the teacher as a loss of control and power and can even lead to feelings of uncertainty, inadequacy and anxiety (Bashir, 1998). Developments in medical education, such as problem-based learning and outcome-based or competency-based education, may be associated with a concern that the teacher's role has diminished. Such perceptions, however, are wrong – they result from a misunderstanding of the role of the teacher. The teacher always has had and continues to have an important and essential role to play in the education of the student (Fig. 1.1). This is not in doubt, and it is now recognised that all doctors have teaching as an important responsibility. We describe in this book how the teacher can have a specific and identifiable effect on the student's learning. One thing that is certain, however, is that the teacher's role is changing dramatically. In *Essential Skills for a Medical Teacher* (Harden and Laidlaw, 2017), we highlighted both the traditional and newer skills or competencies expected of a teacher. In this text, we focus on the changing responsibilities of the teacher in the 21st century and the different roles the teacher now has to play in facilitating student learning.

The teacher is important, and there is good evidence from many sources that student achievement correlates with the quality of the teacher. In school classes taught by a good teacher, students perform significantly better compared with students in classes taught by a teacher who is not so good. It was found in The New Teacher Project (TNTP, 2012) in the USA that the top 20% of teachers in schools helped students learn 2 to 3 additional months' worth of mathematics and reading compared to students with average teachers and 5 to 6 months more compared to students with low-performing teachers. Just as or even more interesting was the finding that students taught by the better teachers were more likely to go to college and earn higher salaries and were less likely to be teenage parents. This long-term effect of a teacher on a student was confirmed when it was shown that the performance of a teacher in the first year of a student's course predicted students' performance in later years (Winters and Cowen, 2013). In another study in elementary education, Luyten and Snijders (1996) investigated student education achievement in different schools and the extent to which the teacher accounted for this. They found that in terms of student achievement, the difference between teachers outweighed the difference between schools. The teacher does matter. Terry Dozier (1998), in advice to the US Secretary of Education, argued that "if we don't focus on the quality of teaching, other reform efforts won't bring us what we are hoping for." (p. A24)

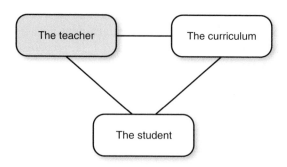

Figure 1.1 The elements in a teaching programme

Many of these studies quoted have looked at secondary school education. In higher education, the teacher matters too, and studies of student satisfaction regularly highlight the importance of the teacher. A European Union high-level group on modernisation of higher education has acknowledged that quality teaching is essential if students are to qualify with the right blend of skills for their personal and professional development (European Commission, 2013). The group recommended that by 2020 all teaching staff in higher education institutions should have received certified pedagogical training, with continuous professional education a requirement for teachers. The group also recommended that decisions about appointment, progression and promotion should take into account assessment of teaching competence alongside other factors.

The findings and conclusions with regard to the importance of the teacher are also applicable to the education of medical students. The UK General Medical Council (2006), in their document *Good Medical Practice*, stated that all doctors should be willing to contribute to educational activities and that all doctors, if they are involved in teaching, must develop the skills, attitudes and practices of a competent teacher. Wright et al. (1998) found that excellent role models identified by junior doctors were more likely to have had training in teaching and to spend more time teaching. Junior doctors in New York identified their clinical supervisor as being of greater importance in their training programme than the hospital to which they were attached, the range of patients they saw or the time they spent with patients (Kendrick et al., 1993). In a study of medical students in Malaysia, Kek and Huijser (2011) found that a teacher as a person and his or her approach to teaching plays a key role in influencing a student's learning style and whether or not they adopt a deep approach to learning. Medical teachers have an important role to play in students' learning: they have the responsibility of shaping the next generation of healthcare professionals and influencing the care they will give to the patients for whom they are responsible.

Sir Derrick Dunlop, a distinguished physician in Scotland, argued in 1963 that:

> It is important to remember that the actual details of the curriculum matter little in comparison to the selection of students and teachers. If these are good any system will work pretty well; if they are indifferent the most perfect curriculum will fail to produce results.

That the teacher is an important factor in the student's learning is as true today as it was in 1963. As Sir Ken Robinson (2013) suggested in his TED talk, "How to escape education's death valley," the teacher is more than just a delivery system, and no education system is better than the teacher. Learning has been defined as "the process whereby knowledge is created through the transformation of experience" (Kolb, 2014). A teacher is important if this transformation of experience is to be effective and efficient. As a teacher, you can have a significant influence on the delivery of health care through the many students you teach and the many more patients for whom each student will be responsible after they enter practice (Fig. 1.2).

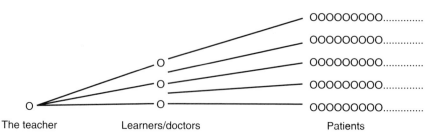

The teacher	Learners/doctors	Patients

Figure 1.2 Each teacher can influence many students who, in turn, will each be responsible for managing many patients

If you reflect back on your own experience as a student, it is likely that the teachers who taught you were more memorable than the teaching method they used. As a student at medical school in Glasgow and a junior doctor at the Western Infirmary, I (RMH) was fortunate to have teachers who have had a lasting effect on my development and career. A highlight of the week was the Saturday morning grand rounds when, after the morning ward round, hospital staff from the different disciplines met in the surgery department lecture theatre to discuss the presentation of patients with features of particular interest. This was a powerful learning experience, led by great teachers such as Sir Edward Wayne, the professor of medicine, and Sir Charles Illingworth, the professor of surgery. I still remember, 50 years later, one animated discussion about the merits of operating on a patient admitted to the surgery wards when Sir Edward pointed out that a more important issue that had been ignored was the patient's aortic stenosis. The different pathological perspectives on patients provided by Professor John Anderson and Professor Robert Goudie and the microbiological perspective from Sir James Howie were illuminating. Occasionally, a patient was presented with an obstetric or gynaecology aspect, and the input from Sir Ian Donald, the father of the use of ultrasound in obstetrics, was fascinating. Going home from the grand rounds with Robert Goudie (we both lived in Bearsden), we often continued the discussion, and I was able to benefit further from his views on the patients who had been presented. I still remember these great teachers who encouraged my passion for medicine and later my interest in teaching. Teachers do matter. It is a sad reflection on medical education today that although they still exist, there are now fewer opportunities for such interactions.

The doctor as a teacher

Although a major responsibility of a doctor is the care of patients for whom they are responsible, to a greater or lesser extent, all doctors and healthcare professionals are also teachers of students, of practitioners in training, of colleagues and of the public and patients for whom they are responsible. Shapiro (1951) highlighted the role of the doctor in educating patients and the need to train students as patient educators. He pointed out that the word "doctor" is derived from the Latin *doceo*, which means "I teach." This represents an important responsibility for the doctor.

Not only does the doctor as a teacher influence his or her students, but the role as a teacher can also affect their clinical performance as a doctor. A study of nearly

8,000 physicians in Canada demonstrated a relationship between clinical performance and teaching. Clinicians with greater involvement in teaching were found to have higher scores in a multisource feedback assessment of the quality of clinical care (Lockyer et al., 2016). The reason for this is not clear but may be explained by the fact that engaging in teaching involves more explicit thinking about the content to be taught and the practices to be followed. When a doctor takes responsibility for teaching, medical practice can be enhanced and excellence furthered, as suggested by Whitman and Schwenk (1997). They quoted Charles Mayo's view that "the safest thing for a patient was to be in the hands of a man engaged in clinical teaching" and encouraged all doctors to pursue excellence in their teaching as enthusiastically and thoroughly as they have in their practice of medicine, because teaching future physicians will be part of their legacy.

What motivates a doctor to teach? According to Budden et al. (2017), five main factors motivate surgeons to teach:

- A sense of responsibility to teach future physicians
- An intrinsic enjoyment of teaching
- The need to maintain and expand one's own knowledge base
- Watching students develop into competent practising physicians and playing a role in their success
- Fostering positive lifelong professional relationships with learners

Teaching may not be a high priority for many doctors, but it is an important responsibility. The doctor can contribute as a teacher in different ways. This is illustrated in the eight different roles for the doctor as teacher, discussed in the chapters that follow.

Challenges facing the medical teacher

Teaching is an important responsibility but it is not easy, and a number of challenges may face you as a medical teacher:

- Research, clinical practice and administration may all compete with teaching for your attention and time
- The culture or climate in the school or institution may not support a commitment of the doctor as a teacher
- Many changes are taking place in medical education in response to outside pressures, to which the doctor as a teacher needs to respond
- Medical education itself is a complex business – it is both a craft and a science

Competing demands on the teacher

Only a small number of teachers in medicine have teaching as their sole responsibility. The great majority have, in addition, other commitments to patient care, research or both. Some have administrative responsibilities. These competing responsibilities represent a problem and an advantage. It is a problem insofar as responsibilities other than teaching may be given a higher priority. This may, in part, be due to the fact that the doctor as teacher has not been recognised sufficiently compared with the clinician and research worker. This has been a common theme in many of the reports that have been written about teachers and teaching in medicine (Calman, 2006). The explicit reward structure of academia favours research and publication compared with teaching in terms of money and status (Leslie, 2002). Teaching, unfortunately, is sometimes perceived as a role only for individuals who have failed to generate a reputation in research and attract research funds. Fortunately, as we discuss in Chapter 11, this attitude is changing.

Clinical responsibilities may also be perceived as a priority over teaching, and clinical commitments may be seen as a reason for cancelling or arriving late at teaching sessions. This too is changing, though, with the need being recognised for clinical cover to be arranged and for time to be allocated to teaching and formal teaching sessions included in an individual's schedule.

The competing roles expected of a doctor as a clinician and teacher should not be seen only as a problem. If managed appropriately, they can enhance the teaching programme. The clinical teacher can bring authenticity to the teaching and, as we will see in Chapter 7, may be an excellent role model for the student.

The teacher who is also a researcher can bring added interest and excitement to the programme, provided that this is in the context of the educational needs of the students. In a non–research-intensive university, faculty research productivity has been reported as being associated with improved student learning. Galbraith and Merrill (2011) found that "research superstars" had 66.6% of their courses with above average student learning outcomes, compared with 61.3% for other "research active" faculty and 45.8% for "research inactive" faculty. The position in a research-intensive university, however, may be different if teaching is not given the priority it deserves.

In an interesting study, Stupnisky et al. (2016) compared faculty members' emotions when they were engaged in teaching and research. They found significantly more engagement and pride but more boredom regarding teaching and more anxiety, guilt and helplessness associated with research. As highlighted by Alan Denison, a radiologist who is the programme leader for medicine at the University of Aberdeen, UK, teaching can provide considerable job satisfaction (Box 1.1).

Both the clinician and the researcher must recognise that teaching is not something to be done without thought in odd minutes, when they are free. It requires dedicated time, serious consideration and the development of the necessary teaching skills.

Lack of a supportive environment or climate

In addition to the competing priorities for the teacher as a clinician or researcher, as described above, a related problem may be that the culture of the school and the

Box 1.1 Personal reflections: a precious and energising activity[a]

Teaching is, for me, a precious and energising activity. Theories can and should underpin what we do but the act of guiding a learner through the uncertain and shifting landscape of medical education cannot be described by frameworks alone. I find teaching both a transient experience, yet one which can leave a lasting memory for both me and the learner. Although I have a senior leadership role, I cherish and defend the opportunities to teach and nurture that professional bond with my students of today as they transition to colleagues of tomorrow. Sharing the joy of clinical and academic curiosity is a gift that is hard to measure, but I find it as energising and worthwhile today as I did 10 years ago.

[a]Alan Denison, Programme Lead for Medicine at the University of Aberdeen, UK.

climate or environment in which the teacher works does not value teaching in the same way as it values research or clinical work. Excellence in teaching may not be recognised and rewarded and may not count towards personal advancement and promotion. This is discussed further in Chapter 11.

It is possible with appropriate leadership, however, to change the climate in a medical school. Teachers can help by enhancing the reputation of the school and the education programme through demonstrating educational excellence. The ASPIRE-to-Excellence initiative discussed earlier is one approach in which excellence in teaching is recognised. The teacher's personal responsibility for creating a culture where teaching is valued is discussed in Chapter 9.

Changes in medical education

Significant changes have taken place in medical education in response to advances in medicine, changing healthcare delivery systems, patients' demands and expectations, developments in educational thinking and new learning technologies. This presents a challenge for the teacher. The teacher's roles in a medical school or postgraduate training programme have almost certainly changed, as highlighted by Valli and Buese (2007).

The revolution that has taken place in medical practice has not been mirrored by similar changes in education. Although there have been some significant developments, the adoption of new approaches in education in the curriculum, particularly in relation to the use of new learning technologies, has been disappointing. This can be attributed at least in part to a reluctance of teachers to accept the new roles expected of them and failure to embrace the new learning technologies. The consequence has been to hold back or slow down many desirable changes in medical education, including the move from an analogue to a digital world. This is a general problem in education, not just in medical education (Valli and Buese, 2007).

The extent to which a traditional approach to education or a new innovation is a success or failure when implemented in practice depends to a large measure on the teacher. As noted by Brown and Manogue (2001) when considering the use of lectures,

"There are no bad lectures, only bad lecturers." The success of problem-based learning (PBL) depends on the teacher's skill in facilitating the work of the student group, the development by the teacher of appropriate problems to be used as the basis for the learning, the integration of PBL into the curriculum, including matching the learning outcomes with PBL and how the students' performance is assessed (Taylor and Miflin, 2008). The teacher's input and performance have a significant impact on the success of PBL, and this makes the interpretation of research in the field difficult, because the quality of teachers' input has often not been described in reported studies. This problem in research is not unique to education and a similar problem arises in the interpretation of research in clinical practice. The result of surgical procedures, for example, depends to a large measure on the skill of the surgeon. As an endocrinologist, I (RMH) have had the responsibility for selecting, in collaboration with the patient with hyperthyroidism, their treatment. The choice included thyroidectomy, treatment with an anti-thyroid drug and radioactive iodine therapy. The decision was influenced by which surgeon would operate on the patient. This was because the end results and incidence of complications, including damage to the recurrent laryngeal nerve and parathyroid glands, both associated with serious consequences, varied considerably, depending on the surgeon's skill and expertise. In the same way, as a teacher you are important to the student's success, and you can affect the student's learning, as noted by Squires (1999, p. 60): "What happens on courses is often due not to rational planning or curriculum design, but to the personal likes, enthusiasms, energies, expertise, prejudices, habits and sheer bloody mindedness of the staff."

Teaching as a craft and a science

Teaching in medicine is both a craft and a science, as argued by Tim Dornan in a presentation at a meeting of the Association for the Study of Medical Education (ASME) in Belfast in July 2016. As we highlight throughout this book, teaching is a highly complex art/science which must be deliberately learned rather than learned by simply practising it.

Undoubtedly, there is an element of craft skills in teaching, as described by Squires (1999):

> Teaching does involve elements of craft skills. These are things that can be demonstrated, observed, imitated, learned, developed and refined, and in this they are no different from skills in technical and vocational fields, or sports and the arts. The good footballer or good musician has to practice, hard and regularly. Teachers may not have to be quite so rigorous in this regard, but they do need to take their skills seriously. This implies plenty of opportunities for observation and practice. (p. 100)

Squires has argued, however, that we cannot regard teaching as simply a craft and to do so trivialises it:

> It is sometimes argued that training for academics to teach should be kept to the bare minimum, and be as practical as possible, because they are more likely to tolerate, if not actually like it, that way. The view taken here

is the opposite. Unless teaching can be shown to have a coherent academic basis, which goes beyond mere tips and techniques, it will never be taken seriously in higher education. It may be built into the structures, but it will never become part of the culture. (p. 139)

There has been built up over the years a science of human learning, although it is still far from perfect. To take simulation as an example, considerable advances have been made in the development and use of simulators in medical education. Simulators are valuable tools that have an important place at all levels of training in medicine. Considerable experience has been gained in their use, and there is undoubtedly a craft associated with their application in practice. As highlighted in the best evidence medical education (BEME) systematic review of the literature, the use of simulators is also a science. There are important evidence-based principles which should be followed when simulators are used in the education programme (Issenberg et al., 2005). This concept of evidence-based or evidence-informed teaching is discussed further in Chapter 9. There is both a craft and a science in teaching, and the use of simulation as a tool to facilitate students' learning is an example of this.

What is a good teacher?

Effective teaching is a result of many factors and teaching, as described by Stronge (2002), is "an extraordinarily complex undertaking." Skelton (2005), in his book *Understanding Teaching Excellence in Higher Education*, discusses what makes a university teacher excellent:

> *...debates rage around whether it is down to subject-knowledge, communication skills, taking a research-led approach or being a technological whiz. Teaching excellence is now part of the everyday language and practice of higher education. Policy makers declare its value to national economies, institutions market themselves through excellent teaching quality scores, and an increasing number of teachers are recognised and rewarded for this excellence at prestigious award ceremonies. ...teaching excellence is a contested concept and...we each need to develop an informed personal perspective on what it means to practice. (p. 3)*

Excellence in teaching may be recognised through local, national and international awards, but what is an excellent teacher? What are the features that distinguish the excellent teacher? In medicine, a number of learning outcomes or competency frameworks have been used to describe the abilities required of a doctor. The three-circle model used to illustrate the attributes of a doctor, as illustrated in Fig. 1.3 (Harden and Laidlaw, 2017), can be adapted to describe the attributes of a teacher (Hesketh et al., 2001).

Technical abilities

The teacher requires a range of **technical abilities**, as highlighted in the inner circle of Fig. 1.3. These include the ability to deliver a lecture, facilitate a small group, plan a curriculum or examine a student's competence. These technical abilities are

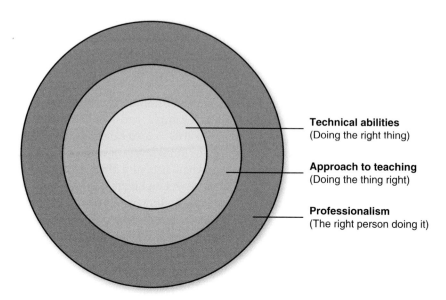

Figure 1.3 The requirement of the excellent teacher, as specified in the three-circle model *(Harden and Laidlaw, 2017)*

reflected in the roles of the teacher as information provider, facilitator, curriculum developer and assessor, and we return to a more detailed description of these in the chapters that follow. Many faculty development programmes, medical education courses and medical texts on the subject concentrate on these technical skills. They are important but, on their own, they are not enough.

Approach to teaching

The good teacher is more than simply a technician. An important additional perspective of the teacher is represented in the middle circle in terms of **how the teacher approaches his or her practice.** This includes the application of basic educational principles, evidence-informed decisions, appropriate attitudes and ethical practices and whether the teacher works as a member of a team.

How the teacher delivers a lecture, runs a small group, organizes an examination or tackles any other educational task can be improved if they have **an understanding of some basic educational principles** such as the FAIR principles for effective learning (*f*eedback, *a*ctive learning, *i*ndividualisation and *r*elevance), as described by Harden and Laidlaw (2017). This is the science of medical education. Excellent teachers need to have an understanding of the basic education principles when they reflect on their teaching as scholars and when they innovate in the area. Wayne Hodgins (2005) used the development of flying as an analogy:

> *We did not learn how to fly by mimicking other examples of success such as birds or animals that can fly. Human flight remained impossible and we were spectacularly unsuccessful while we tried to fly by 'flapping.' Success*

came from understanding what enables things to fly such as air flow and lift and wing design and when we developed innovative ways of achieving flight such as with fixed wing design, propellers, jet engines, new lightweight materials and other creative ways to match our unique conditions. In the end, success came after we stopped trying to flap at all. (p. 251)

In teaching, too, often we are still trying to flap. Just as an understanding of anatomy, physiology, pharmacology and behavioural science is a prerequisite for the practice of medicine, so also is an understanding of educational principles a prerequisite for practice as a teacher.

Excellent teachers adopt an **evidence-informed approach** to their teaching practice, with decisions as to what works and what does not work made on the best evidence available. This, along with an understanding of educational principles, is reflected in the role of a teacher as a scholar and is discussed further in Chapter 9.

The teacher serves as a role model for the learner and should demonstrate **appropriate behaviour and attitudes**. Teachers should be passionate both about their subject and about student learning. The importance of the teacher's behaviour and attitudes is highlighted when the characteristics of the best teachers are studied. These positive qualities, as described by James Stronge (2002) in his book, *Qualities of Effective Teachers*, are given in Table 1.1. Although the context is school education, almost certainly, similar qualities apply to a teacher in a medical school. A shorter set of nine characteristics of a great teacher, listed in Table 1.2, was described by Maria Orlando (2013), a professor in higher education in the USA. There are many similarities to the attributes listed in Table 1.1. Additional perspectives are added in terms of the teacher as a leader (discussed in Chapter 8) and the teacher as a professional (discussed in Chapter 10). George Couros (2010), in his description of the master teacher, also highlighted passion as one of the ten attributes (Table 1.3). His list also includes a focus on "learning goals" as opposed to "performance goals." You may like to look at the three lists and reflect on how many of these features apply to you as a teacher. We asked medical students what attributes they looked for in their teachers. The responses are shown in Table 1.4. Attitudes and passion for teaching feature prominently in all four lists. When the attributes of a good teacher were ranked by students in Singapore, a similar result was found, and the top two qualities of a teacher were the ability to motivate students and to be passionate about teaching (Kua et al., 2006).

Great lecturers give not only a clear, planned and informative presentation, but also pass on their enthusiasm and inspire and excite students, motivating them to learn about the subject. Carl Gustav Jung (1954) suggested:

One looks back with appreciation to the brilliant teachers, but with gratitude to those who touched our human feelings. The curriculum is so much necessarily raw material, but warmth is the vital element for the growing plant and for the soul of the child. (p. 144)

Table 1.1 The positive qualities of an effective teacher[a]

- Assumes ownership of the classroom and the students' success
- Uses personal experiences as examples in teaching
- Understands feelings of students
- Communicates clearly
- Admits to mistakes and corrects them immediately
- Thinks about and reflects on practice
- Displays a sense of humour
- Dresses appropriately for the position
- Maintains confidential trust and respect
- Is structured, yet flexible and spontaneous
- Is responsive to situations and students' needs
- Enjoys teaching and expects students to enjoy learning
- Looks for the win-win solution in conflict situations
- Listens attentively to student questions and comments
- Responds to students with respect, even in difficult situations
- Communicates high expectations consistently
- Conducts one-on-one conversations with students
- Treats students equally and fairly
- Has positive dialogue and interactions with students outside the classroom
- Invests time with single students or small groups of students outside the classroom
- Maintains a professional manner at all times
- Addresses students by name
- Speaks in an appropriate tone and volume
- Works actively with students

[a]As described by Stronge (2002).

Table 1.2 The characteristics of the great teacher[a]

- Respects students
- Creates a sense of community with a supportive, collaborative learning environment
- Is warm, accessible, enthusiastic and caring
- Sets high expectations for all students
- Has his own love of learning, inspiring students with his passion for education in their learning
- Is a skilled leader and provides opportunities for his students to assume leadership roles
- Can "shift gears" and is flexible in his approach to teaching
- Collaborates with colleagues
- Maintains professionalism as a teacher

[a]As described by Orlando (2013).

Table 1.3 The characteristics of a master teacher[a]

- Connects with students and gets to know them individually
- Helps students meet their own individual needs
- Makes the curriculum and what is taught relevant
- Works with students to develop their love of learning, helping students to find their own spark in learning
- Keeps themselves as a teacher up to date. Education and learning will always change
- Focuses on learning goals as opposed to performance goals[b]
- Ensures that "character education" is an essential part of learning. Students need to grow emotionally as well as mentally
- Is passionate about the content they teach
- Is concerned not just with what is taught in their class but with their overall impact on the school culture
- Communicates well with all the stakeholders and not just the students

[a]As described by Couros (2010).
[b]A performance goal, Couros has suggested, is similar to having students wanting to receive an "A" grade in French, whereas a learning goal is a student wanting to become fluent in the language.

Table 1.4 Desirable attributes of a teacher, as identified by medical students

- Passionate
- Enthusiastic about student learning
- Respects students and has a commitment to their learning
- Empathetic, caring and compassionate
- Inspirational, motivating and encouraging
- Understanding and sensitive to learners' needs
- Fair and non-judgemental
- Flexible
- Easily approachable and willing to listen
- Humorous
- Takes a personal approach and knows each student
- Humble and knows limitations

Excellent teachers in medicine do not approach their teaching responsibilities as a chore. They have passion for their teaching and believe that they have a positive effect on students and ultimately on the health care of the community that their students will serve. Teachers demonstrate their passion and enthusiasm in different ways, and all teachers can be passionate or enthusiastic in their own fashion (Harden and Laidlaw, 2017). Tan Chay-Hoon, with 31 years' experience of psychiatry and psychopharmacology in Singapore, has described her attitudes to her students (Box 1.2).

The fourth and final attribute in this middle circle is the ability to **function as a member of a team**. The teacher should recognise the importance of working as a

Box 1.2 Share, lead, learn, impart, encourage and inspire[a]

To teach is to share, to lead, to learn, to impart, to encourage and to inspire students to achieve their fullest potential.

My teaching philosophy has been built upon learning from great teachers and using feedback accumulated from students, peers and family. I feel that the key ingredients for teachers are love, humility and honesty. With these we are able to sharpen our teaching skills first. An important principle as educators is to first train ourselves, and then train the students under our charge. To that end, training of the trainer and continuous professional development of the teacher are indispensable. Then we can inspire our students to soar to greater heights of excellence as our future doctors, dental surgeons, pharmacists, scientists and leaders in the profession.

I find respecting students as individuals is essential. Accord them the respect and dignity as individuals – unique personality, culture, education and experiences that are distinct from others. Some students require reassurance and feedback that they are on the right track. Empathetic teachers can help by giving their listening ear and providing guidance as needed. Sometimes, just listening to them can help to ease their anxieties. Be the "friend in need" as a mentor. Promote students' self-directed learning and taking responsibility.

[a]Tan Chay-Hoon, Associate Professor, Department of Pharmacology, National University of Singapore, Singapore.

member of a team and collaborating with other healthcare professionals, with other teachers contributing to the curriculum and with those providing educational support or expertise. This ability is discussed further in Chapter 8 in relation to the role of the teacher as a manager or leader.

The teacher as a professional

The outer circle in the three-circle model represents **the teacher as a professional,** embracing all the attributes described in the inner and middle circles. Teachers should exhibit appropriate conduct and behaviour, enquire into their own competence, evaluate their teaching, keep themselves up to date with current teaching practice as it relates to the different activities in the inner circle and be responsible for their personal well-being. This is discussed further in Chapter 10.

The attributes of the good teacher

The attributes of the excellent teacher described earlier—combining technical abilities, the approach to practice and professionalism—are represented in the equation shown in Fig. 1.4. The lecture can be taken as an example of how the different elements in the equation interact with each other. To deliver an effective lecture, the teacher should have the necessary technical skills as an information provider (the inner circle). He or she should also understand the relevant education principles that can assist in facilitating the students' learning. With this understanding, the lecturer can make the lecture relevant to the students' needs and transform the lecture from a

$$ET = (I + F + C + As) \times (E \times At \times D \times T) \times (P)$$

ET = Excellent teacher, I = Information provider, F = Facilitator, C = Curriculum developer, As = Assessor, E = Education principles, At = Attitudes, D = Decision making, T = Teamwork and P = Professionalism.

The "+" symbol in the first part of the equation signifies that the excellent teacher may not be excellent in all four domains. The "×" symbol in the second and third parts indicates that these are essential features with a "0" for any one resulting in an overall "0".

Figure 1.4 The attributes of an excellent medical teacher

passive to an active learning experience (the middle circle). The teacher may also give students the opportunity to assess their understanding of the topic covered in the lecture, either during the lecture or afterwards. The teacher should demonstrate passion for the subject and for the students' learning in the lecture. The good lecturer will be familiar with the curriculum and will integrate his or her lecture with other elements of the course. The good teacher will also keep up to date with new approaches to lecturing, such as the use of digital media and the flipped classroom (the outer circle).

Outcome frameworks and the abilities required of a teacher

We have described how the three-circle outcome model can be used to describe the abilities required of the teacher. Ramani and Leinster (2008) applied the three-circle model for teachers working in the clinical environment, as shown in Table 1.5. This included the technical skills required by the clinical teacher (doing the right thing), how the clinical teacher approaches her or his teaching (doing the thing right) and the clinical teacher as a professional (the right person doing it). Other competency frameworks, such as the US Accreditation Council for Graduate Medical Education (ACGME) framework, have also been used to frame the competencies expected of a teacher (Srinivasan et al., 2011).

Anyone can become a good teacher

We have highlighted the importance of the teacher and excellence in teaching and the attributes expected of an excellent teacher, but can everyone be a great teacher? Is the great teacher born or made? Although individuals may have inherent differences in their personality and character, everyone has the potential to achieve excellence in one or more of the roles described in this book if they strive sufficiently and have the appropriate understanding of their role. As a teacher, you require (Fig. 1.5):

- Mastery of the techniques relating to your work as a teacher
- An appropriate approach to your teaching
- Demonstration of professionalism relating to your teaching

Table 1.5 The three-circle outcomes model applied to teachers in the clinical environment

Tasks of a clinical teacher: *Doing the right thing*	Approach to teaching: *Doing the thing right*	Teacher as a professional: *The right person doing it*
• Time-efficient teaching • Inpatient teaching • Outpatient teaching • Teaching at the bedside • Work-based assessment of learners in clinical settings • Providing feedback	• Showing enthusiasm for teaching and towards learners • Understanding learning principles relevant to clinical teaching • Using appropriate teaching strategies for different levels of learners • Knowing and applying principles of effective feedback • Modelling good professional behaviour, including evidence-based patient care • Grasping the unexpected teaching moment	• Soliciting feedback on teaching • Self-reflection on teaching strengths and weaknesses • Seeking professional development in teaching • Mentoring and seeking mentoring • Engaging in educational scholarship

Adapted from Ramani and Leinster (2008).

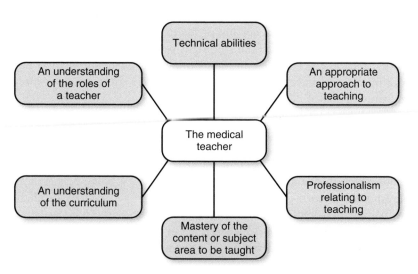

Figure 1.5 The requirements to be a good teacher

- Mastery of the content or subject to be taught
- An understanding of the curriculum in the medical school or education programme, including the expected learning outcomes
- An understanding of the different roles of a teacher and your own role

We have described the first three of these requirements earlier in this chapter. We should be able to assume that as a teacher you have the necessary mastery of the subject, the fourth requirement. Excellence in teaching is the blending of content knowledge and teaching knowledge. You need to consider what content should be covered in relation to your teaching, whether it is a subject such as anatomy or surgery or a theme such as ethics or cultural competency. This is explored further in Chapter 3.

The need for understanding the curriculum in the local context may seem an obvious requirement but it is sometimes ignored. An overview of the curriculum should be included in all induction courses for new teachers. You should have an understanding of the curriculum in your school and how your own teaching is expected to contribute to this. What courses prepare students for your own course, and what courses follow your course? What are the accepted educational strategies in the school? How are students assessed? These curriculum issues are discussed in Chapter 5.

The final requirement, and one that has largely been neglected, is a consideration by the teacher of the different roles and functions of a teacher and of an individual teacher's role as a member of the teaching team. The aim of this book is to provide such an understanding. Some individuals have more natural ability as teachers than others. A consideration of the individual roles of a teacher and how they can be developed can help a poor teacher become a good teacher and a good teacher become a better or excellent teacher. As Pullias and Lockhard (1963) advocated:

> Excellence in teaching means the inclination and the ability to do with high skill the work of a teacher; that is, to play effectively the role of the teacher in the process of learning. (p. 10)

We describe in this book what is expected of you as a teacher and how you can demonstrate excellence as a teacher in each of the eight roles. An appreciation of the roles can also contribute to your job satisfaction as a teacher, as described by John Sexton, a former president of New York University (Sexton, 2004):

> The university teacher often is someone who can operate at a level of creativity and to a very real extent does, especially in the area of teaching... there is an inherent satisfaction in leading students in the discovery of knowledge, in awakening their innate curiosity, in showing them how to learn and even in some cases shaping their lives. That mission can be the heart of a rewarding vocation – one that is immediate in its impact and gratifying in ways that research is not. And the experience of successful university teachers frequently is overwhelmingly positive in character

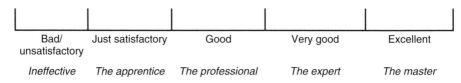

Bad/unsatisfactory	Just satisfactory	Good	Very good	Excellent
Ineffective	The apprentice	The professional	The expert	The master

Figure 1.6 The quality of the teacher

compared to that of even the most successful scholars and researchers, who, by the nature of their role, must subject themselves to criticism, skepticism, and even a certain negativism as their work is scrutinized in the most intense way.

In the next chapter, we introduce the eight roles of the medical teacher. An understanding of these roles can help move the teacher along the path from a "just satisfactory" teacher to an "excellent" teacher (Fig. 1.6).

Take-home messages

1. The teacher has a major influence on how effectively and efficiently students learn.
2. The teacher is important if medical education is to respond positively and adapt to the many changes that are taking place in medicine and healthcare delivery.
3. The teacher should have mastery of the content area, an understanding of the local curriculum and context, the necessary teaching skills, an appropriate approach to teaching, professionalism in his or her teaching and, importantly, an understanding of her or his role as a teacher.

Consider

- Think of the different functions teachers fulfil in your school and why teachers are important.
- How would you rate yourself as a teacher in terms of the descriptions provided in Tables 1.1, 1.2, 1.3 and 1.4?
- Do you have the required abilities of a teacher, as set out in Fig. 1.5?

Explore further

Bashir, T.H., 1998. Dangerous liaison: Academics' attitude towards open learning in higher education. http://www.tandfonline.com/doi/abs/10.1080/0268051980130107.

Brown, G., Manogue, M., 2001. AMEE Guide No 22: Refreshing lecturing: A guide for lecturers. Med. Teach. 23 (3), 231–244.

Budden, C.R., Svechnikova, K., White, J., 2017. Why do surgeons teach? A qualitative analysis of motivation in excellent surgical educators. Med. Teach. 39 (2), 188–194.

Calman, K., 2006. Medical Education: Past, Present and Future. Elsevier, London.

Couros, G., 2010. What makes a master teacher? The principal of change. http://georgecouros.ca/blog/archives/267.

Dozier, T., 1998. Philadelphia Inquirer, July 12th, p. A24.

Dunlop, D., 1963. Medical education in Scotland. In: Goldberg, A. (Ed.), Future of Medical Education in Scotland. Scottish Medical Journal, Glasgow.

European Commission, 2013. Report on improving the quality of teaching and learning in Europe's higher education institutions. High level group on the modernization of higher education. http://ec.europa.eu/education/library/reports/modernisation_en.pdf.

Galbraith, C.S., Merrill, G.B., 2011. Faculty research productivity and standardized student learning outcomes in a university teaching environment: A Bayesian analysis of relationships. Stud. Higher Educ. 37 (4), 469–480.

General Medical Council, 2006. Good Medical Practice. GMC, London.

Harden, R.M., Laidlaw, J.M., 2017. Essential Skills for a Medical Teacher. Elsevier, London.

Hesketh, E.A., Bagnall, G., Buckley, E.G., et al., 2001. A framework for developing excellence as a clinical educator. Med. Educ. 35, 555–564.

Hodgins, W., 2005. Into the future of meLearning: Every One Learning … imagine if the impossible isn't! In: Masie, E. (Ed.), Learning Rants, Raves, and Reflections: A Collection of Passionate and Professional Perspectives. Pfeiffer, San Francisco.

Issenberg, S.B., McGaghie, W.C., Petrusa, E.R., et al., 2005. Features and uses of high-fidelity medical simulations that lead to effective learning: A BEME systematic review. Med. Teach. 27 (1), 10–28.

Jung, C.G., 1954. Development of Personality. In: Adler, G., Hull, R.F.C. (Eds.), Collected Works of C.G. Jung, vol. 17. Princeton University Press, Princeton, NJ.

Kek, M.Y.C.A., Huijser, H., 2011. Exploring the combined relationships of student and teacher factors on learning approaches and self-directed learning readiness at a Malaysian university. Stud. Higher Educ. 36 (2), 185–208.

Kendrick, S.B., Simmons, J.M., Richards, B.F., et al., 1993. Residents' perceptions of their teachers: Facilitative behaviour and the learning value of rotations. Med. Educ. 27 (1), 55–61.

Kolb, D.A., 2014. Experiential Learning: Experience as the Source of Learning and Development. Prentice Hall, Upper Saddle River, NJ.

Kua, E.H., Voon, F., Tan, C.H., et al., 2006. What makes an effective medical teacher? Perceptions of medical students. Med. Teach. 28 (8), 738–741.

Leslie, D.W., 2002. Resolving the dispute: Teaching is academe's core value. J. Higher Educ. 73 (1), 49–73.

Lockyer, J., Hodgson, C., Lee, T., et al., 2016. Clinical teaching as part of continuing professional development: Does teaching enhance clinical performance? Med. Teach. 38 (8), 815–822.

Luyten, H., Snijders, T.A.B., 1996. School effects and teacher effects in Dutch elementary education. Educ. Res. Eval. 2 (1), 1–24.

Orlando, M., 2013. Nine characteristics of a great teacher. http://www.facultyfocus.com/articles/philosophy-of-teaching/nine-characteristics-of-a-great-teacher.

Pullias, E.V., Lockhard, A.S., 1963. Towards Excellence in College Teaching. W.C. Brown, Dubuque, IA.

Ramani, S., Leinster, S., 2008. AMEE Guide no. 34: Teaching in the clinical environment. Med. Teach. 30 (4), 347–364.

Robinson, K., 2013. How to escape education's death valley. http://www.ted.com/talks/ken_robinson_how_to_escape_education_s_death_valley.

Sexton, J., 2004. The common enterprise university and the teaching mission. https://www.nyu.edu/about/leadership-university-administration/office-of-the-president-emeritus/communications/the-common-enterprise-university-and-the-teaching-mission.html.

Shapiro, I., 1951. Doctor means teacher. J. Med. Educ. 2, 125–129.

Skelton, A., 2005. Understanding Teaching Excellence in Higher Education: Towards a Critical Approach. Routledge, London.

Squires, G., 1999. Teaching as a Professional Discipline. Falmer Press, London.

Srinivasan, M., Li, S.T., Meyers, F.J., et al., 2011. Teaching as a competency: Competencies for medical educators. Acad. Med. 86 (10), 1211–1220.

Stronge, J., 2002. Qualities of Effective Teachers. Association for Supervision and Curriculum Development, Alexandria, VA.

Stupnisky, R.H., Pekrun, R., Lichtenfeld, S., 2016. New faculty members' emotions: a mixed-method study. Stud. Higher Educ. 41 (7), 1167–1188.

Taylor, D., Miflin, B., 2008. AMEE Guide No. 36: Problem-based learning: Where are we now? Med. Teach. 30 (8), 743–763.

The New Teacher Project, 2012. The irreplaceables: Understanding the real retention crisis in America's urban schools. https://tntp.org/publications/view/the-irreplaceables-understanding-the-real-retention-crisis.

Valli, L., Buese, D., 2007. The changing roles of teachers in an era of high-stakes accountability. Am. Educ. Res. J. 44 (3), 519–558.

Whitman, N.A., Schwenk, T.L., 1997. The Physician as Teacher. Whitman Associates, Washington, DC.

Winters, M.A., Cowen, J.M., 2013. Who would stay, who would be dismissed? An empirical consideration of value-added teacher retention policies. Educ. Res. 42 (6), 330–337.

Wright, S.M., Kern, D.E., Kolodner, K., et al., 1998. Attributes of excellent attending-physician role models. N. Engl. J. Med. 339, 1986–1993.

Chapter 2

The roles of the teacher

The good teacher wants students to learn more than they are taught.

Anon

This chapter introduces the concepts of what it means to be a teacher and the different roles and responsibilities of a teacher.

The function and responsibilities of a teacher

After refrigerators were introduced in the USA, Wayne Hodgins (2005) studied what happened to companies whose business was the distribution of ice. The ice distributors were so occupied with their day-to-day work of delivering ice to customers in their homes and restaurants that they failed to recognise the key need they met and their function to assist customers in cooling food and drink. Few ice distributors went into the production of refrigerators and almost all, as a result, went out of business. In education, Hodgins argued, we make the same mistake. Teachers are so preoccupied with their day-to-day activities—for example, giving a lecture—that they lose sight of their function, to help students learn. Think for a moment of your function as a teacher and ask yourself how could your students learn if you were not there to teach them? What would they miss most? This book is about your function and roles as a teacher.

We described in Chapter 1 the requirements to be a good teacher (see Fig. 1.5). We argued that an understanding of the roles and functions of a teacher are every bit as important as the teaching skills. When giving a lecture, for example, or using a simulator for teaching, teachers should reflect on their role and how they are contributing to students' learning. What does it mean to be a teacher?

What does it mean to be a teacher?

Here are some thoughts on what it is to be a teacher:

> To teach is to help someone learn something more quickly than he would learn it by trial and error.
>
> **Anon**

> The whole art of teaching is only the art of awakening the natural curiosity of young minds for the purpose of satisfying it afterwards.
>
> **Anatole France**

> To teach is to transform by informing, to develop a zest for lifelong learning, to help pupils become students – mature independent learners, architects of an exciting, challenging future.
>
> **Edgar Dale**

> The man who can make hard things easy is the educator.
>
> **Ralph Waldo Emerson**

> The young man taught all he knew and more
> The middle-aged man taught all he knew
> The old man taught all that his students would understand.
>
> **Arnold Ross**

The quotes represent different perceptions of the responsibility and functions expected of a teacher. You might find it of interest to examine them now and to return to them later when you have studied the eight roles of the teacher and reflect on which roles relate to each quote.

When the question is asked "What does a teacher do?" the answer is often given in terms of delivering a lecture, teaching students in a clinical setting or taking responsibility for a laboratory or practical class. These activities are simply the methods or means used by the teacher. As important is the role or function of the teacher in relation to the activities. Squires (1999) has strongly refuted the view that teaching can be seen merely in terms of methods. Teaching is not methods; methods are the means of teaching. Squires asked the following:

> What are teachers there for? If they were not there, how would we miss them? Would we in fact miss them? What do teachers do for students or pupils that the latter cannot do for themselves? (p. 28)

This leads us to the key question – what is your function or role in the education programme? The answer to the question is at the very heart of teaching and is key to your effectiveness as a teacher.

The work of a teacher is complex. It can be understood better through a consideration of the different roles or functions expected of the teacher. Some of these roles may be familiar to you as a teacher, whereas others you may not have considered in detail. The roles will differ undoubtedly in different contexts. Each role requires a set repertoire of skills and, as a teacher, you will not be expected to have a major commitment to all the roles. It is important, however, that you have an understanding and some input to all of the roles.

The different contributions made by the teacher to students' learning may at first sight not be obvious. The majority of articles published on teaching, texts on the subject and courses for teachers usually address issues such as lecturing, teaching of clinical skills, specifying learning outcomes, organising and implementing an objective structured clinical examination (OSCE) or preparing a multiple-choice question examination. These represent, as we have suggested, only the tools used by the teacher. Teaching is much more than the tools. This preoccupation with and emphasis in education on methods of teaching and learning rather than on what the teacher does is unproductive (Squires, 1999). If, as described in Chapter 1, you have a passion for teaching and a desire for your students to learn, you will wish to consider how as a teacher you can make a difference. Would learning happen without your input as a teacher? There is a need for greater clarity, transparency and reflection on your roles as a teacher.

Unfortunately, the part played by teachers and their role in the learning process is often taken for granted or assumed. This book is a plea for you to consider seriously your roles, responsibilities and functions as a teacher. This will help ensure that the learner's needs are more effectively and efficiently met and that you approach your work in a manner appropriate to a particular situation. If we are to respond to the pressures for change in medical education, we need to look at the roles of the teacher and, through this, gain a fresh insight into teaching. This is particularly important at a time of change in education and the need to move away from seeing the teacher as simply a source or provider of information.

Your purpose as a teacher

In the book *The Purpose Effect: Building Meaning in Yourself, Your Role and Your Organization*, Pontefract (2016) asks us to consider why we are doing the things we are doing – what is the purpose, and is our purpose personally and at work aligned with the purpose of the institution where we work? We are reminded that Peter Drucker wrote about the role of purpose in his article "*The theory of the business*" (1994), and that Simon Sinek's books popularised it with *Start with Why: How Great Leaders Inspire Everyone to Take Action* (Sinek, 2011).

As a teacher, you should have a sense of purpose – why are you teaching? To train doctors who will meet the needs of the patients and communities they will serve is too superficial an answer and provides little insight into our day-to-day activities as a teacher. We return to the question – what is your role, and how would students be worse off if you were not there?

Pontefract (2016) has pointed out that problems may arise if the teacher's and the institution's purposes are not shared. An example would be if the teacher sees as his or her purpose the provision of information to the student, whereas the school sees the role of the teacher as a facilitator of learning, supporting the student on a personal learning journey.

Individuals who have a sense of purpose in what they do in their job have, as Pontefract described, a great commitment to their work and to their institution. They also have greater job satisfaction. A study of the roles expected of you as a teacher and a decision as to which roles as a teacher you will fulfil is an expression of purpose.

Teacher's roles are different from the methods they use or their competencies. The roles relate to the functions performed by the teacher and can be considered as the teacher's identity. In a text on writing behavioural objectives, Vargas (1972) highlighted the importance of considering why we teach students. He described as a key reason the desire to expedite students' learning and to change students' behaviour:

> Just as an artist or scientist is judged primarily by his products, so the measure of a teacher is his product – the change in his students' behavior. Most people would think it absurd to judge an artist by his method of mixing paints, his way of holding the brush, or his way of dressing while painting. Yet in education, teachers are judged by analogous techniques or characteristics. They are rated on use of audio-visuals, lecture style, neatness of displays or bulletin boards, and even on things as remotely related to student learning as their dress. (p. 2)

It is important to consider what is our purpose as teachers. What do we aim to achieve? We trivialise our job if we see it simply as using tools such as lectures or simulators.

Views of teaching and the teacher's roles

Fox (1983) asked teachers the question, "What do you mean by teaching?" From the answers, there emerged four basic views:

> There is the transfer theory which treats knowledge as a commodity to be transferred from one vessel to another. There is the shaping theory which treats teaching as a process of shaping or moulding students to a predetermined pattern. Thirdly, there is the travelling theory which treats

a subject as a terrain to be explored with hills to be climbed for better viewpoints with the teacher as the travelling companion or expert guide. Finally, there is the growing theory which focusses more attention on the intellectual and emotional development of the learner. (p. 151)

The *transfer theory* relates to the teacher's role we describe as information provider, whereas the other roles can be identified more closely with the role of the teacher as facilitator. Fox (1983) found that less experienced and more junior teachers tended to favour the first two approaches—what he has described as "simple theories"—whereas more experienced teachers favoured the last two approaches, described by him as "developed theories".

How teachers think about their teaching will colour their attitude to their work; it will influence the roles they assume as teachers and will in turn be influenced by their roles. We discuss this further in the chapters that follow. In Chapter 10 we examine the implications for the training of teachers and in Chapter 11 how teachers can change their view of teaching over time and the implications this has on their roles.

The roles of the teacher model

The AMEE Guide, The Good Teacher is More Than a Lecturer – The Twelve Roles of the Teacher (Harden and Crosby, 2000) published by AMEE, an International Association for Medical Education, described the responsibilities and functions of the teacher in terms of twelve roles arranged in six groups:

- Providing information in the classroom and work context
- Facilitating learning and mentoring the learner
- Serving as a role model as a teacher and practitioner
- Developing the curriculum and courses within the curriculum
- Assessing the student and the curriculum
- Preparing resource material or study guides to available resources.

Three sources were used to identify the roles – an analysis of the tasks expected of a teacher in the design and implementation of a curriculum in one school; a study of the diaries kept by twelve medical students over a 3-month period and an analysis of their comments as they related to the role of the teacher; and a review of the literature relating to the roles of the teacher. The twelve roles identified were validated by a questionnaire completed by 251 teachers at different levels of seniority in the medical school at the University of Dundee.

The roles identified are illustrated in Fig. 2.1. In this representation of the roles, those at the top right require greater student contact compared with those at the bottom left, where the teacher may work at a distance from the student although engaged in a student-related activity. Those on the right require more medical or content experience, and those on the left require more teaching or education experience.

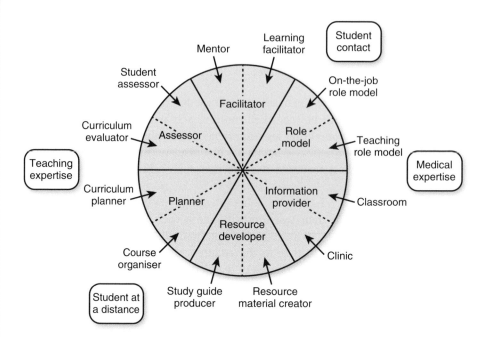

Figure 2.1 The twelve roles of the medical teacher
(Harden and Crosby, 2000).

The model, as described, has been widely adopted by teachers to assess their personal roles, by institutions to plan the education programme, by faculty developers in medical education courses and by researchers studying medical education. Pyörälä (2014), a faculty member at the School of Medicine at the University of Helsinki, used the twelve roles as the basis for a professional development portfolio for university teachers. This was used to chart teachers' development as they participated in a staff development programme (Fig. 2.2).

In the original report (Harden and Crosby, 2000), a five-point scale was used to indicate the extent of the commitment to a role: 1 = none, 2 = little, 3 = some, 4 = considerable and 5 = great. Pyörälä (2014) used a quantitative assessment scale to indicate the type of commitment to the role and the development in the teacher's educational thinking and practice:

- First level: Recognises the role
- Second level: Practises the role
- Third level: Aligns the role with the expected learning outcomes
- Fourth level: Reflects on his or her activities in the role to develop it further
- Fifth level: Adopts a scholarly approach to the role by applying research-based educational knowledge to his or her activities in the role

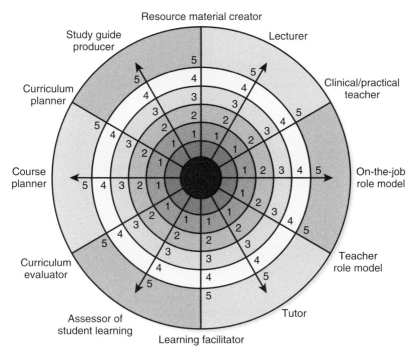

Figure 2.2 Role profile for the twelve roles of a medical teacher
(Pyörälä, 2014).

These stages more closely correspond to the levels of teaching expertise and form of a teacher's commitment to the role, rather than to the extent of the commitment of the teacher to a role as in the initial description of the roles.

Nikendei and co-workers (2016) carried out a survey of how 2,200 medical educators defined themselves. Six descriptions corresponded to the roles of facilitator, information provider, curriculum developer, assessor and assessment creator, role model and resource developer. Other roles defined included professional expert, enthusiast, faculty developer, undergraduate and postgraduate trainer, researcher and administrator.

The roles, as described originally by Harden and Crosby (2000) in Fig. 2.1, reflect the educational responsibilities of a teacher. However, they ignore the responsibilities of a teacher as a leader, scholar and a researcher. In response to suggestions we have received, we have developed and refined the model to include these additional roles.

The eight roles of the medical teacher

We describe in this book eight roles for the teacher, as summarised in Fig. 2.3. We have added to the roles previously described in Fig. 2.1 and combined some of the roles.

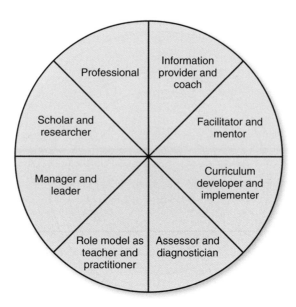

Figure 2.3 The eight roles of the medical teacher

The teacher as an information provider and coach

Students expect to be taught, and they see the traditional role of the teacher as one of provider of information, often in the lecture context. They believe that it is the responsibility of the teacher to pass on to them the information, knowledge and understanding of a topic appropriate to the stage of their studies. This view is shared by many teachers who see their role as an expert who is knowledgeable in his or her field, and who has the responsibility of conveying that knowledge to students, usually by word of mouth.

Although there is a move to emphasise the role of the teacher as a facilitator of learning, as we discuss in Chapter 4, we should recognise that the teacher still has an important role as information provider, as discussed in Chapter 3. With the rapid advances in medicine, information overload is a real problem for the student. The teacher can assist the student to identify the core information necessary for an understanding of a topic and to master the threshold concepts in a subject, which are the concepts necessary for students to understand before they can proceed to the next stage of the education programme.

The teacher should also serve as an information coach to ensure that students develop the skill of searching for necessary information as they require it. This involves asking the right question, knowing where to get the answer, evaluating the answer and stopping their search when they have obtained sufficient information. These different aspects of a teacher as information provider are explored in Chapter 3.

The teacher as a facilitator of learning and mentor

The move in education to a student-centred view of learning has required a fundamental shift in the role of the teacher. This has been described as a move from "the sage on the stage" to "the guide on the side" (King, 1993). The teacher should not be seen predominantly as a dispenser of information but rather as a facilitator or manager of the students' learning, inspiring and encouraging students to take responsibility for their own learning. The more responsibility and freedom given to the student, the greater the shift required in the teacher's role. Today the key responsibility of the teacher is to facilitate students' learning and, as discussed in Chapter 4, this can be achieved in a number of ways. The teacher can also serve as a mentor to learners and to colleagues.

The teacher as a curriculum developer and implementer

To fulfil your responsibility as a teacher, you need an understanding of the curriculum in your school and how your course fits into it. Diamond (1998) has suggested that teachers can undertake few activities that will have greater impact on their students than their active involvement in the design of a curriculum or course they teach. Curriculum planning, as described in Chapter 5, is an important role for the teacher. You can play a part in planning and implementing the curriculum in your school and also contribute to a review of the curriculum and its further development. Most medical schools and institutions have a curriculum committee responsible for the education programme, and you may be asked to serve on the committee or as a member of a group charged with organising one phase or course in the education programme.

The teacher as an assessor and diagnostician

Assessment has a great impact on students' learning and is a distinct area of activity that may dominate the curriculum. All teachers have some role with regard to assessment, but this will vary with their different levels of responsibility. Your responsibility might include selection of the appropriate assessment tool, implementation of the approach in practice, determination of pass/fail criteria, serving as an examiner in an OSCE, or provision of appropriate feedback to the student, identifying any gaps and deficiencies in their learning. As described in Chapter 6, this is an aspect of medical education in which there have been important developments.

The teacher as a role model

A less obvious role for the teacher is that of the role model, which is nonetheless a very important role. The teacher serves as a role model in the classroom and in the clinical context, and his or her example influences students' behaviour, attitudes and career aspirations. As William Osler advocated more than a century ago, we teach by example, whether we choose to do so or not. As described in Chapter 7, teachers serve as a role model for their students as a healthcare professional, as a teacher and through their personal behaviour.

The teacher as a manager and leader

All teachers have to some extent a management and leadership role, but this is frequently ignored. Your role as a manager may relate to the teaching session or the course for which you are responsible or to the curriculum more generally. The teacher's role as a manager has become more important with changes taking place in medical education and with developments such as integrated and interdisciplinary teaching, interprofessional education, problem-based learning, distributed learning and approaches to assessment such as the OSCE. In Chapter 8, we argue that every teacher is not only a manager but also a leader. Problems relating to the education programme that arise can often be attributed to mismanagement or poor leadership.

The teacher as a scholar and researcher

We argue in Chapter 9 that all teachers have a role as a scholar and a researcher in medical education. You should reflect on and evaluate your teaching with a view to enhancing the students' experience and adopt an evidence-based approach where appropriate. As part of your work, you may collaborate with specialists in education research. A few teachers may develop more advanced skills in research in medical education, and their role as a researcher in the field may represent a major activity for them. All teachers, however, have a responsibility to contribute to the advancement of teaching in their own subject and to communicate and share their experiences with others.

The teacher as a professional

As discussed in Chapter 1, the teacher is a professional and not simply a technician. This requires that teachers behave professionally with students, assess and evaluate their own performance as a teacher, keep themselves up to date with developments both in their speciality and in medical education and take responsibility for their own well-being. This is explored further in Chapter 10.

The use of the eight-roles framework

A consideration of the roles of teachers and the eight-roles framework offers major benefits:

- Teachers and the medical school or postgraduate training group are encouraged to think more fundamentally about the education process and the learners' experience and not just from a narrower perspective about the teaching and learning methods adopted. To what extent, for example, is it the intention to move to a more student-centred programme, where a key role of the teacher is to facilitate the student's learning rather than providing the student with the necessary information? What is the position and approach to assessment, and what is the involvement of staff in the assessment programme? What are the requirements and expectations of clinical teachers? Schools that see themselves at the cutting edge of education development will highlight the roles of scholar and change agent.

- The role model framework, as described in this text, provides a model and a language that facilitates discussion about the character of the medical school, the nature of the education programme and the expected roles of teachers. It helps discussion and interaction between the staff and the students. The model provides a basis for the preparation of job descriptions for teachers in the school. A description of the roles expected of a teacher, as defined in the eight-roles model, adds greatly to the value of a job description and complements the description of the tasks expected of the teacher in terms, for example, of lectures to be given.

- The framework highlights how teachers have different roles to play in the curriculum. Staff can then be assigned roles for which they are best suited and from which they will get the greatest satisfaction. Your responsibility for each role may be recognised as a minor one, a major one or you may assume a leadership responsibility.

- The model encourages you to reflect on your role both at the macro level of the school and in relation to your own personal individual teaching sessions, and this is likely to increase your effectiveness as a teacher.

- A staff (or faculty) development programme can be related to the roles assigned to you as a teacher, with an emphasis on the roles with which you are less familiar but where they have an important part to play. You should have an introduction to all the roles as part of an initial faculty development programme. More specialised training may be necessary with regard to specific roles. If, for example, a teacher is to take responsibility for the assessment and running of OSCEs, additional training relating to OSCEs is necessary, including the construction of checklists and global rating scales and information about how decisions are made regarding whether or not a student has achieved a satisfactory level of performance in the examination.

We discuss the uses of the eight-roles framework further in Chapter 11.

A teacher's responsibilities and the different roles

Although you may not be an expert in each area, as a teacher you should have a measure of familiarity and understanding of all the roles. This should be in the context of your medical school or postgraduate programme and should include the expected learning outcomes, the agreed educational strategies, the courses in the curriculum and the assessment methods. You may have a major commitment to selected roles and a minor commitment to others. You may fill each role at a basic level or at an expert or at master level. We have defined this for each of the eight roles. Your role or commitment to a role, however, may change over time.

Two teachers have described their personal roles as teachers and how these have changed over time. Vimmi Passi, an experienced clinical teacher, describes how she

Box 2.1 My roles as a teacher[a]

I have sincerely enjoyed all my varied and interesting roles as a medical educator. My journey begins in undergraduate education. As an assessor in medical student selection, it was a privilege to assess those candidates who in time would become our future doctors. Also, I particularly enjoyed being a facilitator of the small group teaching of communication skills. This was often the first clinical contact that students had with patients and it was fascinating to share their experiences and teach them new consultation and clinical skills.

Moving on, in postgraduate education, I found the one to one relationship with the learner to be quite unique in that it offers the opportunity to role model high standards of patient centred care in clinical practice. My journey then continued as the Director of the Masters in Medical Education Programme, in which my activities involved being a curriculum planner, resource developer, innovator and educational manager. In all these educational roles, I always ensured a student centred approach within supportive and friendly educational environments.

Throughout this journey, I have developed my own interest and passion in medical education research. Reflecting on all these voyages, I have realised that being an excellent medical teacher has similar values to being an excellent physician, in that it involves being compassionate, inspiring and dedicated to maintaining high quality standards.

[a]*Vimmi Passi, Division of Medical Education, Faculty of Life Sciences and Medicine, Kings College, London, UK.*

has assumed a range of roles at different stages of her career in undergraduate and then postgraduate education. The attributes of caring for students, motivating and inspiring them and maintaining high standards as part of a professional approach to her work, as we described in Chapter 1, are the attributes of an excellent teacher (Box 2.1). Matthew Gwee, an experienced teacher in Singapore, describes how his role has evolved from information provider to facilitator, curriculum developer, assessor, manager and scholar (Box 2.2). Both have a commitment to their students and how the students learn.

A competing values framework

Quinn et al. (1996) have used a similar approach to our eight-roles framework for a medical teacher to describe the functions of a manager, as noted in Chapter 8. They described this as a "competing values framework," with the management functions within the quadrants of the framework carrying conflicting messages. In the same way, the different teaching roles appear at first sight to conflict with each other. We see the teacher as a provider of information but also as a facilitator of learning, encouraging the student to take responsibility for acquiring his or her own information. We also see the teacher as a facilitator of learning and as an assessor whose role is to pass judgement on the student. Within the framework, these opposing views of a teacher's role can mutually co-exist. Indeed, different roles may complement each other, such as the facilitator and the role model.

Box 2.2 My journey as a teacher[a]

My journey as a teacher in pharmacology started when the medical curriculum was highly discipline-specific, instruction highly teacher-directed and discipline-silos prevailed. My primary role then was to inform students of factual content knowledge delivered mainly through didactic lectures; students underwent passive learning ("sit, listen, take notes"), often learned by rote ("memorise, recall, regurgitate in exams"), and were also highly teacher-dependent for their learning needs. Assessment focused mainly on factual recall, marking, grading and ranking.

Rapidly changing trends in medical education soon followed, due mainly to the impact of disruptive forces on healthcare delivery. The *BMJ*, The *Lancet* and the *NEJM* also devoted precious space to current issues in health professions education. The Lancet Commission (Frenk et al., 2010) stated that 20th century health professions education "*produces ill-equipped graduates*" and that "*...strategies are not fit to solve 21st century challenges.*" Transformative learning was strongly advocated to educate and equip health professions students with lifelong habits of mind, action and behaviour for 21st century practice.

Thus, from just 'informing', the teacher now needs to involve students actively in the teaching-learning process, and take on the role of planner, designer, manager of the learning environment; to facilitate knowledge acquisition and development of intellectual and interpersonal skills; empower students to take greater initiative and responsibility to direct-manage more of their own learning (to develop the ability for self-directed learning as a foundation for future lifelong continuing self-education); assess more knowledge-processing skills and knowledge-application; provide feedback to help improve student learning; and teach as scholars of education to reflect scholarship in teaching and learning.

[a]*Matthew Gwee, National University of Singapore, Singapore.*

We will return in Chapter 11 to how the roles are interconnected, their significance in curriculum planning, their relevance to individual teachers' portfolios and their importance for faculty development programmes.

Take-home messages

1. Insufficient attention has been paid in healthcare professions education to the roles and responsibilities of the teacher. For the medical school or postgraduate programme, attention to the teachers' or trainers' roles leads to a more effective and efficient learning programme. For the individual teacher or trainer, there is potentially greater job satisfaction and a greater opportunity to make a valuable contribution to the programme and to students' learning.
2. Defining the teacher's roles provides an insight into the institution's approach to education, the education environment and how students learn.
3. The roles of a teacher include information provider, facilitator, curriculum planner and implementer, assessor, role model, manager and leader, scholar and professional.

Consider

- Is sufficient attention paid in your institution to the different roles of teachers or trainers?
- Think about the contribution you personally make to your students' learning. What would your students miss if you were not there?
- Take a few minutes to consider your own role in terms of the eight roles. You can refine your thoughts about what you see as your preferred role, and how you can best contribute to the education programme, as you read a more detailed description of each role in subsequent chapters.

Explore further

Diamond, R.M., 1998. Designing and Assessing Courses and Curricula: A Practical Guide, 2nd ed. Jossey-Bass, San Francisco.

Drucker, P.F., 1994. The theory of the business. Harvard Bus. Rev. Sept-Oct

Fox, D., 1983. Personal theories of teaching. Stud. High Educ. 8 (2), 151–163.

Frenk, J., Chen, L., Bhutta, Z.A., et al., 2010. Health professionals for a new century: transforming education to strengthen health systems in an interdependent world. Lancet 376 (9756), 1923–1958.

Harden, R.M., Crosby, J., 2000. The good teacher is more than a lecturer - the twelve roles of the teacher. Med. Teach. 22 (4), 334–347.

Hodgins, W., 2005. Into the future of meLearning: every one learning imagine if the impossible isn't! In: Masie, E. (Ed.), Learning Rants, Raves, and Reflections: A Collection of Passionate and Professional Perspectives. pp. 243-290 Pfeiffer Publishing, San Francisco.

King, A., 1993. From Sage on the Stage to Guide on the Side. College Teaching 41 (1), 30–35.

Nikendei, C., Ben-David, M.F., Mennin, S., et al., 2016. Medical educators: How they define themselves – results of an international web survey. Med. Teach. 38 (7), 715–723.

Pontefract, D., 2016. The Purpose Effect: Building Meaning in Yourself, Your Role and Your Organization. Elevate Publishing, Boise.

Pyörälä, E., 2014. How we developed a role-based portfolio for teachers' professional development. Med. Teach. 36 (9), 765–768.

Quinn, R.E., Faerman, S.R., Thompson, M.P., et al., 1996. Becoming A Master Manager: A Competency Framework, second ed. Wiley, New York, pp. 9–24.

Sinek, S., 2011. Start With Why: How Great Leaders Inspire Everyone to Take Action. Penguin, London.

Squires, G., 1999. Teaching as a Professional Discipline. Falmer Press, London.

Vargas, J.S., 1972. Writing Worthwhile Behavioral Objectives. Harper & Row, New York.

Chapter 3

The teacher as an information provider and coach

Knowledge is of two kinds. We know a subject ourselves, or we know where we can find information upon it.

Dr Samuel Johnson, Boswell, *Life of Johnson*, 18th April, 1775

The role of the teacher as information provider has changed, but it remains an important role.

- Your role as an information provider
- Your role as a subject expert and transmitter of information
- Your responsibilities as an information provider and transmitter of information
- Core information and information overload
- Threshold concepts
- The information pyramid
- Provision of information
  - The lecture
  - The flipped classroom
  - Handouts and notes
  - Recordings of lectures
  - Clinical context
- The impact of the information provided
- Your role as a curator of information
- Your role as an information coach
- The teacher as information provider, an expert information provider and a master information provider
- Take-home message
- Consider
- Explore further

Your role as an information provider

Bishop (1984, p. 91), winner of the Nobel Prize in Medicine, described the three purposes and practices of teaching as "First, to inspire. Second, to challenge. Third, and only third, to impart information." In later chapters, we discuss your role of inspiring and challenging the student. In this chapter, we explore

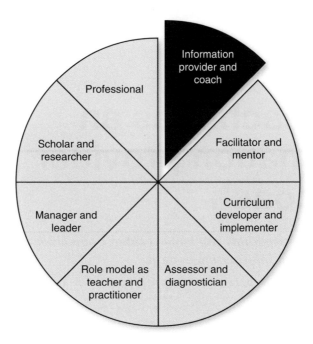

Figure 3.1 The role of the teacher as information provider

your role as an information provider (Fig. 3.1). The elements of this role are (Fig. 3.2):

- As a conduit for information – transmitting information to the student
- As a curator of information – filtering information and making information available from a number of sources
- As an information coach – guiding the student in seeking information

Your role as a subject expert and transmitter of information

This represents the traditional role of the teacher, passing on your knowledge and expertise to the student. The need to provide the student with the required knowledge effectively and efficiently has been seen as a basic function of teachers by virtue of their expertise in an area. Teachers are expected by students to be responsible for transmitting to them the substance of the course, a view that is shared by many teachers. For example, when students in Sri Lanka were asked to rate the different roles of the teacher, the role of information provider ranked higher than other roles, such as being a role model or facilitator of learning (Hettihewa and Karunathilake, 2017). At the University of Glasgow, the senior academic post of Reader was created, reflecting the practice whereby the teacher transmits information in a lecture by reading to the students from a selected text.

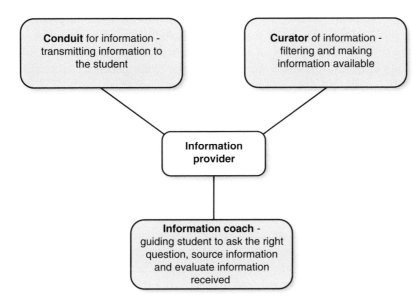

Figure 3.2 The three roles of the teacher as an information provider

In a survey of medical educators, common terms used to describe themselves were *medical expert* and *information provider* (Nikendei et al., 2016). The information provider was defined as "a skilled person who devotes him/herself to passing on knowledge in clinical and non-clinical settings, with the aim to enhance patient care."

The concept of the teacher as someone who imparts knowledge is reflected in Fox's "transfer model" of teaching, as introduced in Chapter 2 (Fox, 1983):

> *People who adopt the transfer theory of teaching see knowledge as a commodity which can be transferred, by the act of teaching, from one container to another or from one location to another. Such people tend to express their view of teaching as 'imparting knowledge' or 'conveying information.' (p. 152)*

Teachers who are information providers may take their work very seriously. As Fox has reported:

> *Conscientious transferrers spend a great deal of time preparing their material and making sure that it is accurate and up-to-date. Some of them also go to great lengths to develop and refine their methods of transfer and they often devise elaborate teaching aids to inject the essence of their subjects accurately into the heart of the container. (p. 152)*

This role of the teacher as an expert who is knowledgeable in his or her field and who passes on this knowledge to students commonly features in descriptions of the "good" or "excellent" teacher, as described in Chapter 1. Even in problem-based learning (PBL), the value of the teacher as an expert has been identified. Groups where the tutor or facilitator is an expert in the topic have been more highly rated by students than groups where the tutor has the skills necessary to facilitate the work of the group, but does not have expert knowledge in the area. The potential disadvantage of the "expert facilitator," however, is that the teacher adopts the role of information provider throughout the session, which deteriorates into a lecture or tutorial on the topic delivered by the teacher – a not uncommon problem in PBL.

This role of the teacher as a transmitter of information features prominently in the literature. Johnston (1996) has reported that although teachers did not speak specifically of teaching as transmitting the content of their subject, disciplinary knowledge was at the heart of their teaching approaches. In a study of distinguished clinical teachers, Irby (1994) has concluded that a key element in teaching is the organisation and presentation of medical knowledge "so that learners can comprehend it to satisfy their learning objects" (p. 340). The importance attached to the role of the teacher as an information provider is partly cultural. Gokcora (1997), for example, has found that Chinese students, more than American students, value the professor's knowledge of the subject and its transmission to the student.

Unfortunately, it is the students who often perpetuate this theory of teaching and learning with their support for the process where knowledge is transferred from the teacher to the student through, for example, well-structured lectures. In their view, it is the teacher's job to teach and theirs to learn.

When you consider your role as information provider, it is important to remember that the information communicated to the student should vary with the seniority of the student. The information required by first-year students when they see a patient with a fractured femur or discuss a patient in a PBL session will be different from the information appropriate for a final-year medical student. One orthopaedic surgeon, I (RMH) observed, treated the first-year students in his PBL group as if they were final-year students. Although the specialist surgical approach to the patient with the fractured femur was of some interest to the students, it could not be fully appreciated because the students still had to master an understanding of the relevant anatomy and basic clinical skills. Students in a spiral curriculum will expand their knowledge and understanding of a topic as they revisit the topic in the education programme (Harden and Stamper, 1999).

Your responsibilities as an information provider and transmitter of information

The role of the teacher as information provider is changing, and other roles of the teacher, as described in Chapter 2, have attracted more attention. The good teacher embraces these changing roles. As a teacher, however, you have a responsibility to ensure that the students directly acquire the necessary information through your teaching or indirectly from available information sources. There are good reasons why this is so.

Your responsibilities as an information provider are to:

- Provide information that may not otherwise be available to the student. This may be up-to-date information about a topic when there have been significant changes or information that is relevant to a specific locality or context.
- Identify the core information that the student should master. With the rapid expansion of knowledge in medicine and the medical sciences, information overload is a potential problem which as a teacher you can help guard against. It is no longer possible for the learner to acquire all the knowledge in a specific area. The *core or essential* information should be specified. This is discussed in more detail below.
- Identify the threshold concepts that are key to mastery of a subject and, as described below, are essential for the learner to grasp if they are to progress.
- Include information that, although not essential, may help motivate the student and add interest to the topic. For example, when thinking about stress and hyperthyroidism, I (RMH) aroused a student's interest by describing the first case of hyperthyroidism or Graves' disease that manifested itself in a patient confined to a wheelchair shortly after he had the misfortune of careering down a hill, having been released inadvertently by his attendant. Macnab (2017) has suggested that such historical accounts offer new and creative avenues for students to explore the art and science of medicine.
- Demonstrate the links and relationships between items of information and, in the process, integrate the basic sciences and clinical medicine. A concept map can be used for this purpose; this can be developed into a curriculum map, as discussed in Chapters 4 and 5.
- Assist the student to move up the information pyramid from awareness to information, knowledge and wisdom, as described below.

Wojciech Pawlina, a renowned anatomy teacher since 1978, highlights what he sees as his role in the curriculum as an information provider in Box 3.1.

Core information and information overload

One of the important challenges facing medical education is information overload. This has been described as leading to an "information fatigue syndrome," with associated anxiety and deficiencies in remembering (D'Eon et al., 2000):

One of the most contentious issues with which faculty struggle concerns how much material to give students to learn. Time after time faculty wonder how they can 'cover' so much material in so little time. The problem is not one of technique (How can I magically get all this information into the heads of students in the time allotted?) nor one of judgement (How do I know, while I am teaching, when I have filled their heads with enough information?). The problem is one of social expectations

Box 3.1 Beyond mere knowledge[a]

Teaching anatomy in medical school used to be simple: lecture, supervise dissection, write and label practical exams, grade the students, repeat. Basic sciences knowledge once seemed to me to be a pure science—mere knowledge packaged for memorization, easily transmitted and acquired. This is no longer true. Being an anatomy teacher today is a complex art. Beyond transfer of content, teachers must carefully create a culture of safe clinical practice and offer many windows for application and integration with the healthcare professions. When I teach anatomy, I focus on concepts and on the most clinically relevant information so that learning may be rewarded with a recognition of their basic science knowledge in the first patient encounters they have. Anatomy should no longer be regarded as a stack of facts to memorize to pass exams; rather, anatomy should be considered to be an essential physician tool vital for patient examination, diagnosis, and treatment. I pride myself that I am a teacher of first skills, first words, and early clinical competency. In addition, basic science educators must share the responsibility for promoting early development of non-technical skills such as situational awareness, decision-making, teamwork, leadership, and professionalism in relation to the delivery of safe clinical practice. Over the years I have learned that to be a successful teacher you must be authentic, you must always look to teach more than your subject, so as to ultimately assess competencies beyond mere knowledge.

[a]Wojciech Pawlina, Professor of Anatomy and Medical Education, Chair of Department of Anatomy, Mayo Clinic College of Medicine and Science, Mayo Clinic, Rochester, USA.

(I am expected to teach this much!) and norms (This is the way that I was taught and this is what most other people seem to be doing.) and purpose (What is it that I am supposed to be doing anyway?). (p. 159)

Knowledge doubled in the 150 years from 1750 to 1900, in the 50 years from 1900 to 1950, in the 5 years from 1960 to 1965 and is predicted to double in 73 days by 2020 (Gilliani, 2000). Although learners are expected to have a breadth of knowledge, it is no longer possible for the student (or the doctor) to have a depth of knowledge across the board. Shumak (1992) has suggested that:

with the proliferation of new medical knowledge and the desire of faculty to try to cover everything the factual overload faced by medical students under the traditional curriculum was becoming absurd. (p. 1152)

The problem of information overload was highlighted in an editorial in the *Lancet* (Anon., 1991):

Especially in good basic science departments and teaching hospitals, the excitement of new knowledge, the presence of research units, conspire to pack the curriculum ever tighter. (p. 1048)

Atul Gawande illustrated the problem during a presentation at an AAMC meeting in Seattle in 2016. He described how the doctor is faced with more than 60,000 different possible diagnoses, 6,000 available drugs and 4,000 possible medical and surgical procedures. The student or doctor cannot be expected to master details of all of these. As a teacher, you should identify the essential knowledge expected and be selective in the information that you assist the learner to acquire or master. For example, in the management of a patient with hyperthyroidism, students must be aware of the therapeutic possibilities, including anti-thyroid drugs, radioactive iodine and surgery and the main side effects. They do not need to be able to recall the dose of the drug or the details of radioactive iodine administration or surgery, nor do they need anatomical knowledge relating to blood supply to the thyroid gland or the details of thyroid hormone synthesis. Some might argue, however, that an understanding of thyroid hormone synthesis can help them appreciate the time lag between the administration of an anti-thyroid drug and the patient's clinical improvement.

The problem of information overload has demanded a fundamental reorientation of the curriculum and this included the strategy of a core curriculum which covered the essential elements of a course that all students should master and options or student-selected components in the curriculum that allowed a student to study a subject in more depth (Harden and Davis, 2001). This concept of a core curriculum and options was a key element of the recommendations from the UK General Medical Council in their report on 'Tomorrow's Doctors" (General Medical Council, 1993):

> Until an attempt is made to circumscribe the requirements of the course in
> respect of factual quantum, the unconfined overload of the curriculum will
> prevail and will continue to deny students the educational opportunities
> to which they are entitled. We therefore recommend the introduction of
> what we will refer to as a 'core curriculum' which defines the requirements
> that must be satisfied before a newly qualified doctor can assume the
> responsibilities of a pre-registration house officer. (p. 7)

The concept of a core curriculum stimulated an interest in the curriculum content and whether important topics were neglected and not addressed. Groups and professional bodies, including physiologists, neurologists, obstetricians and behavioural scientists, have specified what they believed to be the core content for their subject. Agreeing what constitutes a core curriculum and the core information that a student should master is not easy. Who should decide the core information? This should not be left to individual disciplines or specialities but should be addressed jointly by the different stakeholders:

- Specialists in the field
- Practising doctors in hospitals and in the community
- University teachers and educationists
- Students and recent graduates
- Other professions (e.g. nurses)
- Representatives of employers
- Patients and representatives of patient groups
- The public

A number of approaches can be used to elicit the key or core information required of the practitioner and which should serve as the basis for the education programme (Dunn et al., 1985; Laidlaw et al.,1995; Harden and Laidlaw, 2017). Approaches include:

- Focus group discussions and a nominal group technique with representatives of the different stakeholders
- A Delphi technique using a panel representing the stakeholders
- A critical incident survey of good and bad practices
- Studies of errors in practice
- Task analysis based on observation of a practising doctor
- Interviews with recent graduates
- A study of existing curricula and publications, including recommendations from specialist bodies and accrediting authorities

The required core information will change over time with advances in medical practice and with other changes as the learner progresses through the different phases of the education programme. Determining what is core information is an important and difficult task but it is essential if you are to tackle the problem of information overload. We discuss this further when we describe the "information pyramid" later in this chapter.

Threshold concepts

The idea of threshold concepts was introduced recently and merits consideration. It has attracted attention over the past decade in different areas of education but has been relatively neglected in medical education. Threshold concepts are crucial points in a conceptual understanding of a field without which one cannot move forward. They were identified by the Open University as one of the ten new pedagogies associated with trends in education practice (Sharples et al., 2014).

The principle of threshold concepts has been attributed to Ray Land, Professor of Higher Education at the University of Strathclyde, Glasgow, and Jan Meyer, Professor of Education at the University of Durham, UK. In a book co-edited with Caroline Baillie (Land et al., 2010), they describe the idea of threshold concepts:

> ...the approach builds on the notion that there are certain concepts, or certain learning experiences, which resemble passing through a portal, from which a new perspective opens up, allowing things formerly not perceived to come into view. This permits a new and previously inaccessible way of thinking about something. It represents a transformed way of understanding, or interpreting, or viewing something, without which the learner cannot progress, and results in a reformulation of the learners' frame of meaning. (p. ix)

Mastery of a threshold concept can be described as the "Aha" moment, when the student integrates and connects different elements of learning and has a new understanding of the subject (Neve et al., 2016).

Some of the first threshold concepts identified were in science subjects. Examples were gravity in science and evolution in biology. Neve and co-workers (2016) described how the theory of threshold concepts can be applied to medicine. Examples they provide of a threshold concept include:

- Homeostasis
- Empathy
- Ethics
- The nature of evidence
- Uncertainty
- Embodied shared care
- The relationships between inequalities and health

Neve et al. (2016) have argued:

> *It may be that threshold concepts are themselves a threshold concept! Our own experience is that getting to grips with the theory can be troublesome: the notion of threshold concepts can initially seem abstract and hard to understand. Yet it has transformed the way we see and practice our educational work. As the literature continues to expand and develop in other disciplines, we would encourage medical educators to explore the value of applying and researching the threshold concept framework within their own contexts. (p. 852)*

We argue that there are threshold concepts too in the speciality of medical education. Examples are:

- The different roles of the teacher (the theme of this book). The teacher needs not only certain abilities to practise as a teacher but requires also an understanding and appreciation of his or her roles as a teacher.
- Facilitation of learning by the teacher is more important than information transmission.
- Teaching, learning and assessment should be authentic and related to the real world of medical practice (as described in Chapter 5).
- Assessment should be *for* learning as well as *of* learning (as described in Chapter 6).
- Education programmes should be outcome-based rather than time-based.

All these concepts are important and may require teachers to reconceptualise their approach to teaching. They are like "Aha" moments for medical education.

Threshold concepts have been described as having certain features. A threshold concept is:

- Transformative – it brings about a significant shift of the learner's perception as a student; it is a quantum leap in ability which makes possible a greater number of solutions to many problems.

- Integrative – it exposes previous hidden connections across boundaries.
- Irreversible – it is unlikely to be forgotten or unlearned.
- Troublesome – learners may find difficulty in passing through the portal; the concept may be difficult until something clicks.
- Bounded – it is demarcated from other conceptual areas.

These recognise a significant shift in the teachers' perceptions of their work and may be difficult for teachers to grasp and implement. Stephen Loftus, in an Essential Skills in Medical Education (ESME) course report, describes these features in Box 3.2.

The role of threshold concepts in medical education is not yet clear, but the idea looks promising and certainly merits further consideration. It offers a fresh insight into the teacher as information provider.

Box 3.2 Threshold concepts[a]

Threshold concepts are said to be transformative. Once grasped, they change people, and they change people forever. There is as much an ontological change as there is an epistemological change. For example, when learning to cope with complex, ill-structured conditions, such as chronic pain, it can come as a major revelation to some students to find that definitive cure is not always possible (Loftus, 2011).

The simplistic cause/effect mechanistic thinking that many students have, when they begin, turns out to be inadequate. They discover that managing, rather than curing, the complexity may be the only viable option. They may also come to appreciate that such complex management is often best done in a multidisciplinary partnership with other health professionals. Once this has been grasped then patients with complex, ill-structured problems are never seen simplistically again. This highlights another feature of threshold concepts. They are irreversible once learned. This can be a problem for teachers who can, in a sense, forget they know such concepts. In such cases, the concept has become so embodied and so much a part of the experienced practitioner that there is little conscious awareness of the concept, even though it is used in practice every day. Another characteristic of threshold concepts is said to be that they are integrative and expose the relationships with other concepts that might not have been so obvious before. Related to this is another characteristic. Threshold concepts are bounded, in that they are clearly demarcated. Cousin (2006) warns that some threshold concepts can be regarded as the exclusive property of a specific discipline with the danger that they may be accepted uncritically. The implication is that curriculum design should always include the requirement for any concept to be questioned and challenged. Cousin (2006) advises that it is always best to regard threshold concepts as provisional. Finally, threshold concepts tend to involve 'troublesome knowledge'. There can be a common sense or procedural understanding of a concept that can interfere with the ability of students to grasp the concept in the way that their teachers desire. Many students may need to experience a liminal state before coming to a fuller understanding of threshold concepts.

---

[a]Stephen Loftus, Associate Professor, Oakland University William Beaumont School of Medicine, Rochester, Michigan, USA.

The information pyramid

We have described the role of the teacher as **information** provider. But what is "information," and how does it relate to knowledge and wisdom? Information can be considered as the facts or details about a subject. It is what is communicated by the teacher to students. It may be, for example, the anatomy of the bones in the leg, the actions of thyroid hormone or the diagnostic features of melanoma. Information is the second level of what we have described as the information pyramid (Fig. 3.3).

Knowledge is described as the third level in the pyramid. The distinction between information and knowledge may be blurred, however, and the two are sometimes equated, with information defined as knowledge or details of a subject. In the classic DIKW (*d*ata, *i*nformation, *k*nowledge, *w*isdom) hierarchy, knowledge is distinguished from information (Rowley, 2007). Knowledge requires the information to be contextualised and for there to be a measure of familiarity and understanding of the topic gained from experience or study of the subject. It implies that there is an element of expert insight and a measure of accumulated learning. Knowledge of hyperthyroidism, for example, includes an understanding of the combination of symptoms and laboratory investigations required to confirm that the patient's thyroid is overactive. Knowledge relating to a patient with melanoma includes an understanding of the risk factors for a patient and recognising when a patient with a skin lesion should be referred for further treatment.

Wisdom, at the top of the information pyramid, comes through reflection and experience and requires judgements to be made when the knowledge is applied in practice in different contexts, with different patients. The doctor knows the right thing to do in different and difficult circumstances; for example, should the 50-year-old female patient presenting with hyperthyroidism be treated with anti-thyroid drugs, radioactive iodine or surgery?

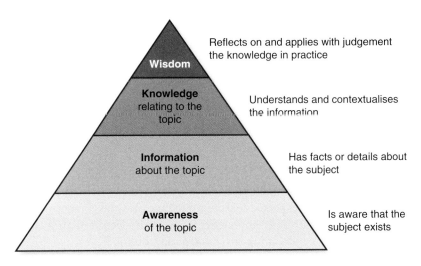

Figure 3.3 The information pyramid

At the bottom of the pyramid, beneath the information level, is "awareness." At the awareness level, the learner has heard about a topic, is aware of it, but does not have significant information about it. This need for a doctor to be aware of a wide range of topics but not have the details of them is an important but relatively neglected concept in medical education. The learner should be aware that many different diagnoses, drugs and practical procedures, as noted by Atul Gawande, exist but they may not have the details. The details can be explored later, if and when they are required – "just-in-time" learning. The challenge is to make the learner aware of a diagnosis, drug or procedure but not require her or him to acquire the sort of information about it, as is often assessed by multiple-choice questions.

As an information provider, you have the critical role of determining the level on the information pyramid expected of the student at each phase of training. The level of awareness, information, knowledge and wisdom expected of a student will vary at different stages in the curriculum. For some topics, it will not rise above the awareness level by the completion of undergraduate training. The student should be aware that the subject exists and, if required later, can acquire further information as necessary. For other topics, the student will be expected to have the relevant knowledge, progressing perhaps later to the level of wisdom.

Provision of information

As we have discussed, the teacher has the responsibility of deciding what information the student should acquire. The teacher also has the responsibility of providing the student with the information in the most effective and efficient way. The teacher can provide the student with information in a range of contexts, both face-to-face and at a distance, in the classroom or in the clinical context, and to large groups, small groups or individual students (Fig. 3.4). The student acquires information by listening, watching or reading.

The lecture

The most traditional approach, and the one still most widely used to transmit information to the student, is the lecture. Many teachers see this as the main function of the lecture. In the lecture, the teacher can be selective as to what information is presented and can personalise this and relate it to the needs of the students in the class. When reviewing the information to be presented in a lecture, you should consider:

- What information do the students already have on the topic?
- What information should you communicate in the lecture, and how does this relate to the expected learning outcomes for the course?
- How will students learn more effectively in the lecture than if they were reading a text or obtaining the information online?
- How does the information to be presented relate to the information students will acquire in other parts of the course?

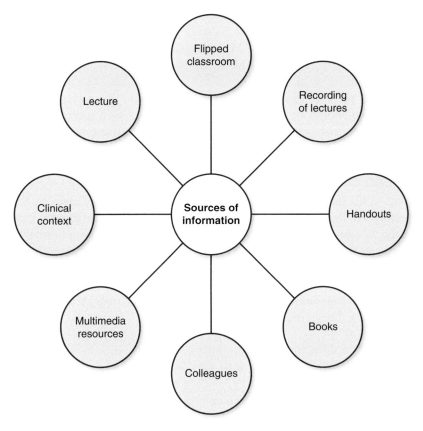

Figure 3.4 Provision of information

- Are you providing the students with a structure or organisational framework for the information provided?
- How can students obtain further details or study the subject in more depth?
- How can students know if they have mastered the information provided?

The lecture can be presented to students in a way that facilitates their learning, as discussed in Chapter 4. Marzano (2009) has suggested five elements to an effective strategy:

- Chunk the new information into small, digestible bites.
- Scaffold the information in a logical order.
- Allow students to interact with the information presented.
- Pace the presentation of the information, not too fast and not too slow.
- Monitor and check students' understanding.

Almost every teacher at one time or another will have the responsibility of delivering a lecture. For some teachers, lecturing will be a major area of activity. The necessary skills can and should be acquired. Not everyone can become a brilliant lecturer but everyone can acquire the necessary skills to be a good lecturer. How to prepare for and deliver a lecture is discussed in AMEE Medical Education Guide no. 22 by Brown and Manogue (2001) published by AMEE – an International Association for Medical Education, and in texts such as *Essential Skills for a Medical Teacher* (Harden and Laidlaw, 2017) and *A Practical Guide for Medical Teachers* (Dent et al., 2017). After your lecture, you should study feedback from students. Much useful advice can be obtained from students' evaluations or from a colleague sitting in and listening to your lecture. The lecture is discussed further in Chapter 5.

The flipped classroom

A variation on the traditional approach to the lecture is the flipped classroom. Students are given access to the information normally presented in the lecture through recordings of the lecture or other learning resources. They study this individually or in small groups. Having done so, the students meet with the lecturer as a large group when they discuss areas of difficulty or apply the information learned to solve clinical or other problems.

The term "flipped classroom" was first used in 2007 by chemistry teachers Bergmann and Sams (2012). They argued that:

- Students need their teachers present to answer questions, to help them apply principles to practice or to provide help if they find areas of difficulty.
- Students don't need their teachers present to listen to a recording of a lecture or review content.

The use of the flipped classroom approach offers a number of advantages:

- Students can study the resource material provided at their own pace, individually, in pairs or in small groups.
- Learning is personalised to the needs of the student, and the time required of them to master the topic can vary. Students may be given a choice of how they can acquire the information (e.g. text, video or interactive programme).
- The classroom time is transformed from a passive to an active experience. The teacher uses the time with the class to tackle issues or problems raised by the class rather than simply communicating the information relating to the topic of the lecture, which has been done by other means. The lecture theatre becomes a "learning space."
- An opportunity is provided in the classroom session for the teacher to provide feedback and remediation to students.

Potential disadvantages of the flipped classroom approach include:

- Time is required to prepare the necessary resources for the students to study before attending the whole class session.
- Students may come to the class session not having used the resources.

- The job of the teacher in the class session is more demanding but also more rewarding.

Before the classroom session, students can study the subject using a range of resources such as:

- A recorded lecture
- Other learning resources prepared by the lecturer
- Online resources and textbooks
- Learning resources prepared by students

You can prepare a study guide to advise the students about the various options available and what is expected of them. In addition to studying the resources provided, students can be encouraged to:

- Write notes
- Identify a question for later consideration
- Discuss with peers

During the classroom session, options include:

- Consideration of questions or issues raised by students
- Consideration of areas of difficulty sometimes experienced by students
- Review of the expected learning outcomes
- In-depth discussion of selected topics or key issues
- Application of knowledge to tackle a problem

The flipped classroom is very different from the traditional lecture. There are a number of implications:

- The teacher must be able to relinquish control of the learning process.
- The teacher must be able to identify or prepare appropriate learning resources for use before the session. A study guide can be prepared to advise the students about their preparation for the whole class session.
- The teacher should be a master of the content to facilitate the classroom discussion. This is challenging but can be enjoyable.
- The teacher must be able to operate in the classroom in a non-linear fashion and have the mental ability to move from one topic to another.
- The teacher must be able to admit when he or she does not know the answer to a student's question and must be willing to research an answer with the student.

What has been learned from the use of the flipped classroom? Strayer (2007), based on experience at Ohio State University, gave the following useful advice:

- Provide students with different approaches to interacting with the content outside the class.

- Avoid too much uncertainty in the class session; support students "meaning making" in the activity.
- Give students the opportunity to reflect on their learning and their mind set towards the activity.
- Consider a less radical flip with the maintenance of some lectures.

How a flipped classroom can be introduced in practice has been described by Jeffries et al. (2017). They have recommended that students should be held accountable in some way for preparing for the class session using a readiness assurance test, where students answer a few questions that count towards their course grade. In the class session, the activities must challenge students at higher levels of learning.

Handouts and notes

The key information relating to a topic presented in a lecture can be summarised for students and presented electronically or in the form of printed notes. Handouts are used frequently to support lectures and can take different forms. They may be complete summaries of the information presented or be in the form of headings, with the student expected to complete the notes during the lecture. Copies of the PowerPoint slides used in the lecture may also be made available to the student. Although this is a common practice, it is a misuse of PowerPoint. When accompanied by audio recordings of the lecture, the slides may be useful. However, if they are used as a stand-alone learning resource, this almost certainly indicates an inappropriate use of PowerPoint as slides should complement the lecturer's commentary, not replace it.

Recordings of lectures

Increasing use is being made of recordings of lectures, and a wide range of software is now available for lecture capture. Students can use the recordings to study the information covered in the lecture instead of attending the lecture or as an aid to revisiting the lecture contents at a later time. The merits of this have been questioned, and concern has been expressed that students will be discouraged from attending the lecture in person if recordings are available and, as a result, not have the advantage of face-to-face contact with the lecturer and not have the opportunity to interact and to ask questions. On the other hand, in terms of information acquisition, the use of lecture recordings has the advantage that students can study the material at their own time, place and pace. This will vary from student to student. In one case, we found that although students took an average of 1 hour to review a lecture recording, some took over 4 hours to study the same lecture. Students can also watch the recording on several occasions to review the content.

Although recordings of lectures are relatively easy to produce and make available to students, they are not ideal as an independent learning resource for either primary learning or revision. The ideal primary learning resource should be more interactive, with students given opportunities to assess their understanding of the subject as they work through the presentation. For the purposes of revision, the recording can be edited and broken down into chunks of information, with each chunk accessed directly, allowing the student a greater flexibility in how it is used. A self-assessment element can be added.

Clinical context

Whether in the hospital or in the community, the clinical setting is a powerful context for the clinical teacher to transmit and the student to acquire information directly relevant to the practice of medicine. This is achieved during:

- Teaching ward rounds
- Ward-based tutorials
- Grand rounds where cases of interest are presented
- More informally, with the student in the role of clinical apprentice

The clinical teacher demonstrates the application of theory to practice and explains the basic skills of history taking and physical examination in clinical practice-based and simulated situations. Good clinical teachers can share their thoughts with the student as a "reflective practitioner," helping to illuminate the process of clinical reasoning and decision making for the student.

The impact of the information provided

A measure of responsibility for the successful transmission of information to the students must rest with the teacher as information provider. The teacher has a responsibility as information provider to make sure that the information is presented in a way that ensures that students successfully acquire the necessary information. All too often, teachers believe that they have done their job and have been successful as information providers, without any reflection or evidence as to whether the learners have processed and understood the information provided. Naïvely, the belief is that what has been taught must have been learned. As Fox (1983) indicated:

> Because the transfer theory concentrates a teacher's attention on the commodity before it is transferred and then on the act of transfer, it often causes him to overlook what happens to the commodity after transfer. ... Thus when it is discovered that, in spite of all the teacher's efforts, the container is not very full, the explanations tend to be in terms of leaky containers. ... Not many lecturers acknowledge that a good deal of the material, although it is being well prepared and 'poured out' is, in fact, missing the target and sloshing over the sides of the container. (p. 152)

However, Bourdieu and Passeron (1990) have argued:

> Teaching is at its most effective not when it succeeds in transmitting the greatest quality of information in the shortest time (and at least cost) but rather when most of the information conveyed by the teacher is actually received.

To be a successful information provider, we need to question whether the student has received and understood the information provided. At a simple and technical level, this may mean questioning, for example, whether the text or diagram in a PowerPoint presentation was legible to students at the back of the classroom or whether the students have had time to read and assimilate all the information on the PowerPoint slide. When I (RMH) was a junior lecturer, the head of department listened to my presentations sitting in the back row of the lecture theatre to ensure my comments were audible and my slides legible.

To gain an understanding of what students have learned in a lecture, it is revealing to examine students' notes at the end of the lecture. Not infrequently, what the lecturer has said has been misinterpreted, and mistakes are found. Particularly worrying is that this is often a greater problem with poorer students who, even at this point in time, as a result of the quality of their notes, are starting at a disadvantage from their more able colleagues.

Giving students the opportunity to ask questions in a lecture and using an audience response system to assess the students' understanding of a concept are ways of checking that students have understood the information provided. As the lecture proceeds, the display on a second screen showing the students' perceptions of their understanding of the information provided by the lecturer is another, perhaps more threatening, approach.

Whatever approach is adopted to providing the student with information, whether it is through a lecture, a set of notes, a learning programme or a clinical teaching session, we can only claim that our role as an information provider is fulfilled if the information presented is received and understood by the students. We also need to pay attention to the relevance of the information provided. Too often, the teacher as information provider pays scant regard to the relevance for the practising doctor of the information provided, having a blinkered view of the subject from their own personal perspective.

Your role as a curator of information

Much of the information needed by the students is available in texts or other learning resources. At an International Association of Medical Science Educators (IAMSE) meeting in San Diego, 2015, Paul Worley, then dean at Flinders Medical School, Australia, held up his iPhone and argued that all of the biomedical science information needed by students was available on the phone. Your role is to filter the resources available and direct the student to appropriate resources so that only helpful resources are included to assist their learning.

Students are often given a list of textbooks or papers they are expected to read – "the reading list" but this is very often ignored by students. If you provide such a list, you should:

- Be specific; advise students what chapter or paper they should read and what figures or illustrations they should study.

- Distinguish core texts considered as essential reading and additional texts to be read if the student has time and is interested.
- Limit what is required to the time available to students. Shaffer and Colbert-Getz (2017) have suggested that 12 pages per hour should be allocated for new or complex material.
- Indicate how the work will be assessed. Satran and Harris (1988) have found that 85–89% of students completed the assigned reading when they were told it would be assessed compared with 31–34% of students who were not given this information.

Some institutions have licences which provide students with free access to a range of texts.

The new technologies have greatly expanded the range of learning materials which students can use as learning and information resources. These provide students with greater opportunities to take responsibility for their own learning. Resources are widely available online, and collections can be found at sites such as MedEdPORTAL. Virtual patients are also available online, and these provide students with the opportunity to apply theory to practice.

Your role in relation to both the electronic and print learning resources used by students can vary:

- You can produce a list of recommended resources that may be consulted by the student but do not comment on how the resources can be used or their value.
- You can provide an annotated list of recommended resources, highlighting their possible value to the student and identifying areas that merit particular attention – for example, "Look at Fig. 1.2 because this gives a clear explanation of the cardiac cycle."
- You can identify specific resources which are embedded into and become part of the students' education programme. One medical school came to the conclusion that most of their requirements in one area could be met by resources available on YouTube.
- You can adapt selected existing resources to make them more appropriate for use by your students, assuming that this is possible within the copyright arrangements.
- You can generate new educational resources, as discussed below.

Not only can you be a curator of learning resources, but you can also be a creator. This offers exciting possibilities, with content experts collaborating with instructional designers in the production of resource material. It may help if an education template for the resource is prepared in advance to facilitate input by the content expert. This strategy was used successfully to assist 39 senior surgeons to contribute their experience to the preparation of a series of modules on surgery for trainee surgeons (Laidlaw et al., 2003).

If wide use is to be made of resource materials, and these are to feature prominently in the education programme as an aid to learning, some teachers should possess the array of skills required to select, adapt or produce materials for use in the institution. Raising awareness and training staff in the role of resource developer may be necessary if technology-supported learning is a feature in an institution (Longstaffe et al., 1996; Ryan et al., 1996).

As a teacher, it is your responsibility as an information curator to help filter the available information, directing the learner to the necessary resources for them to study. In an editorial in the *British Medical Journal*, Smith (2010) highlighted the almost impossible task for the doctor of keeping up to date. He quoted the findings of David Sackett that to keep current in the field of internal medicine, the doctor needed to read 17 articles a day, 365 days a year. Fraser and Dunstan (2010) have shown that even within a narrow specialty, it is impossible to keep up with published medical reports. Trainees in cardiac imaging would require 11 years to bring themselves up to date if they read 40 papers a day, 5 days a week. By that time, however, another 82,000 relevant papers would have been published, requiring another 8 years of reading. Learners need help in filtering this information so that they can direct attention to what is of the greatest importance.

Your role as an information coach

We have discussed your role as a transmitter and curator of information. Equally as important is your role in developing in the learners the ability to find and evaluate information for themselves. Amy Wilson-Delfosse, Curriculum Dean at Case Western Reserve University School of Medicine, describes in Box 3.3 developing in students the skills of asking good questions and identifying resources to answer these questions.

Box 3.3 From content to coaching: the evolving role of the teacher[a]

Technology and the need to train health professionals with well-developed skills in self-directed and lifelong learning have changed the role of the teacher from content provider to coach. Personal computers, tablets and smartphones have allowed learners to access information with the click of a button or tap of the screen. The role of the teacher is now to help their students to make sense of and apply the mass of information that is so readily available. Teachers also become facilitators of learning as they prompt students to develop their skills in asking good questions and identifying evidence-based resources to answer those questions.

While some may mourn the loss of the teacher-centered "sage on the stage" performance that lecturing offers, I have found that facilitating and witnessing the process of learning is a privilege that cannot be surpassed. Eighteen years into my teaching career, I have never felt so lucky to be collaborating with learners who will be our physicians of the future.

[a]*Amy L. Wilson-Delfosse, Professor of Pharmacology and Associate Dean for Curriculum, Case Western Reserve University School of Medicine, Ohio, USA.*

At the AMEE 2017 Conference in Helsinki, in a "Wisdom of Our Crowd" session, 92% of participants rated the role of the teacher as an information coach more important than the role of transmitter or curator of information. As we have argued, it is not possible for students to acquire all the information they will require for a lifetime practice of medicine, and the information provided will often change with time. Some information is best acquired when it is needed. An example is the dose of a drug or the interpretation of a test result. With rapid advances in medical practice and information science, such information is increasingly being made available to inform the work of the doctor on the job – "just-in-time" learning.

To respond to this challenge, you should ensure that your students learn to:

- Formulate a question in a way that increases the likelihood of a relevant response.
- Identify and access relevant sources when seeking an answer to the question specified.
- Evaluate the answers received, and know when to stop the search for an answer.

Friedman and co-workers (2016) cited the oft-quoted advice from the legendary ice hockey player Wayne Gretzky: "Skate to where the puck is going to be." They argue that with health care around the world going digital, this is imperative advice for the medical teacher, given that "in the coming decades, the sophistication, comprehensiveness and accessibility of knowledge to support practice will be sufficient to portray clinical practice as embedded in a virtual 'knowledge cloud'."

The cloud, they predict, will provide answers to requests from the doctor for information, based on a rapidly expanding body of biomedical knowledge. Students need to prepare for the informational future of practice in 2020 and beyond. They need to learn when to ask for help – to know what they know and what they don't know. Friedman et al. (2016) have argued:

> historically, medical education has rewarded students who carry the right answer in their heads. In the information future, we should instead reward students who understand the flaws and limits in their knowledge and appropriately manage their uncertainty. (p. 506)

Students should be taught to ask a good question which will "enable them to address the cloud when necessary to improve their assessment of a problem." To interrogate the cloud and frame a good question, it is necessary to know something to get a good answer. This is where the core knowledge base and understanding of the vocabulary, as well as a measure of familiarity with a range of subjects, are important, as in the "awareness" first level of the information pyramid we have described. Friedman et al. (2016) have argued:

The focus of the curriculum should shift to learning just what is needed in order to find out what one doesn't know – or, alternatively, to learning what one needs to know in order to ask a good question. (p. 507)

It cannot be assumed that students have the necessary information handling skills just because they are digital natives and have grown up around technology. Although students may be technology-literate, they are not necessarily information-literate. Information literacy is an invaluable skill for lifelong learning.

Students must also learn how to evaluate evidence and how to respond when there is uncertainty about the most appropriate actions, whether this relates to establishing a diagnosis, arranging investigations, prescribing treatment or advising about prognosis. A related question is how much information is required. This is illustrated in the case of the family physician who was challenged by a patient about the choice of drug prescribed for his chest infection. When going home that evening, the doctor decided to pursue the matter further and searched on the Internet for advice. He found over 600 references. How many should he consult? Should he stay up late attempting to read as many as possible, or could he resolve his uncertainly more speedily? Students should be prepared for such dilemmas.

Many sources of information are available digitally. The National Library of Medicine now has access to more than 10 million articles on MEDLINE from more than 4,000 medical journals. The Internet has opened up opportunities for knowledge acquisition, but previous ways of navigating and filtering available information may be ineffective. Goldie (2016) has suggested that newer approaches, such as "connectivism," are needed, in which learning and knowledge rest in diversity of opinion and learning is a process of connecting specialised nodes or information sources.

Approaches that you can adopt in the curriculum to help prepare the student for medical practice may include encouraging students to:

- Critically access information online to answer specific problems.
- Access published guidelines and the Cochrane library of evidence-based reviews.
- Obtain information by consulting colleagues or experts, including attending grand rounds and postgraduate meetings.
- Use tools such as UpToDate (http://www.uptodate.com/home).

In the "post-truth" world, students should also be alert to dangers in using the Internet as a source of information. The endless stream of information in today's Information Age is itself a challenge, and students should be taught about the digital world they enter. Filter bubbles are just one challenge. A filter bubble is a result of a search in which a website algorithm selectively queries what information a user would like to see. *The Atlantic* (October 10, 2010) reported an interview with internet activist Eli Pariser:

Since Dec. 4, 2009, Google has been personalized for everyone. So when I had two friends this spring Google "BP," one of them got a set of links that was about investment opportunities in BP. The other one got information about the oil spill. Presumably that was based on the kinds of searches that they had done in the past.

Ideally, in this new information age, the teacher should model appropriate behaviour, acknowledging when they need more information relating to a problem or question raised and seeking the necessary information. Some teachers may be more and others less confident in the process, but transparency with the students is necessary. It is important to remember that you are training students not just to practise medicine today, but also to practise medicine in the future, when the ability to quickly access information is required. A clinician must be able to manage the "e-patient," who may have already have accessed information about his or her condition (Masters, 2017).

The teacher as information provider, an expert information provider and a master information provider

The teacher as information provider

The teacher reflects on and identifies the necessary core information in relation to the element of the course for which they are responsible. They choose an effective and efficient way to present this to the learner. They make appropriate learning resources available. They encourage students to search for and evaluate information obtained from different sources, as required.

The teacher as an expert information provider

The expert information provider has studied in more depth the information that is required by students in relation to their own subject and to the curriculum overall. This includes identifying a core curriculum and the related threshold concepts. The teacher is instrumental in realigning the curriculum, with a greater emphasis on how students find and evaluate information from the wide range of sources available.

The teacher as a master information provider

The master information provider will have gained an understanding of the theoretical principles underpinning information management and will have looked at how these principles can be applied in their own teaching practice. They will have studied how information can best be communicated to students, including the use of curriculum maps and concepts. They will be familiar with developments in the field, such as the use of threshold concepts. Their expertise is likely to be recognised nationally and internationally through their achievements in the field, including publications, presentations at education meetings and courses on the subject.

Take-home message

1. The traditional role of the teacher has been to help the student learn by imparting knowledge relating to their subject. The teacher has an important role in deciding what information should be provided to students and identifying the required core information and threshold concepts in the context of the curriculum.
2. The teacher should present the information to the students as effectively and efficiently as possible, using a range of approaches.
3. Your success as an information provider should not be judged solely on your effectiveness as an expert at transmitting information to the students. It should also be assessed on your role as a curator of information sources for the students.
4. The teacher also has a responsibility as information provider to ensure that the student has the skills to obtain the necessary information when this is required. There should be an unambiguous emphasis placed on the student's ability to learn new conceptual information rather than memorising existing information. This is particularly important in the preparation of students for their lifelong learning as medical practitioners, when the rate of learning needs to be greater than the rate of change in medical practice.

Consider

- Consider your own role as information provider. How effective are you? What value do you add? Could the time spent by you transmitting information to your students be used more effectively, for example, by providing students with opportunities to apply or test their knowledge?
- How effective are you as a curator of information?
- To what extent do your students have the skills necessary to find information for themselves – to ask the correct questions, find an appropriate source and to evaluate the answers they find?

Explore further

Anon., 1991. Editorial. Lancet 338 (8774), 1048–1049.

Bergmann, J., Sams, A., 2012. Flip Your Classroom: Reach Every Student in Every Class Every Day. International Society for Technology in Education, Arlington, VA.

Bishop, J.M., 1984. Infuriating tensions: Science and the medical student. J. Med. Educ. 59 (2), 91–102.

Bourdieu, P., Passeron, J.C., 1990. Reproduction in Education, Society and Culture. Sage, London.

Brown, G., Manogue, M., 2001. AMEE Medical Education Guide No. 22: Refreshing lecturing: A guide for lecturers. Association for Medical Education in Europe, Dundee, Scotland.

Cousin, G., 2006. An introduction to threshold concepts. Planet 17, 4–5.

Dent, J.A., Harden, R.M., Hunt, D. (Eds.), 2017. A Practical Guide for Medical Teachers, fifth ed. Elsevier, London.

D'Eon, M., Overgaard, V., Rutledge Harding, S., 2000. Teaching as a social practice: Implications for faculty development. Adv. Health Sci. Educ. Theory Pract. 5 (2), 151–162.

Dunn, W.R., Hamilton, D.D., Harden, R.M., 1985. Techniques of identifying competencies needed of doctors. Med. Teach. 7, 15–25.

Fox, D., 1983. Personal theories of teaching. Stud. Higher Educ. 8 (2), 151–163.

Fraser, A.G., Dunstan, F.D., 2010. On the impossibility of being an expert. BMJ 341, c6815.

Friedman, C.P., Donaldson, K.M., Vantsevich, A.V., 2016. Educating medical students in the era of ubiquitous information. Med. Teach. 38 (5), 504–509.

General Medical Council, 1993. Tomorrow's Doctors: Recommendations on Undergraduate Medical Education. GMC, London.

Gilliani, B.B., 2000. Using the web to create a student-centred curriculum. In: Cole, R.A. (Ed.), Issues in Web-Based Pedagogy: A Critical Primer. Greenwood Press, Westport, CT.

Gokcora, D., 1997. Teaching assistants from the People's Republic of China and US undergraduates: Perceptions of teaching and teachers. Int. J. Acad. Dev. 1 (2), 34–42.

Goldie, J.G.S., 2016. Connectivism: A knowledge learning theory for the digital age? Med. Teach. 38 (10), 1064–1069.

Harden, R.M., Davis, M.H., 2001. The core curriculum with options or special study modules. AMEE Education Guide No. 5. Med. Teach. 23, 231–244.

Harden, R.M., Laidlaw, J.M., 2017. Essential Skills for a Medical Teacher, second ed. Elsevier, London.

Harden, R.M., Stamper, N., 1999. What is a spiral curriculum? Med. Teach. 21 (2), 141–143.

Hettihewa, A.P., Karunathilake, I.M., 2017. Medical and physiotherapy undergraduates' perception of the importance of roles and qualities of a medical teacher. TAPS 2 (2), 30–33.

Irby, D.M., 1994. What clinical teachers in medicine need to know. Acad. Med. 69 (5), 333–342.

Jeffries, W.B., Huggett, K.N., Szarek, J.L., 2017. Lectures. In: Dent, J.A., Harden, R.M., Hunt, D. (Eds.), A Practical Guide for Medical Teachers, fifth ed. Elsevier, London.

Johnston, S., 1996. What can we learn about teaching from our best university teachers? Teach. Higher Educ. 1 (2), 213–225.

Laidlaw, J.M., Harden, R.M., Morris, A.M., 1995. Needs assessment and the development of an educational programme on malignant melanoma for general practitioners. Med. Teach. 17, 79–87.

Laidlaw, J.M., Harden, R.M., Robertson, L.J., et al., 2003. The design of distance-learning programmes and the role of content experts in their production. Med. Teach. 25 (2), 182–187.

Land, R., Meyer, J.H.F., Baillie, C., 2010. Editors' preface: Threshold concepts and transformational learning. In: Land, R., Meyer, J.H.F., Baillie, C. (Eds.), Threshold Concepts and Transformational Learning. Sense Publishers, Rotterdam, pp. ix–xlii.

Loftus, S., 2011. Pain and its metaphors: A dialogical approach. J. Med. Humanit. 32 (2), 213–230.

Longstaffe, J.A., Williams, P.J., Whittlestone, K.D., et al., 1996. Establishing a support service for educational technology within a university. Assoc. Learning Tech. J. 4, 85–92.

Macnab, A., 2017. History teaches everything. Med. Teach. 39 (9), 997–998.

Marzano, R.J., 2009. Helping students process information. Educ. Leadersh. 67 (2), 86–87.

Masters, K., 2017. Preparing Medical Students for the e-Patient. AMEE Guide No. 116. AMEE, Dundee.

Neve, H., Wearn, A., Collett, T., 2016. What are threshold concepts and how can they inform medical education? Med. Teach. 38, 850–853.

Nikendei, C., Huhn, D., Pittius, G., et al., 2016. Students' perceptions on an interprofessional ward round training – A qualitative pilot study. GMS J. Med. Educ. 33 (2), Doc 14.

Pariser, E., 2010. The Filter Bubble: What the Internet is Hiding From You. Penguin Press, New York.

Rowley, J., 2007. The wisdom hierarchy: Representations of the DIKW hierarchy. J. Info. Sci. 33 (2),163–180.

Ryan, M., Wells, J., Freeman, A., et al., 1996. Resource-based learning strategies: Implications for students and institutions. Assoc. Learning Tech. J. 4 (1), 93–98.

Satran, L., Harris, I., 1988. The relationship of examinations to amount of student reading: The examination as symbol. Med. Teach. 10 (2), 169–174.

Shaffer, K., Colbert-Getz, J., 2017. Best practices for increasing reading compliance in undergraduate medical education. Acad. Med. 92 (7), 1059.

Sharples, M., Adams, A., Ferguson, R., et al., 2014. Innovating Pedagogy 2014: Open University Innovation Report 3. The Open University, Milton Keynes.

Shumak, K.A., 1992. Canada: Medical curriculum changes in Ontario. Lancet 340, 1152.

Smith, R., 2010. Strategies for coping with information overload. BMJ 341, c7126.

Strayer, J.F., 2007. The effects of the classroom flip on the learning environment: A comparison of learning activity in a traditional classroom and a flip classroom that used an intelligent tutoring system. PhD Dissertation, Ohio State University, Columbus, OH.UpToDate. http://www.uptodate.com/home.

Chapter 4

The teacher as a facilitator and mentor

We cannot teach another person directly; we can only facilitate his learning.

Carl Rogers (1961)

Facilitation and helping a student to learn are the key characteristics of good teaching.

- Facilitation of learning
- A key role for the teacher
- Approaches to facilitating learning
- Clarifying the learning outcomes
  - Outcome-based education
  - Outcome-based progression
- Identifying learning opportunities
  - A curriculum map
  - Study guides
- Making learning effective
  - Applying the FAIR principles for effective learning
  - Using concept maps
  - Creating a supportive learning environment
- Engaging the student
  - Engaging the student in the curriculum
  - Motivating the student
  - Self-determined learning: Heutagogy

- Clinical supervision
  - Who is a clinical supervisor?
  - What is expected of the clinical supervisor?
  - Supervisory interventions
  - Different roles for the clinical supervisor
- Mentoring
  - A mentor is different from a coach
  - The duties of a mentor
  - What makes an effective mentor–mentee relationship?
  - Implementation in practice
- The teacher facilitator, expert facilitator and master facilitator
- Take-home messages
- Consider
- Explore further

Facilitation of learning

Alfred Ziegler, a German physics professor, was hired not to lecture or to research but to offer "consulting hours." His responsibility was to help students when they had difficulties and where there were elements of the course they did not understand. "This all raises fundamental and contentious issues about the nature of university teaching," suggested Brian Bloch, writing in *Times Higher Education* (Bloch, 2015, p. 21). Ziegler's role represents an example of the move from the teacher as an information provider to the teacher as a facilitator of students' learning, the theme of this chapter (Fig. 4.1).

The most important role we have as teachers is to facilitate our students' learning – to unlock in the students their potential to learn and to guide them in the process. The teacher as someone who is there to help the student to learn is a very different concept from the teacher as a provider of information. In the previous chapter, we referred to the provision of information by the teacher as reflecting the "transfer" theory of teaching (Fox, 1983). Theories held by experienced teachers who have thought more deeply about their role as a facilitator are the "travelling theory" and the "growing theory" (Fox, 1983):

> In the travelling theory the process of teaching is like helping students on a journey through unfamiliar and often rough terrain. The growing theory on the other hand views teaching as being a matter of encouraging and helping students in their personal growth and development – rather like an

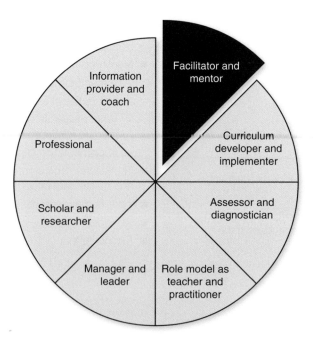

Figure 4.1 The role of the teacher as a facilitator

expert gardener encourages the growth of plants in the various parts of a productive garden. (p. 152)

According to the travelling and growing theories, the teacher guides the student, leads and points the way. This corresponds to the role of a teacher as a facilitator of learning.

Nikendei et al. (2016) have described the facilitator as someone who:

inspires, stimulates, and challenges the learner in order to promote learning in medicine. The facilitator interactively guides and supports students and colleagues in finding their own way of successful learning according to their current stage of education. (p. 718)

Doug Belshaw (2016), in his blog, has captured well the concept of facilitation with his analogy that we stand with our students on one side of a river and give them stepping stones to reach the other side.

A key role for the teacher

The role of teacher as information provider may appear more attractive to staff and students than the role of facilitator. This may be in part due to a lack of what has been termed "individual awareness" (Ballantyne et al., 1999). The subject expert may feel stronger and more comfortable serving as a subject expert rather than responding to the challenge of facilitating the students' learning. The role of information provider may also correspond more closely to how he or she was taught as a student or junior doctor.

To some teachers, having to take on the role of facilitator seems equivalent to asking them to abandon their primary responsibilities. In adopting the role of facilitator, the teacher may be perceived as having less power and authority compared with a role of expert or information provider. This need not be the case. The role of facilitator can empower both the teacher and the student and can have a much greater impact on the students' learning. Teri Turner, a teacher who is passionate about the growth and development of all learners across the continuum of medical education, and Al Dowie, a leader in the design and delivery of ethics in the medical curriculum, describe in Boxes 4.1 and 4.2 a passion for their role as facilitators.

Your role as a facilitator is not an easy one. How much support should you provide for your students or trainees? How much freedom to adopt their preferred method of learning? Returning to the question we asked in previous chapters, what would learners miss if you were not there as a teacher? There is no doubt that learners could more easily do without us as providers of information than they could with us as facilitators of their learning in the ways we describe in the chapter. Alternative sources of information can be found relatively easily. John Cookson highlights this from his own experience as a teacher (Box 4.3).

Box 4.1 Helping each learner to reach his or her full potential[a]

My passion as a teacher is to facilitate reflection and growth so that each learner can reach his or her full potential. Metaphors are powerful tools for understanding the many roles teachers play. As a metaphorical gardener, I seek to find the optimal environment – one that is warm and nurturing, with a balance of support and challenge – in which a learner can take root, grow, and blossom. Plutarch stated, "The mind is not a vessel to be filled, but a fire to be ignited." Accordingly, I also serve as the sun, a catalyst to stimulate a thirst for learning within the trainee's soul; then, I provide springs of intellectual inquiry. Initially, the trainee needs a trellis as a support until the roots are deep and the stems are strong and secure. As the learner matures, I observe and provide feedback on growth and, as needed, occasionally trim weeds and prune when growth is dormant. During this entire process, I, too, grow and learn, becoming thereby a better teacher. In the end, when you give yourself to nurturing, the result is not merely another plant; rather, eventually you have an entire orchard to harvest.

[a]*Teri Turner, Associate Professor of Paediatrics, Baylor College of Medicine/Texas Children's Hospital, Houston, USA and Vice Chair of Education and Director, Center for Research, Innovation and Scholarship.*

Box 4.2 Creating a passion for learning[a]

The deepest accomplishment I know as a teacher is the privilege of being party to the shift in a student's understanding that occurs when learning takes place. Others might value more highly the reward and sense of achievement that comes from contributing to change at a strategic level, and for good reason. Developing the organisation in order to improve the delivery of education is a system enhancement, and reaches farther than localised, operational impact. Nor are the two in opposition; educators can actively participate in both, and better delivery through institutional advances will foster better learning for more students.

But while we can justly have the greatest of pride and tremendous purpose in building structures to benefit learners in the longer term, the satisfaction that follows is at a remove from the thrill of visibly cultivating positive movement in a student's knowledge, attitudes, and skills. We only truly understand a concept, or an experience, or a practice when we are in some way grasped by it; when in our head, heart or habits there is some increment of constructive change; and to catalyse such comprehension in the individual learner can, for educators too, be something that is profoundly personal.

[a]*Al Dowie, Senior Lecturer in Medical Ethics and the Law, University of Glasgow, UK.*

Approaches to facilitating learning

Given its importance, how can a teacher facilitate learning? We describe four approaches (Fig. 4.2). You may find it useful to think about how you can facilitate your students' learning in each of these areas. As a teacher, you can facilitate learning by:

- Clarifying the expected learning outcomes and pointing the learner in the direction of what has to be learned

Box 4.3 The importance of individualised observation and feedback[a]

A key moment in my understanding clinical education was of a few minutes' conversation with a student. She said, "what I need from you is half an hour a week of observation and feedback on my performance with patients. I can do everything else myself, study books, go to clinics and ward rounds and see patients on my own but if I don't have that half hour I don't know if I'm doing it right."

It was a damascene moment; it was suddenly clear that students, however bright, could not learn good consultation skills, including problem-solving skills, without guidance. Observation of others was not enough. Further, if teachers did nothing else, students would flourish; other teaching modalities were no doubt desirable but only if students got their 30 minutes. Since then I have tried to organise curriculum matters so that patient, student and teacher come together with the teacher observing the student, not the other way around.

[a]John Cookson, Emeritus Professor, Hull York Medical School, UK, and Tutor for AMEE-ESME online courses.

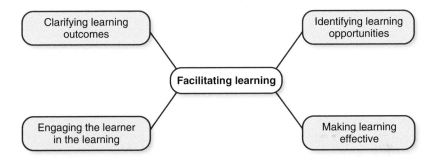

Figure 4.2 Four areas for facilitating student learning

- Identifying and guiding the learners to what are, for them, the appropriate learning opportunities
- Making the learning effective and efficient
- Engaging the learner in the learning process

We give examples of facilitation in each of these areas, but you will develop your own approach to facilitating your students' learning.

Clarifying the learning outcomes

Outcome-based education

There has been a move from an emphasis on process and learning experiences, such as lectures, small group work, practical activities and clinical work, to the product or outcome of the education and the learning outcomes that it is expected the student will master at each phase of the curriculum, by the end of the course, before graduation and by the end of postgraduate training. This move to outcome-based education (OBE) has been described as the most significant development in medical education over the past 2 decades. In OBE, there is an explicit statement of the learning outcomes expected of the learner, and this is communicated to staff and students or trainees. As described in Chapters 5 and 6, an understanding of the expected learning outcomes provides the basis for curriculum development and assessment.

Students and trainees should not see themselves as joining a "magical mystery tour," as in the Beatles' song. They should have a clear understanding of where they are going and the abilities or competencies that it is expected they will master. The first key thing that you can do in facilitating learning, therefore, is to ensure that learners are aware of and appreciate what is expected of them as set out in the specified learning outcomes. As the teaching dean at Dundee Medical School, I (RMH) welcomed the students on their first day at medical school and introduced them to what it was expected they would achieve over the following 5 years, based on the learning outcomes in twelve domains (Harden et al., 1999a):

1. Clinical skills
2. Practical procedures
3. Patient investigation
4. Patient management
5. Health promotion
6. Communication skills
7. Information handling
8. Basic and clinical sciences
9. Ethics and attitudes
10. Decision-making skills
11. Teamwork skills
12. Personal development

Over the following 2 weeks, newly qualified doctors used their experiences as junior doctors to provide the students with practical examples of each domain as related to myocardial infarction, a condition with which students could relate. The examples provided helped the students develop an understanding and appreciation of each of these domains. The students were asked to document in a portfolio their work over the 5-year course, demonstrating their achievements in each of the domains. This contributed to their final assessment. If during the course they found difficulty relating a learning experience to the stated learning outcomes, they were encouraged to ask the teacher for an explanation.

Outcome-based progression

As a teacher, you can help students monitor their progress against each of the outcome domains (Harden, 2007). For example, students may make satisfactory progress relating to their understanding of the basic and clinical sciences but have problems relating to their communication and clinical skills and need further support in these areas. With regard to progression towards the exit learning outcomes, the concept of milestones has gained significant attention in medical education (Englander et al.,

2017). A milestone is a step in the learner's progression to the final expected learning outcomes which can be measured. Achievement of the milestone provides evidence of the learner's progression. A milestone is "a defined, observed marker of an individual's ability along a developmental continuum" (Englander et al., 2017). Milestones have been developed for many postgraduate training programmes.

The learner should have a clear vision of the learning outcomes expected by the end of the educational programme. If learners know where they are going, they can better plan how to get there. Without this, it is difficult for them to plan their studies and to see what learning experiences are necessary or relevant to their learning. By providing learners with the expected learning outcomes, the teacher or trainer facilitates their learning and points them in the appropriate direction of travel, giving them an indication in terms of milestones of how far down the road they need to travel at each stage of their journey. In OBE, you take responsibility for ensuring that learners are aware of and understand the expected learning outcomes and support them in achieving these. Although acknowledging that learning requires effort on the part of the learner as well as the teacher, the statement by Mr. Miyagi, in the film *The Karate Kid* (1984), that "there are no bad students, only bad teachers," has an element of truth. The teacher's responsibility for the learner achieving the learning outcomes is an aspect of OBE that is often ignored.

Identifying learning opportunities

Having ensured that learners understand what is expected of them, your next task as a facilitator is to advise them how they can achieve the expected outcomes. Students and trainees should be guided on the range of learning opportunities and resources available which might best suit their needs and how and where they can access them. These include formal activities such as a lecture and a clinical session and/or opportunities for independent study using available resources. Greater emphasis has been placed on self-directed learning, where learners take responsibility for their own learning. This should be encouraged because it is valuable preparation for their continuing education after graduation and completion of their postgraduate training. Rather than the term *self-directed learning*, however, we prefer the term *directed (or guided) self-learning*. The teacher still has an important role in facilitating and guiding students' learning, particularly in the early years of the course.

Two tools can be used to help direct or guide the learner:

- A curriculum map
- A study guide

A curriculum map

A map of the curriculum is an important tool to:

- Give learners an overall picture of the curriculum
- Help them appreciate the expected learning outcomes

- See how the learning outcomes are addressed and assessed in the educational programme
- Help them plan their own study journey

The curriculum map shows how the different pieces of the education programme jigsaw fit together. It provides a broad perspective of the different learning outcome domains, such as clinical examination, practical procedures and patient management, along with more details of each domain. In the case of patient management, for example, by clicking on the learning outcome, information is provided as to where in the curriculum approaches to management, such as drugs, surgery, psychotherapy, rehabilitation, physiotherapy and alternative medicine, including acupuncture, are addressed. The curriculum map is multidimensional but in its simplest form can be seen as a series of two-dimensional relationships:

- The expected learning outcomes and the courses or phases of the curriculum where the learning outcomes are addressed
- The expected learning outcomes and the range of learning opportunities available to the student where the learning outcomes are addressed both formally and informally, including lectures, practical classes, sessions scheduled in the clinical skills laboratory and other learning resources available
- The expected learning outcomes and where in the programme of assessment the learner's mastery of the learning outcomes is assessed

Some schools have developed their own platform for a curriculum map, and others have built their curriculum map using a commercially available resource or one developed by another school. The curriculum map makes the curriculum more transparent to the different stakeholders, including students, teachers, curriculum developers, accrediting agencies, the public and those undertaking research in medical education. It helps you communicate to students what, when, where and how they can learn. The curriculum map will not only help you to support your students in managing their own learning relating to the course for which you are responsible, but will also help you demonstrate to them how your teaching and your course fit-in with other courses and how the course contributes to their achievement of the expected exit learning outcomes.

The steps in developing a curriculum map and how you might introduce a map in practice have been described in *AMEE Guide No 21: Curriculum mapping: A tool for transparent and authentic teaching and learning* produced by AMEE, an International Association for Medical Education (Harden, 2001). It is suggested:

Faced with curricula which are becoming more centralized and less departmentally based, and with curricula including both core and optional elements, the teacher may find that the curriculum map is the glue which holds the curriculum together. (p. 3)

Study guides

As a teacher, you may have produced notes on a topic, lecture handouts, reading lists, course outlines or even sets of learning outcomes for your course. However, it is less likely that you will have produced a study guide to support your students' learning. If you have, you can skip this section, or you may want to read it to compare your own experiences with our recommendations.

In your role as facilitator, a study guide is a tool you can use that has a powerful impact on the students' or trainees' learning and, at the same time, helps them play an important part in their own learning. It is an electronic or printed aid designed specifically to support students' learning (Harden et al., 1999b). Rowntree (1986) has likened a study guide to a tutor looking over the student's shoulder, giving advice about their studies and being available 24 hours a day, 7 days a week. The study guide pulls together all that learners should know about a course – what is expected of them and the learning opportunities available. It can be seen as providing a guided tour of the relevant areas on the curriculum map.

What constitutes a study guide will vary with the course and stage of training. It might address or include:

- An indication of why the course is important and how the course will help the learner in his or her practice as a doctor.
- What is expected of the learner during the course in terms of clinical work, scheduled teaching sessions or activities, such as attending lectures, participating in problem-based groups or keeping a learning portfolio.
- The expected learning outcomes and what the learner should achieve by the end of the course or postgraduate training programme, including the core or threshold concepts (see Chapter 3). The guide may illustrate the learning outcomes expected as they relate to the tasks performed by the junior doctor (Table 4.1).

Table 4.1 Extract from a grid in a paediatric training guide[a]

| | Task | | | |
Outcome	Convulsions	Dehydration	Pyrexia	Breathlessness
Practical procedures	Administration of rectal diazepam	Intravenous access	Lumbar puncture	Use of peak flow meter
Communication skills	Discuss prognosis of febrile fits	Explain how to give oral rehydration	Counsel parents	Minimize anxiety while giving a maximum of realistic information

[a]Showing the relationship between the tasks undertaken by a junior doctor and the expected learning outcomes.
From Mitchell, H.E., Harden, R.M., Laidlaw, J.M. 1998. Towards effective on-the-job learning: The development of a paediatric training guide. Med. Teach. 20(2), 91-98.

- An advance organiser or framework for studying the topic. The study guide for an endocrinology course, for example, may list the endocrine glands and, for each of the glands, the problems found when the gland is overactive, underactive or producing normal amounts of hormone.
- The prerequisites and the knowledge and skills that the student is expected to master before the start of the course and how the course builds on previous learning.
- How the course relates to other curriculum elements and courses. This is important regardless of whether the curriculum is integrated or discipline-based or the degree of vertical integration, as described in Chapter 5.
- The formal and informal learning opportunities available to the learner and how the learner can interact with them. This is likely to include clinical work, lectures, group discussions, practical work, including with simulators, and a range of online learning resources.
- Key core references to recommended texts, annotated with reference to particular chapters, pages or figures and an indication of their value to the learners, including what they will gain from reading the text. For example:
  - A simple explanation of a difficult concept
  - A good and succinct overview
  - A useful diagram, figure or photograph
  - A more in-depth study of the subject
  - Different views on a controversial issue
- A glossary or definition of terms used. The guide may simply list the new terms which learners may encounter as they study the course or it may provide definitions.
- Information about how the learner's mastery of the learning outcomes will be assessed.
- The provision of opportunities for learners to assess their own achievements.
- How learners can contact a teacher or trainer if they have a problem. Sometimes teachers indicate that they are available to speak with a student at a set time each week. Contact by email can be encouraged but may be problematic and may be seen as placing excessive demands on the teacher.

A study guide may use icons to identify the different elements in a guide. Two examples are given in Figs 4.3 and 4.4 from study guides for postgraduate dental trainees and paediatric trainees.

A study guide is most effective when you write it as a one-to-one personal communication with the learner. You can express your views on controversial issues and indicate what you see as the key issues on a topic. You may introduce personal examples from your practice. You may also recognise areas or aspects where, from your own experience, learners have difficulty in mastering. I (RMH) remember when learning the fingering for the microwriter (sadly, now an obsolete input device!), I was at the point of giving up when I was reassured by the guide provided with the machine that almost everyone had difficulty at this point, and that perseverance for another hour could result in the acquisition of the necessary skill.

Patients with a Caries Problem: Diagnosis

You may like to read the following article which compares the fibre optic transillumination (FOTI) with radiographic and/or clinical caries diagnosis:

Stephen K W, Russell J I, Creanor S L and Burchell C K (1987) Comparison of fibre optic transillumination with clinical and radiographic caries diagnosis. Community Dentistry and Oral Epidemiology, 15, 90–94.

It is pertinent to discuss **methods of caries detection** with your trainer at an early stage of the four-week period allotted to this task.

You may have heard about the videotape entitled "From black to white" which was produced in 1988 by the British Postgraduate Medical Federation (BPMF) on the diagnosis and management of coronal caries in permanent teeth. It is a 30-minute programme and covers three main aspects:

a) examining carious teeth without using probes,
b) remineralisation in dental caries, and
c) sealant restoration.

Although this tape has provoked some controversy in general dentistry on choice of restoration, it is very instructive and convincing regarding (a) and (b). Why don't you view it and see for yourself then discuss the issues with your trainer and peers?

You will find a copy in the practice or with your course organiser.

In general practice you will treat a variety of caries cases – early lesions, approximal caries, occlusal caries, root caries as well as some cases of secondary caries. You have studied the clinical features of each type in your undergraduate education but probably saw a limited number of each category. The situation in your training year is quite different. You will receive more patients and it is here that your trainer's experience in spot-diagnosing different degrees of caries will count. Spend as much time as you can afford in the trainer's surgery while he deals with caries patients. He will pass on useful diagnostic hints.

If the subject of diagnosing caries is to be dealt with in a session of the day-release course, prepare for the discussion by doing some reading.

Kidd E A M and Joyston-Bechal S (1987) Essentials of Dental Caries: The Disease and its Management. Bristol, Wright. pp 41–57 and 158–169

Figure 4.3 A page from the training guide for dental vocational training produced by the Scottish Council for Postgraduate Medical and Dental Education and the Centre for Medical Education, Dundee

(Abdel-Fattah et al., 1991).

Therapy

Strict schedules governing oral intake are not helpful. Discuss with nursing and medical staff when oral fluids or diet should be increased or reintroduced.

Black's *Paediatric Emergencies* has several useful sections:

- Appendix 3, p 766–769 (water and electrolyte requirements)
- Appendix 5, p 773–755 (advice on necessary maintenance fluids)

For an overview of home-based oral rehydration for diarrhoea, Almroth & Latham, *Lancet*, Mar 1995; 345(8951): 709–711.

A Meyes, Modern management of acute diarrhoea and dehydration in children, *Am Fam Phys*, Apr 1995: 57(5): 1103–1118, may also give you some ideas.

Teamwork

Speak to colleagues in the local Public Health Department. Discuss infection-control policies and notification of diseases.

Experienced nursing staff may help you decide on the best method of rehydration. Remember – you can always reassess cases after a few hours and review your decisions.

Professional development

Do you know how to prevent cross contamination?

With each case, consider what measures may be required, e.g. hand washing alone, or additional gloves, masks and gowns.

Think *why* a child is being barrier nursed. Is it to protect the patient or the staff/other patients/environment?

Look at the local infection-control policy for guidance.

Microbiology in Clinical Practice (p 602–607) contains a short section on different standards of isolation, with suggested isolation procedures.

Figure 4.4 A page from a study guide for paediatric trainees, "Learning paediatrics: A training guide for senior house officers"
(Harden et al., 1999b.)

Although the main aim of a study guide is to provide advice and suggestions to facilitate learning, it can also be used to provide the learner with information about the content of the topic when this is not readily available from other sources (Harden et al., 1999b). It can also be used as a workbook for student activities, such as documenting information about patients seen or problems addressed, and can contribute to a student's portfolio.

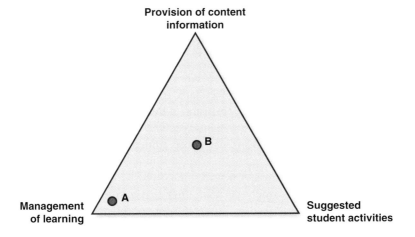

(A) a guide exclusively devoted to facilitating learning, with no
content information and no suggested student activities.

(B) a guide concerned equally with management of learning, provision
of content information and suggested student activities.

Figure 4.5 The study guide triangle

The study guide triangle is a visual representation of the extent to which a study guide serves these three functions as a management tool, a source of information about the topic and suggestions for student activities (Fig. 4.5).

Making learning effective

As a teacher, you can facilitate learning by adopting a number of approaches to make learning more effective for the student. We have already described the use of curriculum maps and study guides. Approaches include:

- The application by you of education principles that are known to improve learning. We describe four of these (the FAIR principles).
- The use of concept maps, which can be seen as elements in a curriculum map.
- The creation of an educational environment or climate that is supportive of learning.

Applying the FAIR principles for effective learning

Much has been written on theories of learning (e.g. see the series of AMEE guides on theories of medical education). Here we describe four key evidence-based principles which can be applied by any teacher or trainer and, which, if applied, will lead to more effective learning. We have highlighted these principles in our face-to-face and online Essential Skills in Medical Education (ESME) courses and have found that they resonate with course participants. Many put them into practice in their own teaching.

The four FAIR principles are as follows: (1) provision of *f*eedback to learners; (2) *a*ctive rather than passive learning; (3) *i*ndividualisation of learning; and (4) making learning *r*elevant (Harden and Laidlaw, 2017).

Feedback to learners

A lack of feedback or inappropriate feedback to the learner is a common complaint of students and doctors in training. There is often a gap between the feedback that learners perceive they have received and the feedback that teachers believe they have provided. Here are some guidelines to make feedback more effective:

- Feedback should be timely (as soon after the learning or assessment event as possible). We described in *The Definitive Guide to the OSCE* (Harden et al., 2016) the value of providing feedback to learners during the objective structured clinical examination (OSCE) and immediately after the examination is completed.
- Feedback should be frequent and should be provided on a number of occasions during the programme. We describe in Chapter 6 how this is part of the move to assessment *for* learning.
- Feedback should be specific. Address where the learner has achieved the learning outcomes and where there remain gaps or misunderstandings. It may be that the learner has not fully appreciated the range of learning outcomes expected of them, and this can be clarified in the feedback. For example, the learner may have neglected health promotion or the development of communication skills.
- Feedback should be concerned not only with the learners' mistakes but should also compliment the learner when a good performance is identified. This helps motivate the learner. Many years ago, I (RMH) entered a local garden competition and, to my surprise, received first prize. This stimulated me to take a greater interest in gardening.
- Feedback, as well as identifying any gaps or deficiencies, should also address how the learner can remedy these – "smoothing the pebbles." Learners should express their learning intent following receiving the feedback. You also have a responsibility for the higher achiever and advising them about further study – "polishing the diamond."
- The provision of feedback should be seen as a two-way process and not a unidirectional transmission of information from the teacher to the learner. Feedback should be an active conversation between the teacher and the learner (Boud, 2015; Murdoch-Eaton and Bowen, 2017). This has been described as "feedback through an educational alliance." Increasing attention is being paid to this aspect of feedback.
- The learner and the teacher have a mutual responsibility for feedback, and teachers need to invest time in this relationship if they are to be a credible source of feedback (Telio et al., 2016). Learners may need help in understanding the need for and value of feedback and how they should respond to the feedback provided. Better students may make efforts to

engage with available feedback about their performance. Poorer students may ignore the feedback and not take the opportunity to try to improve (Sinclair and Cleland, 2007). Learners should be encouraged to reflect on the feedback received and what they will do following their receipt of the feedback.

- Feedback should be seen from a longitudinal perspective as it is provided across the curriculum, with learners reflecting on feedback previously provided and understanding the future opportunities for feedback.
- In addition to feedback provided through the teacher, learners should be encouraged to assess their own performance.

Medical professionals are notoriously bad at self-assessment. The ability for a graduate to assess her or his own competence, however, is important for continuing professional development and lifelong learning, and the skill of self-assessment should be developed in the curriculum. This should become increasingly important as students progress through the undergraduate and postgraduate training programmes.

Here are examples from a recent ESME course where learners considered why the provision of feedback to them was important:

"I want to know where I stand in my strengths and weaknesses."

"I want to improve my performance and need to know how to do this."

"Feedback is a road sign to where I am going and where I am at a particular moment."

"Feedback reinforces good behaviour and performance."

"Feedback provides a signpost to further learning strategies."

Active learning

Learning is facilitated if learners are actively engaged in the learning process. This activity can take a number of forms. You can ask learners to:

- Reflect on their experiences and learning. The curriculum may even have time scheduled formally for learners to reflect on their learning. Roger Strasser highlights the importance of reflection in Box 4.4.
- Apply what they already know to a new topic. This has been described as a constructivist approach to learning.
- Apply their theoretical knowledge to solving practical problems.
- Assess their own competence in an area – for example, through multiple-choice questions (MCQs) or a checklist.
- Engage in a practical exercise or project.

Box 4.4 Challenging learners to learn[a]

Learning is the process whereby knowledge is created through the transformation of experience.

David Kolb, 1984

The term *experiential learning* is often misunderstood. We all have experiences all the time; the issue is what we do with these experiences. The excellent medical teacher *challenges* the medical student or trainee to learn. It is not enough to facilitate learning; rather teaching is about confronting the learner to develop new insights, new knowledge and new competencies. In this context, the teacher/challenger encourages reflection and exploration of experiences to ensure that they become "learning experiences" resulting in real change in the learner's performance.

The teacher/challenger approach is particularly important with learners who are performing poorly and lack awareness of their inadequacies. Having said that, this approach is equally important for learners who are high-performing. It is very frustrating for them to be told that they are "very good" without any guidance as to how they can learn more and be even better.

Another misunderstood term is *self-directed learning* (Knowles, 1975). Rather than leaving learners to their own devices, self-directed learning requires the teacher to challenge the learner to learn. Specifically, learners "don't know what they don't know or need to know" so that the teacher must provide a learning environment which challenges the learner to discover what they need to know and be able to do.

[a]*Roger Strasser, Professor of Rural Health, Dean and CEO of Northern Ontario School of Medicine, Lakehead and Laurentian Universities, Canada.*

- Build over time their learning portfolio, which describes their learning experiences and demonstrates their achievement of the expected learning outcomes.
- Share their knowledge with colleagues; peer-to-peer learning is of value not only to the peer tutee but also to the peer tutor.

In Boxes 4.5, 4.6 and 4.7, Bill Jeffries, Martin Fischer and Jonas Nordquist share their approaches to making learning active for their students.

All activities are not necessarily valuable; the activity must be meaningful. Simply clicking on the computer to change the page does not contribute to the student's learning, nor does the completion of a logbook of patients seen unless this is part of a learning portfolio highlighting what the learner has learned in the process, and the result is reviewed by the teacher, with feedback to the learner.

Examples of teaching with active learning embedded are:

- Problem-based learning (PBL) and other small-group activities. By their nature, these should involve students in active learning.

Box 4.5 From information provider to learning facilitator[a]

As a young teacher I strived to deliver essential information. To enhance retention, I peppered my lectures with colorful stories and analogies. These evolved into well-crafted monologues. My students had magnificent recall on examinations, and I became an award-winning teacher – a diva! However, mounting evidence suggested that I could do better. For example, despite demonstrable short-term knowledge gains, many students didn't remember my content later in the clinic. Published data about "active" learning suggested that other teaching modalities might produce better long-term retention, depth of learning, critical thinking and application. Therefore, I put my ego aside to embrace other learning formats such as the flipped classroom. In this setting, student groups apply knowledge to solve problems right before your eyes. The focus is on the student's learning, rather than the teacher's delivery. My initial fears that students would not get all the information needed were unfounded and students actually moved well beyond simple recall. I sometimes mourn the loss of the diva on the stage, but I now recognize that the teacher's role is to maximize student learning beyond the short term, which is ultimately a greater reward.

[a]William B. Jeffries, Senior Associate Dean for Medical Education and Professor of Pharmacology, Robert Larner M.D. College of Medicine, University of Vermont, USA.

Box 4.6 Question and reflect[a]

The longer I teach clinical medicine in our endocrine block in Munich the less I seem to know about why things are as they are. Instead of providing answers I stimulate my students to question what I present. I also tell them about the mistakes and misunderstandings I encountered at the bedside myself. I also stimulate my students to recall erroneous examples they have observed themselves and reflect on those with me. I have to admit that we still teach some clinical methods nobody in real clinical life ever applies, like using a Tip Therm device to test for peripheral neuropathy. When I make my students question what they observe, and when they compare my and other teaching with actual professional behavior in "clinical wild life," I hope to have contributed to their growth and learning.

[a]Martin Fischer, Director of the Institute for Medical Education, Associate Dean for Clinical Studies, Medical Faculty and University Hospital of LMU Munich, Germany.

- Practical laboratory and clinical work provide active learning opportunities.
- Lectures turned into an active experience by introducing questions and an audience response system.
- Online learning programmes with activities built into the learning programme.
- Simulators and virtual patients. These provide an active learning experience for the learner and can be used not only in the mastery of clinical skills, but also in gaining an understanding of the basic medical sciences (Issenberg et al., 1999).
- Educational games with active engagement of the user as a key feature. Prensky (2006) has advocated the use of games as an educational tool. In

THE TEACHER AS A FACILITATOR AND MENTOR

Box 4.7 Designing the classroom[a]

It is all worth it when the learners experience the world in a different light, suddenly realizing a new depth in the understanding of a phenomenon. The learners are never a tabula rasa. In fact, they always bring tons of previous knowledge and experience. It is my role to challenge their assumptions, to make them reflect, to stimulate debate and to introduce new perspectives. I first and foremost see my role as someone stimulating the learners' thinking – asking challenging questions and stimulating dialogue. I identify myself as a learning facilitator, using dialogue as a central tool for learning. I therefore also need to pay close attention to how my learning space is physically organized.

My classrooms needs to be designed so the learners are visible and can read each other's faces. I need plenty of space on the walls to be able visualize the dialogue. Such classrooms are flipped; the center of the room is one of the longer walls. The distance between the first and last row is minimized with higher seating in the back rows, with lower seating in front. All learners now become visible and swivelled chairs are to be preferred in order to easily connect with each other. Together we are exploring new dimensions of learning.

[a]Jonas Nordquist, Director, Medical Case Centre, Karolinska Institutet; Associate Director, Residency Programs, Karolinska University Hospital, Stockholm, Sweden.

his book, *"Don't Bother me Mom, I'm Learning,"* he described how game developers, by making learning active, individualising the experience and relating progress to the achievements of the player and the level of play, are more adept at facilitating learning than many teachers.

Individualised learning

A challenge for the teacher is to personalise the learning to the needs of the individual learner. As clinicians, we match the management of patients to their individual needs. We should do the same for our students. Each student is also different in terms of:

- Their previous knowledge and understanding. Fig. 4.6 shows the results of students' response to an MCQ test of their knowledge of endocrinology. What is interesting is that the test was given on the first day of a third-year endocrine course, before the students had started the course. Some students demonstrated little understanding of endocrinology, whereas one student almost passed the examination (the passing mark was 50) before commencing the course. Each student required a course of study that took account of his or her individual endocrine knowledge.
- Their goals, aspirations and motivation. Some students may have aspirations for a career in family medicine and others for a career in surgery or another specialty. When chairing the endocrine system course, I (RMH) arranged for students to have time scheduled each week to look at

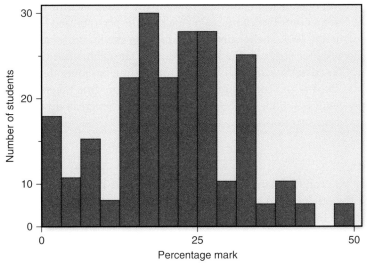

Figure 4.6 Students' responses to a multiple-choice question test of their knowledge of endocrinology

endocrinology from their specialty choice – for example, to attend a diabetes clinic in the community, to assist in theatre for a thyroidectomy or to work in a pathology or biochemistry laboratory looking at endocrine function tests.

- Their abilities to master a specific learning outcome. Some students may have better communication skills and others have better procedural skills.
- Their learning style, pace and preferred time of learning. Although learning style is a controversial topic, there is no doubt that given the choice, students will choose to learn in different ways – such as on their own, with a colleague or as part of a group. Some students may take as much as four times as long as others to study the same subject.

The teacher can facilitate students' learning by helping them develop a learning plan in line with their personal learning needs. Part of this process of individualisation is the provision of feedback, as described above. The teacher reviews the learner's progress and, based on this, recommends further learning, tailoring the education programme to the needs of the individual learner.

Facebook founder Mark Zuckerberg and his wife used the occasion of their daughter's birth to announce that they were investing their fortune in good causes. Personalised learning was the first item on their wish list. The assumption was that learning could be improved and made more widely available by the use of software programmes that act like automatic tutors – giving feedback, allowing students to go at their own pace and recommending lessons based on a student's previous work. There has been a rapid expansion of education software that provides such facilities. Although such programmes have a contribution to make, adaptive or personalised learning requires a more fundamental look at the curriculum, relating the learning experience offered and time allocated for study to the learner's needs. Individualisation is reflected in a competency-based approach, with a move from a time-based model to an approach where what is fixed is the competency achieved, not the time taken to do so. Some learners may require 1 hour in the simulation centre whereas other learners may require 2 or 3 hours to master the same skills.

Relevance

As a teacher, you can facilitate a student's learning as we have described by providing feedback to the students about their progress, by making the learning active rather than passive and by personalising the learning to the needs of the individual students. All of these are important, but more important is that we ensure that what learners have to learn is understood by them as being relevant in their studies to be a doctor. Although some may want to become a basic scientist, the majority will want to become a medical practitioner who is managing patients. What they are asked to learn and the learning experiences provided must have this objective in mind.

In a recent ESME course, students highlighted a number of reasons why relevance as to what is taught is important to them:

"I learn better and found it easier to understand if case studies are used to show relevance."

"If it is relevant, I get more involved and encouraged."

"I am more motivated if I see the subject is relevant to me as a future doctor."

"It is always interesting if it is relevant."

"Clinical correlation is a must for medical science teaching."

"The introduction to patients in the early years helps me to see the relevance of what I am learning."

Cooper (2014) has described six common mistakes in the classroom that undermine motivation. One was failure to provide practical examples demonstrating the relevance of the topic: "Telling students to study simply because they must or making narrow pitches to a subject's future utility typically fail to generate student interest." She showed that, although relevance of content did not feature prominently in classroom teaching, when present it resulted in the greatest level of student engagement.

Relevance is discussed further in Chapter 5 in relation to the "authentic curriculum." Brown et al. (1989) emphasised what they described as "situated cognition" and the importance of authentic learning:

...authentic learning contexts are vitally important if students are to acquire and develop cognitive skills that are transferable to real world living...learning knowledge and skills in contexts that reflect the way the knowledge will be useful in real life....

Krajcik and Blumenfeld (2006) have suggested that "authentic academic tasks ask students to engage with content as though they were practitioners in that field." Relevance is important.

Using concept maps

A practical tool that you can use to facilitate learning and make learning effective is the concept map, which is a visual representation of items of information or concepts with links and relationships between the items displayed (Novak and Gowin, 1984; Novak and Cañas, 2006). The map shows the network of related concepts. The learner thinks and learns by linking new concepts to what is already known. The ability of the learner to relate one concept to another in the map and see them as pieces of a larger jigsaw, with an understanding of how each piece relates to other pieces, can be thought of as moving up the information pyramid from information to knowledge (see Fig. 3.3). It represents congruence between knowledge and information.

The display of information items on a concept map can help integrate new and old information explicitly. In an account of how concept maps can create meaningful learning in medical education, Daley et al. (2016a) have noted:

In medical education, part of what one needs to learn is how to deal with vast amounts of information so that the information is actually usable when providing care to patients. Committing information to memory is one skill. However, medical students typically need additional abilities to function in clinical practice. (p. 3)

They went on to propose that the ability to integrate various pieces of information can be supported by the use of concept maps, in which information items are shown along with the links between the items.

Fig. 4.7 shows part of a concept map relating to the cardiovascular system. It represents how the creator thought about the topic, with hierarchies and interconnectivity included. By using concept maps with your learners, you demonstrate your interest in students gaining an understanding of the relationships between facts, not just knowing the facts. Instead of asking "What do I want to teach?" the emphasis is on "What do I want my students to learn?" As has been described, the concept map can be used as an advance organiser to provide an overview and structure for what is to be studied. It represents the picture on the jigsaw, with the information items as the individual pieces that make up the picture.

Using concept maps can help learners organise their knowledge, which is as important as the knowledge itself. The concept map may also serve as an efficient access to

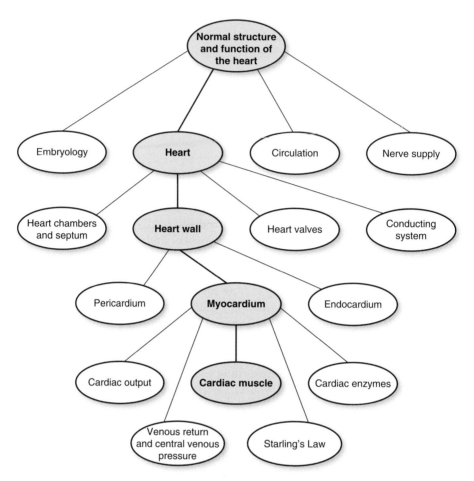

Figure 4.7 Part of a concept map relating cardiac muscle to normal structure and function of the heart

Web-based information resources (McDonald and Stevenson, 1998). Schmidt (2004) have noted:

> It has been clearly shown that knowledge organisation influences the efficiency and the effectiveness of recall and problem solving within a domain and that domain experts have more coherent, well-structured knowledge than novices. (p. 251)

Through the use of concept maps, learners can acquire problem-solving and critical thinking skills (Hsu and Hsieh, 2005). In medical education, concept maps are of value (Daley et al., 2016a, b) to:

- Promote meaningful learning and integration of learning across disciplines.

- Assist learners in linking basic science to clinical practice and promote clinical reasoning.
- Make thought processes more visible and specific.
- Provide a means whereby groups of learners can share their thinking and understanding (e.g. in PBL).
- Specify different and complementary roles of healthcare professionals and help students understand these roles as part of interprofessional education.
- Assess a learner's understanding and mastery of an area.
- Teach evidence-based medicine.

Highlighting the value of concept maps as a means of representing information, Novak and Cañas (2006) have noted:

While at first glance concept maps may appear to be just another graphic representation of information, understanding the foundations for this tool and its proper use will lead the user to see that this is a truly profound and powerful tool. It may at first look like a simple arrangement of words into a hierarchy, but when care is used in organizing the concepts represented by the words, and the propositions or ideas formed with well-chosen linking words, one begins to see that a good concept map is at once simple, also elegantly complex with profound meanings. (p. 31)

You may still not be clear as to how to best make use of concept maps in your teaching. The tips in Table 4.2 may help. The review by Daley et al. (2016a) has provided more detailed information.

Table 4.2 Tips for using concept maps

1. Remember that concept maps are both theory-driven and an evidence-based teaching and learning strategy.
2. Emphasize that the creation of the maps is not an "add-on" assignment but an integral part of learning to think like a physician.
3. Concept maps can have multiple roles in your teaching practice.
4. Introduce and show how to construct a concept map.
5. Make sure students use linking words in constructing a concept map.
6. Show the different map techniques related to learner tasks.
7. Continue to use concept maps as learning tools, even after completion of the map.
8. Have students create longitudinal maps of disease processes, and then have them build on that same map later in the course.
9. Have students construct maps of their patients, including pathophysiology and differential diagnosis.
10. Use concept maps to foster collaborative learning.
11. Use concept maps to assess critical thinking and a learner's ability to organise knowledge.

From Torre, D.M., Durning, S.J., Daley, B.J., 2013. Twelve tips for teaching with concept maps in medical education. Med. Teach. 35(3), 201–208.

Creating a supportive learning environment

A less obvious way you can facilitate students' learning is the contribution you make to creating a supportive learning environment:

- Does the learning environment encourage students to approach you when they have a problem?
- Does the environment encourage students to collaborate and support each other or to compete?
- Does the environment encourage students to acknowledge their mistakes?

Little attention was paid in the past to the concept of the education environment or climate. As we describe in Chapter 5, the education environment in which the student operates has an important influence on behaviour and learning. As a teacher, you can help create a learning environment that is conducive to the student's learning, both in the school generally and in your own course. Fortunately, one only rarely encounters an educational climate in which the education programme is seen as a test of survival and it is considered that students who need support from the teacher do not deserve to qualify.

Engaging the student

Engaging the student in the curriculum

Learning is a partnership between teachers and students. Supporting and developing this partnership is an essential role for you as a facilitator. Traditionally, the relationship between learners and the teaching programme was very different. The student was there to be taught and had no role or contribution to make to curriculum development, the evaluation of teaching or the delivery of the teaching programme. The situation today is very different, with students engaged in all the activities. Student engagement with the curriculum, however, is not a new concept. John Dewey, in *Democracy and Education* (1916, p. 14) argued: "Making the individual a sharer or partner in the associated activity so that he feels its success as his success, its failure as his failure, is the completing step."

There has been renewed interest in student engagement, in the "student voice" and in staff working in partnership with students to deliver the education programme and to facilitate change. On today's agenda is co-owned education, with an expectation that students will take greater responsibility for learning. Student representation in teaching and learning committees is now standard practice in many schools, and there is a high level of commitment to the student voice in committees in the school.

Mahatmya et al. (2014) have used metaphor to help us understand the changing perception of the students' role in education:

- The student as product. Students receive instruction and are assessed as they move through the education programme. This is the 19th century equivalent of students as parts in a product assembly line.

- The student as consumer. Students here are not identified as the product but as consumers of education, with the programme responsive to consumer demands. This is the 20th century approach, in which the emphasis is on what consumers want to buy.
- The student as client. Here students are partners in the learning process. They are engaged dynamically and contribute to the success of the education programme. It is suggested that the student as a partner in the learning process should be the 21st century education model.

Student engagement in the curriculum is one of the areas where excellence in medical education is recognised in the ASPIRE-to-Excellence initiative (www.aspire-to-excellence.org). Four spheres of engagement are recognised:

- Student engagement with the management of the school, including matters of policy and the mission and vision of the school.
- Student engagement in the delivery of teaching and assessment.
- Student engagement in the academic community eg. the school's research programme and participation in meetings.
- Student engagement in the local community and the service delivery.

It has been recognised that cultural, social and other issues are likely to have an influence on the engagement of learners in an education programme, and how learner engagement manifests itself will vary from programme to programme. Medical schools and postgraduate programmes vary in how they respond to the challenge of engaging learners as partners in the learning. The inaugural *Wall Street Journal-Times Higher Education* college ranking in 2016 found that the elite research universities rated poorly. Only eight of the top 20 overall institutions were in the top 100 for student engagement, with Harvard and Princeton University languishing in the 601 to 800 bracket (*Times Higher Education*, 2016).

A continuum of student engagement in the medical school and in the curriculum is given in Table 4.3. This ranges from a failure to engage students to involvement of students in governance issues.

Table 4.3 Continuum of student engagement in the curriculum

1. Students are not engaged
2. Feedback is given, and students are encouraged to assess their own competence
3. Students share ideas and have an impact on the curriculum through membership in curriculum committees
4. Students have responsibility for specified extracurricular and curricular activities
5. Students participate in the teaching programme through peer-assisted learning
6. Peer assessment contributes to the assessment programme
7. Students are involved in decisions about staff appointments and promotions
8. Students are involved in governance issues through membership in committees and the faculty board

Motivating the student

Student motivation is the *product* of good teaching and not a prerequisite. Without motivation, there is no learning. Motivation is a predictor of students' learning and academic success. A motivated student uses more effective learning strategies, perseveres in case of difficulties or failure and achieves a higher level of performance than a less motivated student (Pelaccia and Viau, 2017). As a teacher or trainer, you can facilitate learning by motivating the learner. This was described by a respondent in a survey of university teachers in Australia (Ballantyne et al., 1999):

> *I think one of the greatest skills an educator can have is the skill to inspire students, to motivate them, to get them excited. That's what I enjoy. I think you can stimulate their minds, enthuse them, send them on a quest for learning. I think we do, in a way, send them off on a voyage of discovery to broaden their knowledge and open new doors. (p. 244)*

True motivation, however, comes from within the learner – intrinsic motivation. Students want to learn about a subject or develop a skill because they have an interest in the topic or see that this learning will help them in some way (e.g. to be a better doctor). Medical education relies heavily on learners' motivation to become doctors. At a serious rail accident near Dundee, medical students on the train were embarrassed to find out that they were less well-equipped to be of assistance compared with nursing students who were present. Following the accident, the students were motivated to request that a class be included in the first-year course that equipped them to respond to such accidents. External motivation, where the motivation is on studying for passing examinations or meeting other school requirements, is less effective than motivation that comes from within the student. Intrinsic and extrinsic motivation, however, are complementary and often co-exist.

What can you as a teacher do to help motivate students? The following points are derived from the recommendations of Mann (1999) and Pelaccia and Viau (2017) and from our own experience.

- First, and most important, demonstrate your own passion and enthusiasm for the subject you are teaching and for the students' learning. A bored and uninterested teacher will result in bored and uninterested students. That you care for the students and their learning really does matter. The importance of passion and enthusiasm have been highlighted by Joel Felner, a senior clinical teacher in the USA, and Moira Maley, an experienced teacher from Australia, in Boxes 4.8 and 4.9.
- Enhance the students' perception of the value of an activity by showing how it relates to the expected learning outcomes. We discussed this earlier in the chapter.
- Pay attention to what is rewarded in the course and ensure that the assessment matches the expected learning outcomes. A powerful factor driving the students' learning is the need to pass examinations; examinations drive student learning. As Don Melnick, former

Box 4.8 My passion for teaching[a]

I touch the future – I teach.

Sharon Christa McAuliffe

Of the many hats I wear as Professor of Medicine/Associate Dean for Education, my greatest passion is for teaching. The ability to teach in several settings enables me to maximize students' learning. Whether in a small group setting of six to eight students around "Harvey's" bedside (the Cardiology Patient Simulator), that I helped develop, or in a large auditorium with more than 100 students, I feel the message that I deliver is that learning is enjoyable.

I teach two large courses at the medical school: a freshman Cardiovascular Module for the entire class of 138 students and a month-long senior elective, entitled "Harvey," with usually eight students per month. When I realized that freshmen learn a great deal and enjoy being taught by senior students, I coordinated the one month of my senior elective that runs parallel with the freshman module, so that the seniors can teach and interact with the freshmen, around Harvey's bedside and during small group discussions. Since the senior elective month starts one week before the Cardiology Module, it gives me ample time to prepare the seniors for their teaching responsibilities. The comments by both the freshman and the seniors are always very positive.

I believe that I have a unique teaching style. I try to teach by laying things out in as plain a manner as I can, but do not always share the entire story. I often leave just a little bit out, and tell the students that I am doing so, challenging them to come up with the rest of the story. In the small group setting, I use the Socratic teaching method by asking and answering questions to stimulate critical thinking to draw out ideas and underlying presumptions, whereas in a large group setting I utilize my own "live" drawings, more than written words on PowerPoint slides, since I believe students pay more attention to active learning as I build my drawings sequentially. This method allows me to stay in direct contact with the students. I also think that my personality and position as the Dean of Education helps motivate them to study what they are taught. I bring a lot of emotion to my teaching and hope my passion shines through. In the end, I hope the students are motivated as they see how much I care about them and about the subject matter.

[a]*Joel Felner, Professor of Medicine and Associate Dean for Education, Emory University School of Medicine, Atlanta, USA.*

President of the National Board of Medical Examiners, said: "The curriculum instructs the teachers what to teach, the examinations instruct students what to learn." In Dundee, when an OSCE was introduced in the final examination, which students had to pass to graduate, the librarian noted that students spent less time in the library reading books. Instead, they spent more time in clinic-related activities. The alignment of assessment with the teaching programme is discussed in Chapter 6.

- Make learning enjoyable and rewarding. The FAIR principles described earlier in the chapter can contribute to this. Students are more motivated to learn in an authentic curriculum in which the learning is seen as

Box 4.9 What makes a good teacher[a]

These are actions that I feel have been best practice in my teaching and most rewarding for me: listening to students to determine how they may be best engaged; paraphrasing their understanding; providing an optimal template for a task; being enthusiastic and confident; responding quickly to concerns; conveying belief in the student's ability; communicating goals clearly; always being there for consultation; enjoying the student's success; providing sufficient challenge but not too much; letting go; illustrating concepts within a relevant context; thinking out loud; providing a missing link for understanding personal reflection.

These are situations I have witnessed and learned most from: listening to a dialogue between a student and a good teacher; watching two keen students collaborate; reflecting on a series of teaching and learning experiences and synthesising those into a scholarly piece.

[a]*Moira Maley, Australia.*

relevant. The learning should be challenging – not too easy and not too hard.

- Use teaching and learning strategies that are inherently motivating. PBL, integration of clinical medicine and the basic sciences and community-based learning all help motivate the learner. Having the opportunity to put into practice what they are learning through on-the-job or work-based learning shapes what students learn and their motivation to learn.
- Provide regular feedback on progress. This was also discussed earlier in the chapter.
- Encourage self-efficacy. Learners should be assisted to gain confidence in their competence. Encouraging students to undertake teaching responsibilities can act positively on their perceived self-efficacy.
- Enhance learners' perception of controllability by providing them with opportunities to plan their own study programme and progress on a curriculum map. When we first introduced a self-learning programme in endocrinology, students valued the opportunity to choose when and where they would study.

In Box 4.10, Subha Ramani, a general internist and medical education specialist, illustrates the importance of motivating students. Debbie Jaarsma, a teacher and researcher with many years' experience in health professions education, highlights in Box 4.11 motivation and self-regulation. In their book, *The Motivated Brain*, Gregory and Kaufeldt (2015) described the problem of lack of motivation in school education as they saw it:

In today's fast-paced digital world, students often see school as very much an unstimulating entity. For the most part, teachers and parents see school as the traditional teacher-led, top-down, "listen to me" place that they experienced growing up. School is probably the least responsive evolving

Box 4.10 Motivating students[a]

My perspective of learner-centered teaching requires moving away from informing young minds to transforming them, and being a facilitator of learning rather than a provider of knowledge. I need to kindle their internal motivation, without which adult learners are neither likely to understand nor retain content. Internal motivation is stimulated when the learning is commensurate with learners' goals, relevant to their professional practice and directly applicable to patient care. As independent and reflective practice are ultimate goals for clinical trainees, I enjoy guiding, supporting and challenging them during their journey from novices to competent clinicians, encouraging them to reflect on their strengths and areas for improvement and helping them develop action plans for professional growth.

[a]Subha Ramani, Director of Education Innovations and Scholarship, Internal Medicine Residency Program, Brigham and Women's Hospital, Assistant Professor of Medicine, Harvard Medical School, Boston, USA.

Box 4.11 Motivation and self-regulation[a]

As a supervisor of many talented research and Ph.D. students, one of the main challenges for me in this role is to optimise the balance between supporting their autonomy so as to maintain their motivation and build on their capacity for self-regulation and on the other hand giving them enough structure and guidance so as to support their feeling of confidence and competence.

The balance between autonomy and structure has been described in literature on honours students as 'bounded freedom.' An interesting scientific topic which has yet to be researched more profoundly at the teacher and student level is the mechanisms for how to provide such 'bounded freedom' in supervisory practice. In my opinion, this is dependent on the individual in front of you, the stage he or she is at in the research learning trajectory and the teacher's own beliefs and experiences.

[a]Debbie Jaarsma, Professor of Innovation and Research in Medical Education, University Medical Center, Groningen, The Netherlands.

> institution in today's society, clinging to the factory model instead of the thinking model. (p. 146)

How different is the experience in medical school? In our classrooms, are our students bored or motivated to learn?

Even motivated and well-intentioned learners may struggle to meet their learning targets. This intention–action gap was highlighted by Saddawi-Konefka et al. (2016). A strong commitment by the student to change behaviours may not be enough. What has been described in their study as implementation intentions may help:

> Implementation intentions are 'if-then' plans that specify an anticipated future situation and a planned response – 'If I encounter situation X, then

I will respond with action Y.' They differ from simple goals, which specify only a desired behaviour or outcome – 'I intend to perform action Z.' Despite this subtle difference, they have shown substantial effectiveness over goals alone in increasing goal attainment. (p. 1211)

After seeing a patient with hypertension, rather than having a goal of learning about the clinical features and diagnostic approach to a patient with hypertension, the implementation intention would be to read the relevant section in the text or use the appropriate online learning tool after finishing dinner later in the day. Another example of an implementation intention where social media is a distraction for a student is, "If I receive a WhatsApp message, I will silence my smartphone and ignore it until I have completed the study session." The powerful effect of implementation intentions has been replicated in different studies and should be considered when you advise students about their learning strategies.

Self-determined learning: Heutagogy

Heutagogy is a relatively recent term which has found a place in the education literature and was introduced by Hase and Kenyon (2001). It places learners at the centre of their learning and empowers them by allowing them to take control of their own learning and develop their own learning approach. In this sense, it can be seen as the ultimate step in student engagement with their learning.

We have argued for the concept of "directed self-learning" rather than "self-directed learning," with the teacher having an important role in guiding or facilitating the student's learning. As Dron (2007) has suggested, however, the teacher can become less important as students progress through the curriculum, becoming more autonomous and taking more responsibility for their own learning, a situation that reflects the reality of lifelong learning and continuous professional development.

In heutagogy, the teacher's role is to encourage in students the capability to take responsibility for their learning (Abraham and Komattil, 2016). We need to move from a position where the role of education is to provide the learner with the necessary knowledge and skills to one where the learner can ask the appropriate question, knows where to get the answer and can evaluate the answers they receive (Friedman et al., 2016). Addressing these student capabilities is a challenge to the traditional teacher. In heutagogy, the teacher still has a role, even if a very different one from that to which we have become accustomed.

Clinical supervision

Who is a clinical supervisor?

The described approaches to facilitation of learning have relevance to facilitating the students' or trainees' learning in the clinical situation, as well as in the classroom and more generally. The clinical context has some unique features, and the responsibilities of the clinical teacher differ to some extent from those of the teacher in other situations. One obvious difference is the teacher's responsibility to patients and their care. The clinical supervisor is important, and the quality of on-the-job learning is only as good as the quality of the supervisor(s). The school of experience is no school at all; without supervision, the trainee may go on practising his or her mistakes.

Kilminster and Jolly (2000) defined clinical supervision as:

> *...the provision of monitoring, guidance and feedback on matters of personal, professional and educational development in the context of the doctor's care of patients. This would include the ability to anticipate a doctor's strengths and weaknesses in particular clinical situations in order to maximize patient safety. (p. 828)*

What is expected of the clinical supervisor?

As a clinical supervisor, you need to:

- Be committed to the role, and ensure that sufficient time is allocated in your schedule to meet with the student or trainee to discuss and assess his or her progress. Clinical supervisors should have protected time for this purpose.
- Plan with the student or trainee about how they will achieve the expected competences and the milestones on their journey to this end. The learning should not be simply opportunistic, dictated by the service commitment.
- Help the student or trainee make sense of her or his experience and reflect on it by monitoring and working with them. They learn not simply by osmosis. The clinical supervisor should help fuel the student's learning.
- Provide constructive feedback at the level of the management of an individual patient or engagement in a particular task. Lack of feedback or inappropriate unhelpful feedback is one of the most common complaints of students and trainees with regard to on-the-job learning. We discussed earlier in this chapter how to provide effective feedback. It is important to tell the learner how he or she is getting on. Give credit when it is due.
- Review with learners their progress and achievement of the expected milestones, at the same time advising the learner about his or her personal and professional development.
- Ensure that patients and patient safety are considered. This is paramount.
- Help the learner relate theory to the practice. A task-based approach can be adopted, as described in Chapter 5. As described earlier in this chapter, a study guide relates the common tasks in which the learner is engaged to

the learning outcomes and to what it is expected that should be learned. An example for the paediatric trainee is given in Table 4.1.

Your responsibility to assist a student or trainee to master a specific competence or complete a specific task can be addressed in the following steps:

- Show the learner how to do the job.
- Explain the key points.
- Let the learner watch you do it again.
- Let the learner do simple parts of the job.
- Help the learner do the whole job under your supervision.
- Let the learner do it on his or her own.

Heidi Chumley and Athol Kent, both experienced clinical teachers, describe their experience of facilitating learning in the clinical setting in Boxes 4.12 and 4.13.

Supervisory interventions
Interventions by the supervisor can take different forms:

- Prescriptive. The supervisor gives instructions and directs the learner.
- Informative. The supervisor gives advice, information or possible ideas from their own experience.
- Supportive. The supervisor reassures the learner of their care, attention and willingness to help and support.
- Confronting. The supervisor directly challenges the learner with the nature of their actions or achievements. Occasionally, feelings of sadness or anger may challenge the supervisor's own emotional competence.

Box 4.12 Facilitating learning in clinical practice[a]

I had been teaching for some time before I better understood how to facilitate learning in my clinical practice. I knew the guidelines – orient the learner, work in some direct observation, provide specific feedback – but it was later that I learned to create deliberate practice and to set students up to succeed. Short directions often help a new clinical learner know what to practice in a given patient encounter. Do you know the Ottawa ankle rules? Look them up and apply them to the next patient you are seeing. She's following up on her diabetes; make sure you get a sense of what she understands about diabetes and her treatment plan. This patient is more challenging. Try to ascertain the underlying reason for his visit. Giving a student a specific task allowed me to focus my feedback on that task, and to determine when I needed to find a similar task for repetitive practice or when I could increase the complexity.

---

[a]Heidi Chumley, Executive Dean, American University of the Caribbean School of Medicine, Cupecoy, St. Maarten, Netherlands Antilles.

Box 4.13 My best tutorial ever![a]

After a lifetime in clinical medicine, I now give one tutorial a week. I meet 12 bright young things in a quiet room next to the ward where they will be learning history-taking skills from real patients for the first time.

They are a third of my age and give me the benefit of their attention. I ask them to sit in a circle and spend 5 minutes introducing myself and interacting with them in a convivial way. I then start asking them, one by one, if I may ask them how they learn.

Each has my undivided attention, my best listening skills, with respect at the top of my list. Gently checking, probing how they learn about medicine, and after 5 minutes I move to the next. I stop after half the students have been questioned.

The rest of the group are then asked, pair-by-pair, to articulate what they have observed. It slowly becomes apparent to them that they have experienced a session of history taking – usually to their great mirth and delight.

Oh, yes! Your introduction of yourself, permission to ask questions, open-ended style, checking you had understood correctly, eye contact, body language, humour, polite respect for younger and less experienced colleagues, any questions and thanks.

The evaluation forms (open-ended) suggest being a role model can result in "My best tutorial ever!"

[a]*Athol Kent, Obstetrician and Clinical Teacher, Department of Obstetrics and Gynaecology, University of Cape Town, Cape Town, South Africa.*

The good clinical teacher also serves as a role model. Ineffective supervisory behaviours have been described by Watkins (1997):

> *Rigidity, low empathy, low support, failure to consistently track supervisee concerns, failure to teach or instruct, being indirect or intolerant, being closed, lacking respect for differences, being noncollegial, lacking in praise and encouragement, being sexist, and emphasising evaluation, weakness and deficiencies. (p. 168)*

Different roles for the clinical supervisor

In addition to the role as facilitator of learning, the clinical supervisor is likely also to assume other roles, as described in this text. These include the roles of information provider, role model, curriculum planner, assessor and manager. Occasionally, some of these roles, such as the supervisor's role as facilitator and assessor, as we suggest in Chapter 2, may appear to conflict, and this is a challenge that has to be addressed. A good clinical supervisor has many of the features of a good mentor, as described in this chapter.

Mentoring

A mentor is different from a coach

We have described the move from the teacher as information provider to the teacher as a facilitator of learning. The teacher guides the student's learning by clarifying the expected learning outcomes, identifying appropriate learning opportunities, taking steps to make the learning process effective and engaging for the student, and assisting the student to assess her or his own progress. Challenging learners to take responsibility for their own learning takes student engagement a step further. In this way, as a coach, you encourage students to reflect on their learning and take charge of their own development, and you serve as a sounding board for the student.

Sometimes the term *coach* is used interchangeably with the terms *mentor* and *clinical supervisor*. Although there are similar elements, it is useful to distinguish these responsibilities. In mentoring, you have a different role from that of a coach. As a mentor, you are actively engaged in an explicit two-way relationship with a student or future colleague. In Greek mythology, Mentor was the older friend and tutor chosen by Odysseus to take charge of his son Telemachus when he left for the Trojan War. The Standing Committee on Postgraduate Medical and Dental Education in England (SCOPME) (Bligh, 1999) defined mentoring as:

> ...*a voluntary relationship, typically between two individuals, in which the mentor is usually an experienced, highly regarded, empathic individual, often working in the same organisation, or field, as the mentee; the mentor, by listening and talking with the mentee in private and in confidence, guides the mentee in the development of his or her own ideas, learning, and personal and professional development. (p. 2)*

John Gill (2015), writing in the *Times Higher Education*, highlighted the value of a teacher as mentor:

> *A particularly well made observation about the advent of massive open online courses is that universities no longer have a monopoly on knowledge. The internet has blown it to pieces. What they do have, however, which remains of real value, is wisdom, the ability to mentor and inspire.*

Can you think of someone who has had a positive and long-lasting effect on your own career development? This person may or may not have been formally assigned to you as a mentor, and the person may not have been trained as a mentor. However, the person is likely to have been a caring teacher or colleague who provided you with support as a student, trainee or doctor. Hesketh and Laidlaw (2003) captured the concept of mentorship:

> *a relationship that encourages the holistic development of a person... often an exemplary role model, a confidante who will support the mentee through any personal stresses and strains, a teacher, a developer of talent and an opener of doors. (p. 9)*

Box 4.14 A "teacher of teachers"[a]

As Chief of Pedagogy for the Academic Medical Education Institute (AMEI, our in-house, education-based faculty development program), I have a rather unusual educator role from most who may read this book or perhaps even contribute to this book. I view myself as a "teacher of teachers." My main role is to create the learning environment for our health professions' educators that helps them to become outstanding educators in their own right and to help them exemplify the roles, values, and characteristics of a great teacher. And in turn, they then create the positive learning environment for their students. To achieve that, I felt that it was critically important that I "practice what I preach." So, I attempt to role model best practices in each of the eight roles when designing, delivering or mentoring our educators. And above all, I attempt to help them approach their work in a scholarly fashion as well as reflect on and continually improve their own competence as a teacher and foster a culture of trust and empowerment. This has been a very rewarding experience, knowing that my reach and impact goes way beyond just those who come to our programs.

[a]Sandy Cook, Deputy Head, Office of Education, Duke-NUS Medical School, Singapore, Chief of Pedagogy for Academic Medicine Education Institute.

Sandy Cook, a senior teacher in Singapore, describes her role as a mentor in Box 4.14. Mentoring is recognised as important for the acquisition of clinical and research skills. Senior residents mentoring interns can enhance patient safety, particularly when new graduates take up their posts in hospital. Mentored faculty have a significantly greater satisfaction with their department and institution, and the absence of mentoring has been found to be an important factor for unsatisfying careers in academic medicine (Mylona et al., 2016; Schafer et al., 2016).

The duties of a mentor

A mentor has a number of responsibilities or duties in relation to the mentee. The roles of the mentor include (Ramani and Gruppen, 2013):

- Teacher
- Adviser
- Role model
- Advocate
- Coach
- Agent
- Confidant
- Sponsor

The mentor embraces for an individual student or doctor (the mentee) all of these roles, as required. The required roles will depend on the needs of the mentee.

What makes an effective mentor–mentee relationship?

Mentoring has evolved from a casual arrangement between the student and the teacher to an important recognised role for the medical teacher. People are not born with the skills necessary to be a mentor. These are acquired over time. Simply matching mentors with mentees and leaving them to get on with it is not acceptable. Mentors need to know what they should be doing and why they are doing it. Experience has shown the factors that influence and contribute to a successful mentor–mentee relationship (Hesketh and Laidlaw, 2003; Long, 2014; Ramani and Gruppen, 2013; Rowley, 1999; Sng et al., 2017). Here we suggest ten requirements if you wish to be a successful and effective mentor.

Commitment

The first requirement for a successful mentorship is that you (and the mentee) are committed to making it work, with generosity on both sides. You should recognise that you can make a significant difference to your mentee but that this may be challenging and may require an investment of your time and effort.

Individualisation

Remember that each mentee is unique, with different abilities, problems and career aspirations.

Respect

There should be respect and mutual trust between you and the mentee. This may take time. It includes listening to the mentee and his or her views and aspirations. Maintaining confidentiality is essential.

Approachability

You need to be easy to approach and available to your mentee, as necessary. It is important that you are not seen as intimidating or threatening. Does your mentee feel able to tell you, for example, about a mistake they have made?

Empathy

Empathy is essential for the establishment of your relationship with your mentee. You should be caring and compassionate. Remember the problems that you may have had as a student or trainee and that your mentee is also human.

Successes

Take pride and rejoice in your mentee's successes. You should be committed to your mentee's success. Hope and optimism are important attributes of the mentor. You should discuss not only the mentee's problems and difficulties but also their successes, no matter how small. In *Mentors: They Simply Believe*, Lasley (1996) has argued that a crucial characteristic of a mentor is the ability to communicate the belief that a person is capable of transcending present challenges and of accomplishing great things in the future.

Feedback

Provide honest advice and feedback to your mentee, as necessary. Honesty is an important part of the relationship.

Challenge

As a mentor, you should challenge the mentee to reflect on his or her progress and future plans and to think in new ways. You can pose your advice as questions, requiring mentees to think for themselves. Be willing to argue and discuss with the mentee in a constructive way.

Matching

This may be outside your control but, where possible, the mentor and mentee should be matched. The chemistry between the two is important. The nature of mentoring pivots on the compatibility of mentors and mentees (Sng et al., 2017).

Culture

Be aware that culture and context may have a central role to play in mentoring (Sawatsky et al., 2016).

Institutional arrangements

The approach of the school to mentoring is important. Is mentoring valued? Are there clear goals and expectations of staff? Is a staff development programme in place? Are guidelines available?

Implementation in practice

We know that a critical and negative mentoring style by trainers is detrimental to the trainee's acquisition of the necessary skills. Misunderstanding about mentoring is common, and the application in practice often is lacking. This may be because of a failure of teachers to understand the concept of mentoring or, if they do, it may be the result of a failure of the teacher to accept or prioritise the relevance in their own situation. This was illustrated in one school, in which mentoring was seen as an important element in the education programme. A staff development activity was organised to familiarise the teachers with mentoring, but the result was a mixed success. Some teachers who attended the staff development sessions and some who did not successfully undertook their roles as mentors for the students. Others who attended the training programme, however, did not implement what they had learned. This is an example of when the pedagogical knowledge of the teacher does not necessarily translate into action. The problem is explored further in Chapters 9 and 10, when we consider scholarship and professionalism, and in Chapter 11, when we review the implementation of the roles of teachers in practice.

The teacher facilitator, expert facilitator and master facilitator

The teacher facilitator

The teacher understands and is committed to her or his role as a facilitator and applies in his or her teaching a range of approaches to facilitate students' learning.

An expert facilitator

The expert facilitator is committed to facilitating students' learning and has given particular consideration to and explored and developed ways of facilitating learning for use in their own institution.

A master facilitator

The master facilitator is committed to facilitating students' learning and has studied and researched different approaches. He or she has developed particular skills in one or more aspect and is recognised nationally and internationally for this.

Take-home messages

1. Facilitation of learning is the most important role for the medical teacher.
2. Facilitation involves clarifying for student and trainee what is expected of them in terms of the learning outcomes.
3. Learners should be guided to appropriate learning opportunities and resources and when and how they should be used or accessed.
4. A study guide and a curriculum map are useful tools in facilitating a student's learning.
5. Incorporating the FAIR principles (*f*eedback, *a*ctivity, *i*ndividualisation and *r*elevance) into your teaching can facilitate the student's learning.
6. Learning is facilitated if learners are engaged in the curriculum and are partners in the process, not just consumers.
7. Facilitation of learning in the clinical context is also important and has some unique features.
8. The teacher as a mentor can have a powerful influence on the student's or doctor's learning, personal development and career choice.

Consider

- Have you considered the importance of your role as a facilitator, rather than simply an information provider?
- Do your students fully understand the expected learning outcomes for your course?
- Do your students make the best use of the learning opportunities and resources available?
- Have you explored providing learners with a study guide to support and facilitate their learning?
- Is a curriculum map available for learners relating the learning outcomes to the learning experiences and the assessment?
- To what extent are the FAIR principles for effective learning (*f*eedback, *a*ctivity, *i*ndividualisation, *r*elevance) incorporated into your teaching?
- To what extent are students engaged in your curriculum, as specified in the ASPIRE-to-Excellence criteria (www.aspire-to-excellence.org)?

- As a mentor for students or colleagues, do you meet the requirements for an effective mentor, as described in this chapter?

Explore further

Abdel-Fattah, A.M.A., Harden, R.M., Laidlaw, J.M., 1991. A new approach to vocational training. Med. Educ. 25, 166.

Abraham, R.R., Komattil, R., 2016. Heutagogic approach to developing capable learners. Med. Teach. 39 (3), 295–299.

ASPIRE-to-Excellence. www.aspire-to-excellence.org.

Ballantyne, R., Bain, J., Packer, J., 1999. Researching university teaching in Australia: Themes and issues in academics' reflections. Stud. Higher Educ. 24 (2), 237–257.

Belshaw, D., 2016. How to use metaphors to generate badge-based pathways. http://dougbelshaw.com/blog/2016/06/28/badge-pathway-metaphors.

Bligh, J., 1999. Mentoring: An invisible support network. Med. Educ. 33 (1), 2–3.

Bloch, B., 2015. A little explanation goes a long way. https://www.timeshighereducation.com/comment/opinion/a-little-explanation-goes-a-long-way/2018271.article.

Boud, D., 2015. Feedback: ensuring that it leads to enhanced learning. Clin. Teach. 12 (1), 3–7.

Brown, J.S., Collins, A., Duguid, P., 1989. Situated cognition and the culture of learning. Educ. Res. 18 (1), 32–42.

Cooper, K., 2014. 6 common mistakes that undermine motivation. Kappan. 95 (8), 11–17.

Daley, B.J., Durning, S.J., Torre, D.M., 2016a. Using concept maps to create meaningful learning in medical education. https://www.mededpublish.org/manuscripts/380.

Daley, B.J., Morgan, S., Black, S.B., 2016b. Concept maps in nursing education: A historical literature review and research directions. J. Nurs. Educ. 55 (11), 631–639.

Daley, B.J., Torre, D., Stark-Schweitzer, T., et al., 2006. Advancing teaching and learning in medical education through the use of concept maps. In: Cañas, A.J., Novak, J.D. (Eds.), Concept Maps: Theory, Methodology, Technology, vol. 1, 24–31. Universidad de Costa Rica, San José, Costa Rica.

Dewey, J., 1916. Democracy and Education: An Introduction to the Philosophy of Education. Free Press, New York.

Dron, J., 2007. Control and Constraint in e-Learning: Choosing When to Choose. IDEA Group Publishing, London.

Englander, R., Frank, J., Carraccio, C., et al., 2017. Toward a shared language for competency-based medical education. Med. Teach. 39 (6), 582–587.

Fox, D., 1983. Personal theories of teaching. Stud. Higher Educ. 8 (2), 151–163.

Friedman, C.P., Donaldson, K.M., Vantsevich, A.V., 2016. Educating medical students in the era of ubiquitous information. Med. Teach. 38 (5), 504–509.

Gill, J., 2015. Cooking in an open kitchen. Times Higher Ed., 17 December 2015.

Gregory, G., Kaufeldt, M., 2015. The Motivated Brain. http://www.ascd.org/professional-development/webinars/the-motivated-brain-webinar.aspx.

Harden, R.M., 2001. AMEE Guide No. 21: Curriculum mapping: A tool for transparent and authentic teaching and learning. Med. Teach. 23 (2), 123–137.

Harden, R.M., 2007. Learning outcomes as a tool to assess progression. Med. Teach. 29 (7), 678–682.

Harden, R.M., Crosby, J.R., Davis, M.H., 1999a. AMEE Guide No. 14: Outcome-based education: Part 1 – An introduction to outcome-based education. Med. Teach. 21 (1), 7–14.

Harden, R.M., Laidlaw, J.M., 2017. Essential Skills for a Medical Teacher. 2nd edn. Elsevier, London.

Harden, R.M., Laidlaw, J.M., Hesketh, E.A., 1999b. AMEE Medical Education Guide No 16: Study guides—their use and preparation. Med. Teach. 21 (3), 248–265.

Harden, R.M., Lilley, P.M., Patricio, M.F., 2016. The Definitive Guide to the OSCE. Elsevier, London.

Hase, S., Kenyon, C., 2001. Moving From Andragogy to Heutagogy: Implications for VET. https://epubs.scu.edu.au/cgi/viewcontent.cgi?article=1147&context=gcm_pubs.

Hesketh, E.A., Laidlaw, J.M., 2003. Developing the teaching instinct, 5: Mentoring. Med. Teach. 25 (1), 9–12.

Hsu, L., Hsieh, S.I., 2005. Concept maps as an assessment tool in a nursing course. J. Prof. Nurs. 21 (3), 141–149.

Issenberg, B., McGaghie, M.C., Hart, I.R., et al., 1999. Simulation technology for health care professional skills training and assessment. JAMA 282 (9), 861–866.

Kilminster, S.M., Jolly, B.C., 2000. Effective supervision in clinical practice. Med. Educ. 34, 827–840.

Knowles, M.S., 1975. Self-Directed Learning: A Guide for Learners and Teachers. Prentice Hall, Upper Saddle River, New Jersey.

Kolb, D.A., 1984. Experiential Learning: Experience as the Source of Learning and Development. Prentice Hall, Upper Saddle River, New Jersey.

Krajcik, J.S., Blumenfeld, P., 2006. Project-based learning. In: Sawyer, R.K. (Ed.), The Cambridge Handbook of the Learning Sciences. Cambridge University Press, New York.

Lasley, T., 1996. Mentors: They simply believe. Peabody J. Ed. 71(1), 64–70.

Long, K., 2014. Eight qualities of a great teacher mentor. http://www.edweek.org/tm/articles/2014/09/30/ctq_long_mentor.html.

Mahatmya, D., Brown, R.C., Johnson, A.D., 2014. Student-as-client. Kappan. 95 (6), 30–34.

Mann, K.V., 1999. Motivation in medical education: How theory can inform our practice. Acad. Med. 74 (3), 237–239.

McDonald, S., Stevenson, R.J., 1998. Navigation in hyperspace: An evaluation of the effects of navigational tools and subject matter expertise on browsing and information retrieval in hypertext. Interacting Computers 10, 129–142.

Mitchell, H.E., Harden, R.M., Laidlaw, J.M., 1998. Towards effective on-the-job learning: The development of a paediatric training guide. Med. Teach. 20 (2), 91–98.

Murdoch-Eaton, D., Bowen, L., 2017. Feedback mapping – the curricular cornerstone of an "educational alliance. Med. Teach. 39 (5), 540–547.

Mylona, E., Brubaker, L., Williams, V.N., et al., 2016. Does formal mentoring for faculty members matter? A survey of clinical faculty members. Med. Educ. 50 (6), 670–681.

Nikendei, C., Huhn, D., Pittius, G., et al., 2016. Students' perceptions on an interprofessional ward round training – a qualitative pilot study. GMS J. Med. Educ. 33 (2), Doc 14.

Novak, J.D., Cañas, A.J., 2006. The theory underlying concept maps and how to construct and use them. Technical report. Pensacola, FL, Florida Institute for Human and Machine Cognition.

Novak, J.D., Gowin, D.B., 1984. Learning How to Learn. Cambridge University Press, New York.

Pelaccia, T., Viau, R., 2017. Motivation in medical education. Med. Teach. 39 (2), 136–140.

Petrilli, C.M., Del Valle, J., Chopra, V., 2016. Why July matters. Acad. Med. 91, 910–912.

Prensky, M., 2006. Don't Bother Me Mom – I'm Learning! Paragon House, Saint Paul, Minnesota.

Ramani, S., Gruppen, L., 2013. Mentoring: "Getting Started." University of Dundee, UK, Centre for Medical Education,.

Rowley, J.B., 1999. The good mentor. Educ. Leadership 56 (8), 20–22.

Rowntree, D., 1986. Teaching Through Self-Instruction: A Practical Handbook for Course Developers. Nichols Publishing, Asbury, IA.

Saddawi-Konefka, D., Schumacher, D.J., Baker, K.H., et al., 2016. Changing physician behaviour with implementation intentions: Closing the gap between intentions and actions. Acad. Med. 91 (9), 1211–1216.

Sawatsky, A.P., Parekh, N., Muula, A.S., et al., 2016. Cultural implications of mentoring in sub-Saharan Africa: A qualitative study. Med. Educ. 50, 657–669.

Schafer, M., Pander, T., Pinilla, S., et al., 2016. A prospective, randomised trial of different matching procedures for structured mentoring programmes in medical education. Med. Teach. 38 (9), 921–929.

Schmidt, H.J., 2004. Alternative approaches to concept mapping and implications for medical education: Commentary on reliability, validity and future research decisions. Adv. Health Sci. Educ. 9 (3), 251–256.

Sinclair, H.K., Cleland, J.A., 2007. Undergraduate medical students: Who seeks formative feedback? Med. Educ. 41 (6), 580–582.

Sng, J.H., Pei, Y., Toh, Y.P., et al., 2017. Mentoring relationships between senior physicians and junior doctors and/or medical students: A thematic review. Med. Teach. 39 (8), 866–875.

Standing Committee on Postgraduate Medical and Dental Education (SCOPME), 1998. An Enquiry into Mentoring: Supporting Doctors and Dentists at Work. London, Department. of Health.

Telio, S., Regehr, G., Ajjawi, R., 2016. Feedback and the educational alliance: Examining credibility judgements and their consequences. Med. Educ. 50 (9), 933–942.

Times Higher Education 2016. 13 October, pp. 30–69.

Torre, D.M., Durning, S.J., Daley, B.J., 2013. Twelve tips for teaching with concept maps in medical education. Med. Teach. 35 (3), 201–208.

Watkins, C.E., 1997. The ineffective psychotherapy supervisor: Some reflections about bad behaviours, poor process and offensive outcomes. Clin. Supervisor 16 (1), 163–180.

Chapter 5

The teacher as a curriculum developer and implementer

As educators, we are only as effective as what we know. If we have no working knowledge of what students studied in previous years, how can we build on their learning? If we have no insight into the curriculum in later grades, how can we prepare learners for future classes?

Heidi Hayes Jacobs

Teachers should be familiar with the curriculum in their institution and actively engaged with elements of it relating to their own teaching responsibilities.

- The role of the teacher in the curriculum
- What is a curriculum?
- Ten questions to ask about the curriculum
- What is the vision or mission of the medical school?
- What are the expected learning outcomes?
- What content should be included?
- How should the content be organised?
  - The spiral curriculum
- What educational strategies should be adopted?
  - Student-centred and teacher-centred approaches
  - Presentation-based and information-based approaches
  - Integrated and interprofessional education
  - Community-based and hospital-based approaches
  - Core curriculum and electives
  - Systematic and opportunistic approaches
  - Curriculum map
- What teaching methods should be used?
  - The lecture
  - Small group work
  - Clinical teaching
  - Independent learning
  - A blended curriculum
  - Development of e-learning resources
- Integrating assessment and the curriculum
- Communicating information about the curriculum
  - Curriculum map

The role of the teacher in the curriculum

A teacher has an important responsibility relating to the curriculum (Fig. 5.1).

Developing a curriculum is in some respect like building a house. Both have their size specified – a set number of square metres for the house and 4 or 5 years for the curriculum. The house has a number of rooms and the curriculum a number of courses. In the house, each room has a special purpose such as a kitchen, bathroom or dining room and, in the curriculum, each course addresses specific learning outcomes. In the house, each room connects with other elements in the home and, in the curriculum, each course connects with other courses. The house may be open plan or have separate rooms, eco-friendly or traditional, a modern design or conventional and may be situated in a city or a rural area. The curriculum too offers a range of options such as outcome-based, community-oriented and integrated. You

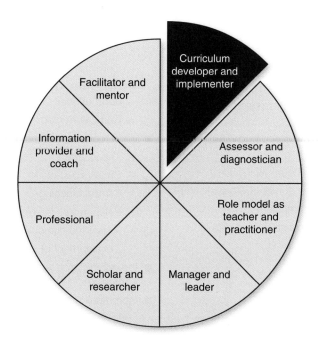

Figure 5.1 The role of the teacher as a curriculum developer and implementer

are likely to have thoughts about the sort of home you wish to live in. In the same way, as a teacher you will have ideas about the curriculum in which you would like to operate.

An architect is responsible for designing a house. Some teachers will be responsible for developing the curriculum and may chair a curriculum or curriculum phase committee. Others will be responsible for developing a course within the curriculum, such as endocrinology or another system-based course, for the teaching of physiology or another subject or for an element in the curriculum, such as electives or student-selected components (Fig. 5.2).

Every teacher, however, has some responsibility relating to the curriculum in his or her institution. As a teacher, you are a stakeholder in your school's curriculum, and you have a responsibility for your institution's curriculum policy, as well as for the course you teach. You can bring to the discussions your own education experience and philosophy and your specialty perspective – for example, as a family physician, an accident and emergency doctor or a basic scientist. Two teachers, Jeni Harden, a sociologist with 20 years' experience teaching in higher education and 6 years teaching social science to medical students, and Peter McCrorie, a medical educationist with considerable experience in curriculum development, share their perceptions of their roles in the delivery of the curriculum (Boxes 5.1 and 5.2).

As a teacher, your curriculum responsibilities include the following:

- You should be familiar with your school's curriculum, including the vision or mission of the school, the different elements and courses that make up the curriculum, the teaching and learning approaches adopted and the policies and practice relating to student assessment. Where does the school sit, for example,

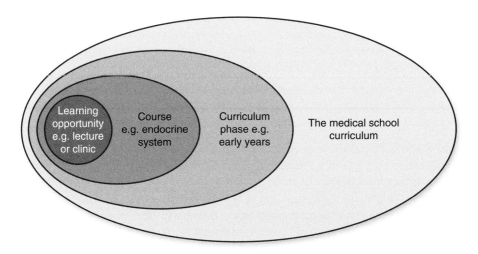

Figure 5.2 Levels of curriculum planning in a medical school

Box 5.1 Being a teacher[a]

There is a beautiful short book by a French author, Jean Giono, *The Man Who Planted Trees*, which tells the story of a shepherd's effort, over four decades, to reforest an Alpine valley by planting seeds as he went about his work. This allegorical tale resonates strongly with my thoughts on being a teacher. From curriculum development, planning teaching sessions, to developing assessment tools, I consider first and foremost how to cultivate the students' learning. This is perhaps less of the opportunistic planting of the shepherd but rather constant consideration: of types of seeds (e.g. knowledge, reflection, critical thinking); of what seeds will grow best in each season (year of study); and of what conditions will foster or hinder their growth. By the end of the story, the valley is full of trees as a result of the shepherd's efforts. Perhaps this is the hardest part of being a teacher; unlike the shepherd, what I identify as success, or my part in achieving it, is not always easy to define or see. I may witness the initial stages of growth as tentative shoots develop and begin to establish and thrive by the time students graduate, but I have to share some of the shepherd's belief that I am embarked on a worthy exercise and faith that in the end I will succeed.

[a]*Jeni Harden, Senior Lecturer, University of Edinburgh, UK*

Box 5.2 Developing the curriculum[a]

I guess at some time or another I've undertaken the roles of the teacher described in this book. Perhaps the one that stands out for me is the Curriculum Planner. In 1999, I was offered the job of a lifetime, – Course Director of the Graduate Entry Programme at St George's in London. It was the most exciting event of my academic career, without doubt – a chance to lead the development of an innovative 4-year programme for graduates in any discipline – science, law or arts. Of course, teamwork was the answer, and I had the privilege of appointing and working with some of the most stimulating people I have ever met, both academic and administrative. Together we created a totally novel programme, based on sound educational principles, which took medical education to a high level – and even got us on prime time BBC TV. Since then, I have worked in a number of other countries helping them develop their own programmes – Brunei, Ireland, Portugal, Malta and most recently Cyprus, who run a franchised, updated version of the original programme. Life has been kind to me. I simply love my job and would recommend it to anybody.

[a]*Peter McCrorie, Professor of Medical Education, University of Nicosia Medical School, Nicosia, Cyprus.*

---

on the SPICES continuum of **s**tudent-centeredness, **p**roblem orientation, **i**ntegration, **c**ommunity orientation, **e**lectives and a **s**ystematic approach? We discuss this later in the chapter.

- You should have an understanding of how your own course, lecture or other contribution to the education programme fits in with the school's curriculum. What have students learned before your course, and what will they learn after it? You should make decisions as to what you teach, how you expect students to learn and how they are assessed. As discussed in Chapter 8, you can no longer develop and deliver your teaching programme in isolation; this should be done in collaboration with colleagues in the context of the curriculum overall.

Medical educators, when asked to define themselves, referred to their role as curriculum developer in the following terms:

delivery of educational programmes, curriculum development, course implementation, design, and evaluation. He/she specializes in arranging the learning environment and in implementation of instructional activities in theoretical and clinical settings. (Nikendei et al. 2016) (p. 718)

The fact that in higher education teachers have a measure of control of the curriculum has been highlighted by Toohey (1999):

Teachers in higher education retain a very significant advantage over teachers in other branches of education: their control of the curriculum. In much of primary, secondary, technical and vocational education, course design has been handed over to 'experts', to the impoverishment of the role of classroom teachers. Yet course design is an advantage of which many teachers in universities seem quite unaware. Much of the creativity and power in teaching lies in the design of the curriculum: the choice of texts and ideas which become the focus of study, the planning of experiences for students and the means by which achievement is assessed. These define the boundaries of the experience for students. Of course the way in which the curriculum is brought to life is equally important, but the power of good teacher–student interactions is multiplied many times by course design. (p. 4)

Much of the literature on change in medical education has focussed on the importance of teamwork and teachers working together to bring about curricular reform. This is important, but as an individual teacher, you can act as a pioneer of reform. Tong and Adamson (2008) have described how in a conservative school a teacher who enthusiastically displayed the characteristics of a pioneer was able to serve as a change agent. I (RMH) have had the privilege of working in Dundee with pioneers who, in their own individual way, had a significant impact on the medical education programme: Peter Stoward revolutionised the teaching of histology, Alex McQueen the teaching of clinical anatomy, John Beck the teaching of pathology and Peter Howie introduced an interprofessional approach to the curriculum. Change can happen from the bottom up as well as top down, and you could be part of it or even an initiator or pioneer. Tong and Adamson (2008) also pointed out that "teachers are the gatekeepers of reform and can determine whether innovations take the high road to fulfilment or turn into a cul-de-sac of frustration."

Pioneers are important but so also is the culture and leadership style of the school. What is expected of you as a teacher in today's medical curricula with integrated programmes, problem-based learning (PBL) and outcome-based education (OBE) is more demanding, but it is generally accepted that this extra effort is worthwhile, given the advantages gained. Time spent in curriculum planning does require the dedication of time from you as a teacher, and this should be recognised. It is no longer reasonable to measure a teacher's workload in terms of the time spent in face-to-face contact with students: time spent on curriculum planning should be factored in.

What is a curriculum?

We have argued that the teacher has an important role to play in the curriculum. We should define the concept of a curriculum and what the term covers. In the past, a curriculum was defined in terms of the syllabus or content and the set of subjects covered. It is now defined more broadly as everything that is planned for the students by the school staff. It covers the education environment and encompasses the set of experiences designed to achieve the learning outcomes. It includes:

- The specified learning outcomes
- The curriculum content
- The courses and sequence of learning
- The education strategies adopted and the planned teaching and learning methods
- Student assessment
- The education environment or climate.

The curriculum that is planned may differ from the curriculum that is delivered. A teacher may not implement aspects of the curriculum as specified for a number of reasons. There may be logistical problems, including insufficient time, or there may be a lack of understanding or acceptance of what is required on the part of the teacher. A teacher may choose to ignore the planned curriculum and go her or his own way, usually with unsatisfactory results.

There may be a difference not only between the planned and delivered curriculum but also between the planned curriculum and educational experience as interpreted and lived by students. Students can acquire knowledge, skills and attitudes from an unofficial or "hidden curriculum," as well as from the official or formal curriculum (Hafferty and Castellani, 2009). The hidden curriculum is the collective messages that students unknowingly pick up in the school's education programme and culture. As Hafferty and Gaufberg (2017) stated: "It differentiates between what is formally/intentionally taught versus the range of other lessons students informally and tacitly acquire during training."

Sometimes these informal messages don't match the school's stated goals and educational programme. The attitudes and values conveyed by teachers in an implicit and tacit fashion may differ from what is intended and may be responsible for students' unprofessional behaviour and a decrease in empathy as they proceed through the education programme.

Ten questions to ask about the curriculum

There are ten questions that, as a teacher, you should ask about the curriculum (Harden and Laidlaw, 2017; Table 5.1). Your role in relation to each of these elements of the curriculum, as summarised in Fig. 5.3, is to:

- Contribute to establishing and influencing the curriculum approach in your school. For example, with regard to teaching and learning methods, should there be a blended approach integrating e-learning and face-to-face teaching? If there are lectures, should attendance be compulsory? To what extent should community-based education or interprofessional education

Table 5.1 Ten questions to ask when planning or evaluating a curriculum (Harden and Laidlaw, 2017)

1. What is the medical school or training programme's vision or mission?
2. What are the expected learning outcomes?
3. What content should be included?
4. How should the content be organised?
5. What educational strategies should be adopted?
6. What teaching methods should be used?
7. How should assessment be carried out?
8. How should details of the curriculum be communicated?
9. What educational environment or climate should be fostered?
10. How should the process be managed?

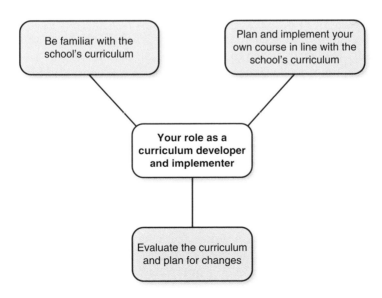

Figure 5.3 The teacher and the curriculum

THE TEACHER AS A CURRICULUM DEVELOPER AND IMPLEMENTER

(IPE) feature? For assessment, should there be a programmatic approach? To what extent should students be engaged in planning and delivering the curriculum?

- Make decisions about the course you teach. For example, how many lectures should be scheduled, and should some be replaced by a "flipped classroom"? What form should the community-based or IPE element in your course take? How does the course student assessment contribute to the overall assessment of the student?
- Implement the decisions in practice. This may include delivering a lecture, running a small group, planning and delivering a community-based education element, collaborating with others in the IPE and preparing the assessment elements for the course.

It is important that you have a broad understanding of the curriculum in your school or institution. Teachers often do not appreciate and make false assumptions about the course outside the components for which they have a particular responsibility. A better curriculum and student experience in your school is not necessarily the result if you simply improve the course for which you are responsible; you do not make a better curriculum just by improving your own course. It helps, but what you need to do is to contribute to making the curriculum better overall. You should not wait until a problem emerges. Debra Klamen, an educator deeply involved in medical education at Southern Illinois Medical School in the USA, urged all teachers to engage in improving the curriculum: her message was, "if it ain't broke, make it better" (Cianciolo et al., 2017).

What is the vision or mission of the medical school?

You should have an understanding of the needs that your school aims to meet:

- Is an aim of your school to train doctors who will choose to work as family physicians in the community?
- Is the aim to produce the next generation of academics and researchers?
- Does your school aim to broaden access to medical studies and to admit to the medical course students from a diverse background who may not have the academic ratings you would normally expect?
- Does your school have an international vision?

Answers to these questions should determine your school's approach to the education programme offered. The school's vision will influence the students admitted, the teaching staff appointed and the education experiences offered to the students.

Almost all schools have set out a vision and a set of values for the school. Such vision and mission statements frequently relate to both teaching and research and often highlight aspirations to excellence in these areas. The statement may describe the qualities of the graduates produced, the characteristics of the staff appointed to the school and the impact of the school on the delivery of health care. Values described

Table 5.2 Extracts from two medical schools' mission statements

Monash University

The Faculty is committed to maintaining Monash University as a leading international medical research university, recognised for the breadth and depth of its research, for its opportunities and commitment to postgraduate training, and as a thriving biotechnology hub.

University of Maryland

The School recognizes that its responsibilities include the disease prevention and health care needs of its West Baltimore community and the state of Maryland. The School will serve as a significant resource for addressing local, state, national and international health and public policy issues.

in mission statements often relate to ethical behaviour, collaboration, communication, inclusiveness, social and local community responsibility, innovation, fiscal responsibility and accountability. Two examples are given in Table 5.2. From their mission, as stated in the extracts, one school appears to place greater emphasis on research, the other on meeting community needs. How does your school's mission statement compare? Is your school's vision reflected in the school's curriculum? We should not overpromise and underdeliver in the mission statement. Couros (2017) has suggested that we should ask three questions about our school's mission statement:

- Who created the mission and vision statement? Staff and students are more likely to work towards the vision or mission statement if they have ownership in its creation.
- Do teachers and students know what it is and identify with it, or is it simply made for public relations purposes?
- Is it available and easily accessed by staff and students and reflected in the education programme?

What are the expected learning outcomes?

In education, there has been a preoccupation with teaching and learning methods:

- How many lectures should be scheduled and should attendance be compulsory?
- Should anatomy teaching require dissection of the body?
- Should face-to-face and online learning be blended?
- What is the role of simulation?

Teaching and learning methods are the means to achieve the educational goals and not the end. What matters are the knowledge, skills and attitudes gained by students as a result of the education programme. Over the past decade, there has been a move from an emphasis in a curriculum on the process (the delivery and teaching and learning methods) to the product (the results and expected learning outcomes and competencies achieved). A consideration of teaching methods, including the adoption of educational strategies such as PBL and the use of new learning technologies, is important. What matters, however, as reflected in the move to Outcome-based Education (OBE), are the learning outcomes that the learner achieves. This move to OBE or competency-based education is not simply an educational fad; it is probably the most important development in education in recent years and has been widely adopted in undergraduate and postgraduate education. The June 2017 issue of *Medical Teacher* had competency-based education as its theme.

During a recent Essential Skills in Medical Education (ESME) course, two students commented with regard to their outcome-based curriculum:

"The curriculum at my medical school was entirely OBE and I actually find it hard to understand what the alternative is! If the outcomes aren't outlined how do I know what is expected of me?"

"I couldn't imagine what the alternative would be if you didn't have outcome-based education …?"

You have an important role to play in implementing an OBE approach. The adoption of OBE requires:

- The learning outcomes for the educational programme are identified, made explicit and communicated to all concerned. The specified learning outcomes represent a statement of what the school values and should reflect the school's vision or mission.
- Decisions about the curriculum made by you and other teachers are in line with the agreed learning outcomes. This includes the content addressed, the teaching and learning methods, the educational strategies and the assessment, as illustrated in Fig. 5.4.
- As a teacher you are responsible for ensuring that the student achieves the learning outcomes. Unfortunately, this element of OBE is often forgotten or ignored.

OBE offers significant advantages and reduces ambiguities as to what is expected of students and should be included in the curriculum. A concern expressed by some teachers, however, is that OBE imposes a rigid structure and removes their freedom and autonomy. Certainly, OBE does give the teacher clear targets to aim for but this is no bad thing given that the responsibility of the school is to train students who will have the necessary abilities to practise as health professionals and be responsible for the care of patients. As described in Box 5.3 by John Cookson, an educator who played a major role in the development of a new medical school, a range of stakeholders should be involved.

The learning outcomes may be specified by a national regulatory body, such as the General Medical Council in the UK. The twelve outcome domains in The Scottish

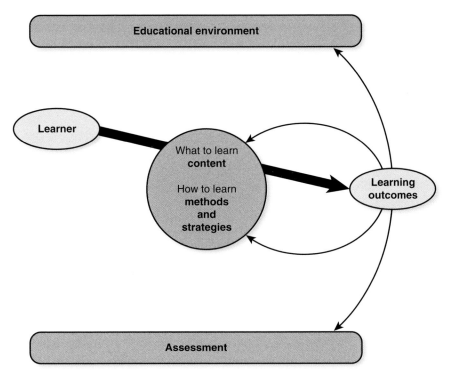

Figure 5.4 In outcome-based education, it is the learning outcomes that dictate the content of the teaching, the teaching and learning methods, the educational strategies and the assessment

Doctor outcome specification were agreed to by all five Scottish medical schools (Simpson et al., 2002). However, it was left to the individual schools and the teachers in the schools to specify in more detail the outcomes in each domain.

In addition to a statement of the overall expected learning outcomes for the course, learning outcomes should be specified for each lecture, clinical teaching session or other learning opportunity offered in the curriculum. The learning outcomes should be considered both in terms of how the teaching session contributes to a mastery of the subject or field of knowledge (e.g. anatomy, clinical medicine) and also how it contributes to the student's progress to achieving the school's agreed final exit learning outcomes. A cardiovascular system course, for example, typically addresses the normal and abnormal structure and function of the cardiovascular system and the assessment and management of patients with a cardiovascular problem. It can also address more generic learning outcomes relating to health promotion and disease prevention and competencies such as communication skills, teamwork, self-assessment and priority-setting. Ethical issues can also be addressed – for example, with regard to a patient with hypertension, should the general practitioner reveal to an insurance company that the patient has a raised blood pressure or has had a myocardial

---

Box 5.3 Ensuring minimum standards[a]

Medical schools are in universities but not wholly of them. Medical schools bring advantages to universities; they usually attract many of the brightest students and mature schools have large income streams. Nevertheless, their undergraduate medical courses have distinct differences. They must ensure that graduates have reached minimum standards, so they are likely to spend considerable effort in addressing the lower end of the ability range, not the top.

There are many stakeholders so 'ownership' of the course is not with individual academics or even departments but is shared with employers and regulators situated outside the university. Academics are uncomfortable with a process where the learning outcomes, learning framework and assessments have been taken away from them.

The greater proportion of undergraduate courses take place outside the university in the health services. The university thus has responsibility but not control. Health services are not designed for education, and their staff members, expert though they are, are not necessarily able to convey to others why they do what they do. Successful curriculum delivery depends on recognising these forces. It is sometimes not clear that either universities or health services do so.

---

[a]*John Cookson, Emeritus Professor, Hull York Medical School, UK, and Tutor for AMEE-ESME Online courses.*

---

infarction? The holistic management of the patient can be highlighted, not "the patient with chest pain" but an individual who may have significant financial and other problems that affect his medical condition. This broader perspective is important, as argued by Callahan (1998):

> *The most glaring deficiency of the 'diagnose and treat' model, as with the biomedical research paradigm on which it rests, is that when simplistically interpreted it fragments the patient as a person into a collection of organ and bodily systems. Sometimes such fragmentation does not matter, as with emergency surgery, but often it fails to capture the full psychological and spiritual dimensions of a patient's illness. Too frequently it alienates patients from physicians, who can seem only concerned about patients as the bearers of pathologies to be eliminated. A rich and strong doctor–patient relationship, historically at the core of medicine, remains a basic and enduring need. (p. 44)*

As a teacher, you should have both a narrowly focussed view from your specialist professional perspective and also a wide-angle lens perspective of the overall expected exit learner outcomes, including those relating to the behavioural sciences. There is increasing recognition of the importance of generic competencies as an outcome of the education programme. These include the 4Cs:

- Communication skills
- Collaboration skills

- *Critical thinking skills*
- *Creativity skills*

Different terms have been used to describe these learning outcomes not specifically related to the mastery of content or a particular skill – generic skills, non-cognitive skills, 21st century skills or soft skills. The Asia-Pacific Education Research Institute Network used the term *transversal competencies* and described six domains (Table 5.3; Care and Luo, 2016):

- Critical and innovative thinking
- Interpersonal skills
- Intrapersonal skills
- Global citizenship
- Media and information literacy
- Physical health and religious health

You almost certainly feel more comfortable addressing your subject's specific learning outcomes rather than tackling these broader learning outcomes. This is likely to require an approach to the curriculum that involves collaboration with a range of specialties and healthcare professions.

Table 5.3 The Asia-Pacific Education Research Institute Network's framework on transversal competencies

Domains	Examples of key skills, competencies, values and attitudes
Critical and innovative thinking	Creativity, entrepreneurship, resourcefulness, application skills, reflective thinking, reasoned decision making
Interpersonal skills	Communication skills, organizational skills, teamwork, collaboration, sociability, collegiality, empathy, compassion
Intrapersonal skills	Self-discipline, ability to learn independently, flexibility and adaptability, self-awareness, perseverance, self-motivation, compassion, integrity, self-respect
Global citizenship	Awareness, tolerance, openness, responsibility, respect for diversity, ethical understanding, intercultural understanding, ability to resolve conflicts, democratic participation, conflict resolution, respect for the environment, national identity, sense of belonging
Media and information literacy	Ability to obtain and analyse information through information and communications technology (ICT), ability to evaluate information and media content critically, ethical use of ICT
Other (physical health, religious values)	Appreciation of healthy lifestyle, respect for religious values

Adapted from Care, E., Luo, R., 2016. Assessment of Transversal Competencies. United Nations Educational, Scientific and Cultural Organization, Paris.

To implement an outcome-based curriculum in your school, it is necessary to:

- Establish and agree to the expected learning outcomes.
- Prepare a grid or blueprint that matches the agreed learning outcomes with the phases of the curriculum, the courses in the curriculum and the learning opportunities. This may be represented on a curriculum map, as described later. As Spady (1988) has suggested: "Exit outcomes are a critical factor, in designing the curriculum. You develop the curriculum from the outcomes you want students to demonstrate, rather than writing objectives for the curriculum you already have."
- Relate the learning outcomes to entrustable professional activities (EPAs) where these have been identified. EPAs are units of professional practice that can be entrusted to a sufficiently competent learner or professional (ten Cate et al., 2015).
- Prepare a grid or blueprint that relates the outcomes to the assessment procedures, such as the outcomes assessed in a multiple-choice question examination or in the stations in an objective structured clinical examination (OSCE).
- Review your own course in terms of the exit learning outcomes and the capabilities expected of the students. You have a responsibility to ensure that students can achieve the expected outcomes through the learning opportunities provided.

The rewards of adopting an outcome-based approach are high. However, the adoption of an outcome-based approach by you as a teacher is not a trivial matter and may require you to change the content of your course and how you present it. "Outcome-based does not mean curriculum-based with outcomes sprinkled on top. It is a transformational way of doing business in education" (Spady, 1993).

Consideration should be given in OBE to a move to time-variable training, in which what is fixed in the education programme are standards and what is variable is the time taken by the learner to achieve them. This is perhaps the most difficult element of OBE to deliver. It is certainly true in respect of the whole course but may be easier to implement for parts of it, such as the time scheduled in the clinical skills centre.

What content should be included?

A major challenge you face as a teacher is the problem of information overload. Knowledge in the biomedical sciences has expanded exponentially, as we discussed in Chapter 3, doubling every 18 months. You need to be highly selective as to what it is you expect your students to learn. They cannot remotely learn everything there is to know about your subject. Moreover, new knowledge will continue to become available during their studies and after they leave medical school. As a teacher, you need to identify the core or essential knowledge required by the students for which they should be expected to demonstrate mastery. In an assessment of core knowledge, it would not be unreasonable to set 90% or more as a pass mark (more generally, in a written assessment, the pass mark is usually about 60%). This is discussed further in the chapter on the teacher as an assessor. The core information may include threshold concepts, as described in Chapter 3.

Subjects and topics identified by respondents in the European Union–funded MEDINE project that should be addressed in the medical curriculum are given in Table 5.4. Many of these do not feature in a traditional curriculum.

Table 5.4 Subjects and topics to be addressed in the medical curriculum for the 21st century[a]

Professionalism

Communication skills

Critical thinking

Evidence evaluation

Research skills

Drug prescribing

Patient safety

Teamwork

Health promotion

IT skills

Complementary and alternative medicine (CAM)

Teaching skills

Lifelong learning

Global citizenship

[a]As identified by respondents in the EU MEDINE2 initiative.

The content addressed in the curriculum should match the expected learning outcomes. Approaches to specifying content include (Dunn et al., 1985; Harden and Laidlaw, 2017):

- A wise men approach – a consideration of opinion among the stakeholders in the area.
- A job analysis – an analysis of the tasks facing a doctor and of the knowledge and skills necessary to carry out the tasks.
- A study of recommendations from governing, accrediting and assessment bodies as to what should be included in a curriculum.
- Recommendations from specialist bodies in medical practice – for example, for behavioural sciences by the behavioural science network.
- An analysis of the performance of recent graduates in practice and where deficiencies are identified.

- A study of the knowledge of star performers in clinical medicine whose practice is seen as exemplary.
- Studies of errors in practice and consideration of the implications for the curriculum.
- A study of existing curricula and publications.
- Critical incident studies of good and bad practice.

How should the content be organised?

The stage in the curriculum at which subjects are addressed and the sequence in which they are considered is important. In the traditional curriculum, there was a divide between the "preclinical teaching" in the early years that addressed the "basic medical sciences" and the "clinical teaching" in the later years that addressed "clinical medicine". The introduction of students to clinical medicine early in the curriculum has now been widely adopted, with the integration of basic science and clinical medicine. This offers major advantages and motivates students to study (Dornan et al., 2006). Less attention has been paid to the integration of basic science with clinical medicine in the later years, and this deserves consideration.

If you are a clinical teacher, consider how, with your colleagues responsible for teaching in the early years, you might introduce students to clinical medicine and clinical skills early in the curriculum and determine how you can help them develop appropriate attitudes and their identity as a doctor. If you are a basic science teacher, consider how you might work with clinical teachers in the early years relating clinical medicine to the basic sciences and how you might continue to interest students in the basic sciences, as applied to medicine in the later years.

The spiral curriculum

Rather than considering the course as a series of discrete parts which students master independently, you will find it helpful to think of what has been described as a spiral curriculum, where students visit a theme or topic on a number of occasions, adding new learning at each visit and relating this to previous learning (Harden and Stamper, 1999). You have a responsibility as a teacher to guide students as they progress through the different phases of the curriculum or loops in the spiral, highlighting what they should have learned already and how they will now build on and add to this.

For example, students may study the cardiovascular system:

- In the early years, where there is an emphasis on normal structure, function and behaviour, perhaps taught in the context of clinical cases and with the development of basic clinical skills, such as measurement of the blood pressure and auscultation of the chest.
- In later years, where there is emphasis on abnormal structure, function and behaviour as they relate to the cardiovascular system and on the further development of relevant clinical skills.

- During clinical clerkships, where students apply what they have learned in practice while at the same time refining their existing knowledge and skills and extending these to develop their competencies relating to clinical reasoning, priority-setting, teamwork and patient safety.

A key feature of a revised Dundee curriculum was its spiral nature, as described in Box 5.4. Managing patients with a cardiovascular problem in an informed manner developed as the student progressed through the course.

Box 5.4 A successful spiral curriculum

The spiral Dundee curriculum was successfully introduced at the medical school in Dundee (Davis and Harden, 2003). Factors in the success of the model included:

- Clinicians and basic scientists were represented on both the phase and the main curriculum committees.
- The organisation of the curriculum and the time allocated to topics was the responsibility of the curriculum committees and was not a departmental responsibility.
- Opportunities were provided for students to undertake clinical, basic science or more integrated electives at all stages of the curriculum.
- A portfolio was adopted as a learning and assessment tool that required the student to demonstrate an integration of basic sciences and clinical medicine in the later years.
- Basic scientists served as examiners in the later and early stages of the curriculum, including as examiners for the final portfolio assessment, which played a major role in the decision as to whether a student should graduate (Davis et al., 2001), in the Objective Structured Clinical Examinations (OSCEs) and in the progress test (Hunter et al., 2002).
- A set of learning outcomes was clearly defined and applied to each element and phase of the course (Simpson et al., 2002). In this way, the clinical teachers were aware of what knowledge and skills the students should have at each phase in the spiral.
- Students had hospital- and community-based clinical experience from day 1 of the course.

Unlike in a traditional curriculum, where students' knowledge of the basic sciences frequently declines in the later years, the students' responses in the progress test showed that this was not the case with the spiral curriculum.

You may find it helpful to think of the progression in the student's learning during the spiral curriculum in four dimensions (Harden, 2007):

1. Increased breadth, with extension to more topics and to different practice contexts, such as paediatrics or care in the community
2. Increased difficulty, with more advanced or complicated or complex aspects of the subject. An example relating to communication skills is breaking bad news.

3. Application to practice, with a move from managing a patient in a teaching setting to managing a patient in the real world, where there are competing demands and pressures
4. Increased accomplishment, with more efficient performance and less need for supervision

How does your course contribute to this progression?

Transitions between different phases in the curriculum should be as seamless as possible. Additional support may be necessary when students are given greater clinical responsibility and following graduation, when they start work as a trainee doctor.

What educational strategies should be adopted?

As a stakeholder in the curriculum, you should consider the educational strategies adopted both at the level of the institution and for individual courses, including your own course. It may be left to you as a teacher, in some measure, to decide the education approach you adopt for the teaching for which you are responsible. You should be clear about the amount of freedom you have with regard to your own course and also take up opportunities to influence the school's policy with regard to the educational strategies that are adopted in the curriculum.

The SPICES model described in 1984 (Harden et al., 1984) and recently updated (Harden and Laidlaw, 2017) provides a framework around which you can assess the educational strategies for the curriculum on six dimensions, as represented in Fig. 5.5.

Student-centred	Teacher-centred
Problem-based/presentation-based	Information-based
Integrated	Discipline-based
Community-based	Hospital-based
Electives	Uniform programme
Systematic	Apprenticeship-based/opportunistic

Figure 5.5 The SPICES model

Student-centred and teacher-centred approaches

In a student-centred approach, what matters is what the student learns, rather than what you teach as a teacher. At the student-centred end of the continuum, teaching is seen as facilitating the students' learning. At the teacher-centred end, it is a way of teaching in which the emphasis is on students as the passive recipients of information transmitted from the teacher to the student.

A student-centred approach requires a different mind-set. You should not assume, for example, that all students will require the same amount of time to master the different elements in the education programme. It has been suggested that 10,000 hours of practice are required to master a skill, whether this is playing chess or playing a musical instrument. In reality, however, some people will require more than 10,000 hours and others will require less. Students are likely to need different amounts of time scheduled in the simulation laboratory to master the technical skill being taught, with some students requiring longer than others to acquire the necessary level of proficiency.

In most schools, the duration of the overall education programme is fixed, although this may change. The fast learner, however, can have additional electives or student-selected component sessions with which they can be credited. When this concept was introduced in the curriculum in Dundee, however, the Scottish Higher Education Funding Council and the General Medical Council both expressed concern that a weaker student would not have the same opportunities for options as the more able student; they invited "the school to consider ways of ensuring that students who fail to perform well on the core elements of the course have the same opportunities to undertake SSCs (student selected components) as their more successful peers." The school stuck to its principle that curriculum time at present is finite, and how students can best make use of this time may vary from student to student. The priority for the school was to enable all students to achieve the core required standard in all outcome domains and to undertake some student-selected components while allowing the better student to complete additional student-selected components (Davis and Harden, 2003).

There is no consensus view about the extent to which students should be allowed to select the learning approach best suited to their individual needs. Should students be compelled or even expected to attend a lecture, or might they choose an alternative approach to studying the topics covered in the lecture? This may include engaging with a recording of the lecture or online learning resources. It has been argued that a student who is struggling may be the one who does not attend the lecture but who would most benefit from the discipline of attending. A compromise may be to have attendance required at some key lectures while leaving students free to choose whether they attend the other lectures or not. There is, however, the obligation in this case to provide alternatives to the lecture.

In medicine, each patient is managed according to his or her particular needs. The same should be true in education, with each student having a personalised or adaptive learning programme. Of the practical suggestions in this text, this is likely to be the most difficult to implement, particularly if you are responsible for large numbers of students. You should not be discouraged – progress can be made.

Presentation-based and information-based approaches

In the original description of the SPICES model, the P represented *p*roblem-based. Many schools have adopted PBL, some only recently for the first time. In PBL, the learning is focussed around a problem, frequently a clinical problem, to be addressed by students, usually but not always working in small groups. Different approaches to PBL have been reported (Taylor and Miflin, 2010). A continuum between PBL and a more conventional information-based approach has been described (Harden and Davis, 1998).

Some schools have moved away from a PBL approach as a basis for their curriculum. We have been impressed with a presentation-based approach to a curriculum and, in the SPICES model, have replaced problem-based with presentation-based. This presentation model is highlighted in the Calgary clinical presentation curriculum (Mandin et al., 1995) and the Dundee task-based curriculum (Harden et al., 1998, 2000). It offers many advantages as part of a move to a more authentic curriculum targeted at equipping the student with capabilities necessary to practise medicine. In a clinical presentation, task-based approach to the curriculum, clinical presentations are identified that reflect how a patient commonly presents to the physician. Medical schools that adopt the approach usually generate about 90 to 150 clinical presentations as a focus for the curriculum. The Dundee curriculum is based on 104 presentations, as described in Table 5.5, and the Calgary curriculum had 120 clinical presentations.

Student learning relating to each presentation becomes more advanced as the student progresses through the curriculum. In the presentation of abdominal pain, for example, the student's attention is focussed in the early years on issues such as the relevant anatomy and physiology of the abdomen, on the understanding of the mechanism of pain and on abdominal pathologies, and in the later years on decision making and the different approaches to the investigation and management of a patient with abdominal pain.

Rubrics or blueprints are produced that identify how a study of each presentation contributes to the learning outcomes and how the presentation is addressed in the range of learning experiences in which the students engage. A clinical presentation or task-based approach in medical education has attracted less attention than it merits, given its potential as an educationally sound, effective and efficient strategy for delivering a medical curriculum. A presentation-based approach offers a number of significant advantages that are likely to be relevant in your teaching programme:

- It provides an organisational and conceptual framework for planning and delivering the curriculum.
- It serves as a scaffold for students to which they can add new information.
- It motivates students by relating theory to practice and helps them understand the relevance of what they are learning.

Table 5.5 Clinical presentations that provide a framework for the curriculum in task-based learning

Problem	Clinical presentations	Problem	Clinical presentations
Pain	Pain in the leg on walking	Paralysis and impaired mobility	Loss of power on one side
	Acute abdominal pain		Tremor
	Loin pain and dysuria		Peripheral neuropathy
	Joint pain		Muscle weakness
	Back and neck pain		Immobility
	Indigestion		Falling over
	Headache	Lumps, bumps and swelling	Lump in the neck
	Cancer pain		Lump in groin
	Earache		Lump in breast
Bleeding and bruising	Bruising easily		Swollen scrotum
	Pallor		Joint swelling
	Haemoptysis		Swollen ankles
	Vomiting blood		Skin lump
	Rectal bleeding	Nutrition, weight	Thirsty and losing weight
	Blood in urine		Difficulty swallowing
	Anaemia		Weight loss
	Postoperative bleeding		Seriously overweight
Fever and infection	Chest infection	Change in body function	Wheezing
	Rash and fever		Pleural effusion
	Urethral discharge		Shortness of breath
	Pyrexia of unknown origin		Cough
	Immunisation		Change in bowel habit
	Sweating		Cannot pass urine
	Hypothermia		Incontinence
	Sepsis		Raised blood pressure
Altered consciousness	Immobility		Palpitations
	Falls		
	Collapse		
	Confusion		
	Dizziness		
	Fits		

Continued on next page

Table 5.5 Clinical presentations that provide a framework for the curriculum in task-based learning—cont'd

Problem	Clinical presentations	Problem	Clinical presentations
Skin problems	Skin rash		Bereavement
	Itching		Alcohol dependence
	Psoriasis		Schizophrenia
	Mole growing bigger, bleeding		Tiredness
			Depression
	Blistering		Adolescence
	Photosensitivity	Reproductive problems	Premenstrual syndrome
	Bedsore		Infertility
	Jaundice		Normal pregnancy
	Burn		Menstrual problems
	Wound		Contraception
Life-threatening, accident and emergency	Shock		Sterilisation
	Involvement in accident		Smear results
	Fracture		Painful intercourse
Eyes	Loss of vision	The child	Child abuse
	Painful red eyes		Down syndrome
	Squinting in child		Prematurity
	Foreign body in child		Poor feeding
Ear, nose and throat	Ringing in ear		Failure to thrive
	Going deaf		Respiratory distress syndrome
	Earache		Developmental delay
	Sore throat		Sudden infant death syndrome, near-miss
	Hoarseness		
	Stuffy nose	Priority-setting, decision-making and audit	Dying patient
Behaviour	Anger		Population screening
	Anxiety		Waiting lists
	Phobias		Triage
	Drug addiction		Acute vs chronic
	Suicide		
	Sleep problems		

Adapted from Harden, R.M., Crosby, J.R., Davis, M.H., Howie, P.W., Struthers, A.D., 2000. Task-based learning: The answer to integration and problem-based learning in the clinical years. Med. Educ. 34 (5), 391–397.

- It supports integrated teaching and learning in the early and later years of the course.
- It introduces the student to clinical practice and helps establish their personal identity as a doctor.
- It provides a basis or framework for lifelong learning.
- It facilitates knowledge retrieval by the practising doctor because the situation where the knowledge is learned more closely resembles the context in which it is applied.

The task-based approach has been described by Phil Race as "a very useful approach to integration of the medical curriculum and, not least, a time-efficient and cost-effective approach to developing highly relevant skills, attributes and competencies for the profession" (Race, 2000).

If you are a basic science teacher, using a task-based approach, you can demonstrate how the knowledge and skills related to your discipline help students understand and manage the range of problems presented in practice, such as abdominal pain or breathlessness. If you are a teacher in the later years, perhaps responsible for a clinical clerkship, a task-based approach is also useful. You can show how the students' experience with you contributes to their capabilities relating to the tasks specified.

Even if your school has not formally adopted a presentation- or task-based approach, you can select from the presentations described in Table 5.5 and use these to highlight the relevance of your teaching.

Integrated and interprofessional education

In the metaphor of the house, the building does not work if each room is separate and is not connected and integrated with other elements in the house. In the same way, the curriculum is not effective if each course operates in isolation from other elements of the programme. An integrated approach to planning a curriculum is now fairly standard, both bringing together subjects normally taught in the same phase of the education programme, such as anatomy and physiology or medicine and surgery (horizontal integration), and the clinical and basic science disciplines (vertical integration). When participants in an ESME course are asked to indicate what for them is the most important educational strategy described in the SPICES model, integration is frequently selected.

Interest is also being shown increasingly in integrating not just the disciplines within medicine but in integrating the different healthcare professions. Students from different professions such as medicine, dentistry, nursing and pharmacy may learn together for part of the course. The argument for interprofessional education (IPE) is that if doctors are to function effectively and practise as a member of a team, they should learn the necessary team skills as a student and gain an understanding and appreciation of the different professions and their role in the delivery of health care. A Best Evidence Medical Education (BEME) systematic review identified the benefits of introducing an interprofessional element to the curriculum (Reeves et al., 2016):

Learners respond well to IPE, their attitudes and perceptions of one another improve, and they report increases in collaborative knowledge and skills. There is more limited, but growing, evidence related to changes in behaviour, organizational practice, and benefits to patients/clients. (p. 656)

Regardless of whether integrated or IPE is the policy in your school, you can adopt elements of the approaches in your programme and move up the interprofessional ladder, as illustrated in Fig. 5.6, from isolation to at least a recognition of other disciplines and professions. This interprofessional ladder is a modification of the curriculum integration ladder previously described (Harden, 2000; Harden and Laidlaw, 2017).

Community-based and hospital-based approaches

An authentic curriculum is designed to equip the student with the knowledge, attitudes and competences required to practise medicine (Harden, 2016). The students' experience should not be restricted to the hospital context but should include the community. This is now standard practice in many medical schools, but the proportion of time in hospital and in the community varies in different schools. The experience in the community should not be seen as an optional extra or as the icing on the cake; it is an essential part of the curriculum. The hospital and the community experiences will each contribute in different ways to the expected learning outcomes. The community-based experience can highlight, among other things, the need for health promotion, the provision of the early manifestations of disease, the indications for referral and how to cope with uncertainty. Experience in the community early in the education programme is valuable and helps the student to develop their identity as a doctor (Dornan et al., 2006). If community-based experience is not a feature of the curriculum in your institution, with some imagination, you can incorporate elements of a community experience in your own teaching.

Students in a recent ESME course highlighted, from their personal perspectives, the advantages of community-based teaching early in the medical course:

"It helps students prepare for real-world practice."

"It is motivating."

"Students can understand better the relevance of what they are learning."

"We learn about people we will care for."

"It is more practical and realistic."

"An expanded base of teachers is provided."

"Students learn better if they have a context."

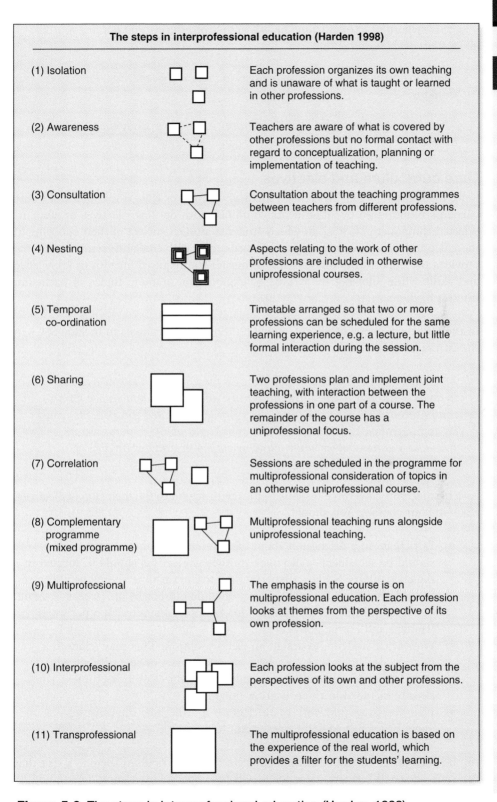

Figure 5.6 The steps in interprofessional education (Harden, 1998)

"It is important to understand health in the community and not just in a tertiary level hospital."

"Early exposure to clinical aspects helps to build a concept map of thinking."

"The more students learn in the community, the more likely they are to choose to work in the community as a career choice."

Core curriculum and electives

Since highlighted by the UK General Medical Council in 1993, the concept of a core curriculum addressed by all students combined with options, electives or student-selected components (SSCs), in which students study a subject of their choosing in more depth, has been widely adopted. A curriculum with core and optional elements provides the opportunity for students to master the required breadth of knowledge and skills while allowing them time to explore one or more topics of particular interest to them.

In the UK, the General Medical Council (2009) requires schools to include SSCs in the curriculum:

> *The curriculum will include opportunities for students to exercise choice in areas of interest ... the curriculum must allow for student choice for a minimum of 10% of course time. SSCs (student-selected components) must be an integral part of the curriculum, enabling students to demonstrate mandatory competences while allowing choice in studying an area of particular interest to them. (p. 47–50)*

As a teacher, you have three responsibilities with regard to the inclusion of electives/ SSCs in your courses. You should:

- Participate in a discussion about what proportion of the curriculum should be scheduled as electives and where electives should be located in the curriculum. No less than 10% of curriculum time should be allocated. Consider whether SSCs should be scheduled in blocks of 2 weeks or more or embedded in the curriculum – for example, one afternoon per week (Harden and Davis, 2001).
- Work with students to design an elective option. This may relate to a more in-depth study of an aspect of your subject or specialty already included in the curriculum or a study of a subject or area of interest not already included in the education programme.
- Plan how students' work in an elective and the how the learning outcomes achieved will be assessed.

As the need arises to add additional subjects to the curriculum there is a risk that the time allocated for options or SSCs will be eroded. This temptation should be resisted. Any proposal to make an addition to the curriculum should be accompanied by a suggestion about what should be removed to make the necessary space available.

Systematic and opportunistic approaches

Of the different education approaches described in the SPICES model, the move from an opportunistic to a systematic approach is almost certainly the most important. There is undoubted value, particularly in the clinical context, in taking advantage of unforeseen training opportunities as they arise. However, there is also the need for a more systematic planning of students' experiences in line with the expected learning outcomes. It is no longer acceptable to define the clinical training in terms of periods of time in a series of clerkships on the assumption that by so doing, students will receive all the necessary clinical education. If you are a clinical teacher, you should specify how each clerkship contributes to the student's training and the expected learning outcomes, including the types of patient seen and the clinical and practical procedures mastered. The same applies if you are a teacher in the early years of the course. It is no longer acceptable for you to base your teaching on aspects of the subject that are of particular interest to you. How a lecture or other learning situation contributes to the expected learning outcomes for the curriculum should be specified.

The adoption of OBE, as described earlier in this chapter, is key to a systematic approach to the curriculum. Integrated teaching and a presentation or task-based curriculum also make a contribution to a more systematic approach, where the whole is greater than the sum of the parts.

A curriculum map is a valuable tool that supports a systematic approach to the curriculum.

Curriculum map

We are all familiar with geographical maps. A map of the UK, for example, shows possible destinations and the location of the different cities and towns, with their relationship to one another. It also shows the roads and railway access links. In the same way, a curriculum map shows the courses, the learning outcomes, the curriculum content, learning experiences and their relationships. It can be examined from any of these windows or perspectives. For example, where in the curriculum do students learn about diabetes, drug addiction, care of the dying or professionalism and ethics, and where are these assessed? Each node on the map provides direct links to available learning resources, learning opportunities, including lectures and practical sessions, and assessment.

More attention should have been paid in the past to curriculum mapping. However, this is now being remedied, and schools are adopting a range of approaches to visualising their curriculum in this way. Is your teaching represented on a curriculum map in your school? If your school does not already have a map of the curriculum, you should consider initiating one. You can get ideas from the many examples available online.

Curriculum mapping is described in more detail in the frequently cited AMEE Guide on the subject, *A Guide to Curriculum mapping: A tool for transparent and authentic teaching and learning* (Harden, 2001).

What teaching methods should be used?

There is likely to be an agreed-on policy in your school with regard to the teaching methods adopted and the blend of:

- Large group, whole-class sessions in the form of lectures or flipped classes
- Small group work as part of problem-based or team-based learning
- Learning in practical laboratories or simulation and clinical skills centres
- Learning in the clinical context in hospital, ambulatory care or community
- Independent learning, with students using a range of learning resources.

If you are responsible for organising the teaching programme, you may be able to influence the blend of different approaches used:

- What reliance should be placed on lectures and should there be a move to the flipped classroom, as described below?,
- How much time should be allocated for independent learning?
- To what extent should students be provided with a menu of different methods from which they can choose (e.g. attendance at a lecture, listening to a recording of a lecture or using alternative learning resources)?
- How can students best be supported in their learning during the course? Different options are described in Chapter 4.
- To what extent should students be given the opportunity to assess their own competence as they work through the course?
- Should peer or near-peer learning be adopted, where students learn from each other in planned sessions?
- How can new technologies such as simulation be used most effectively?
- Should team-based learning be used?

The optimum blend of teaching and learning methods to be adopted will depend on the aims of the curriculum and the expected learning outcomes, the education philosophy of the school and the teachers and resources available. In your own teaching, you may have a measure of freedom as to your use of the different approaches.

The lecture

The lecture has dominated many education programmes. It has been estimated that the average student might have attended as many as 1,800 lectures by the end of the undergraduate course. As described in Chapters 3 and 4, we have seen a move from an emphasis on the teacher as an information provider to the teacher as a facilitator. The use of the lecture has been criticised as a passive and relatively ineffective learning experience, with the assertion that with the wide availability of other learning resources, better options now exist. The continued use of the lecture in education has even been equated to the use of blood-letting in medical practice. To some extent, there is merit in these criticisms of the lecture, which are not new. In 1932, the Final Report of the Commission on Medical Education in New York noted that "there has been much criticism against the excessive use of lectures, particularly those which attempt to supply facts and information which can be better secured through reading and other means."

However, despite these criticisms, most medical schools still feature the lecture as a key instrument in their education programme. Used properly and not excessively, the lecture can be a useful aid to learning. To hear a good lecturer brilliantly summarise a subject, explain a difficult concept and share his or her passion for the subject with the student is of undoubted value. The problem, as Brown and Manogue (2001) have suggested, is misuse of the lecture, "What students disliked was *not* lectures but poor quality lecturing."

New technologies, such as simulators, audience response systems and presentation aids such as PowerPoint, can help you make your lecture more interactive and the content more relevant. When used badly, however, PowerPoint can be a disaster, with the text difficult to read and the amount of information presented impossible to assimilate in the time that the frame is on the screen.

If you have to give a lecture, here is a checklist for you to consider:

- What learning outcomes are addressed in my lecture?
- How does my lecture integrate with other elements of the course that the students have already covered and that they will cover in the following parts of the course?
- Have I allowed enough time to prepare for a lecture? This could be 4 hours or more. For an international presentation at a conference, I (RMH) might spend as much as 30 hours on preparation time.
- Have you planned the different stages of your lecture? These include:
  - The introduction to capture the students' attention and highlight why the lecture is important (Box 5.5)
  - A summary of what you will cover
  - The content covered
  - A summary of the key messages
  - A final suggestion about something, perhaps controversial relating to the subject, for students to think about
- Is the content you address clearly relevant to medical practice?
- Have you made the lecture an active rather than passive experience for the student, with the opportunity to think during your lecture about what you are covering?

Box 5.5 Gaining the attention of your audience[a]

The first few minutes of a lecture are most important and I try to capture the attendees' attention. This was a particular challenge for one presentation I had to make many years ago at an international meeting on the subject of change in medical education. The audience included many conservative senior professors and the lecture was scheduled after a heavy lunch with alcohol served. How was I to interest and engage them in my presentation? During the lunch break, I attached two strings to the ceiling, hanging down onto the stage. At the start of the lecture, I asked one professor to join me on the stage and to try to catch one string in his left hand and the other string in his right. This he found impossible as the second string was just outside his reach. I asked the audience whether it was possible to grasp the two strings at the same time. The answer was a clear 'no'. I then produced a bunch of keys which I attached to one string and started it swinging. I then asked the professor to try again to grasp the two strings and on this occasion he was able to do so, catching the second string as it swung toward him. The message was that what had seemed impossible was possible with a minor adjustment. The same, I argued, could be true of changes in medical education.

Other less dramatic but still attention-grabbing openers can be provocative headlines from a newspaper on the subject of the lecture, a short one-minute recorded interview or a short piece of music with a relevant message.

[a]*Ronald M. Harden, General Secretary, AMEE, Professor of Medical Education (Emeritus), University of Dundee, Dundee, UK.*

- Have you timed your lecture so that it can be completed comfortably in the time available, leaving a few minutes at the end for questions and comments?
- Have you provided advice as to sources of information on the topic that the student can use as a revision tool or to study the topic in more depth at an advanced level?
- Will you have your lecture recorded and made available to the students?
- How will you evaluate the students' response to the lecture?

The good lecturer is not simply a teacher who is an expert in the area and has understood the mechanics of delivering a lecture, including, for example, providing a structure, pacing the lecture and using appropriate audio-visual aids. The good lecturer has considered and understood the different roles that he or she can play in relation to the lecture. These may include:

- Address core information on the subject (information provider).
- Facilitate learning by clarifying common misunderstandings, identifying the expected learning outcomes and providing a scheme on which the student can build her or his further learning (facilitator).
- Encourage students during the lecture to discuss with their colleagues and to respond to issues raised (facilitator).

- Give the students an opportunity to assess their understanding of the subject through the use of questions (assessor).
- Put the lecture in the context of the curriculum by reviewing how the topic fits and integrates into the curriculum (curriculum planner).
- Communicate your enthusiasm for the subject and its importance to medical practice (role model).
- Ensure that the arrangements for the lecture are appropriate in terms of time, location and resources (manager).
- Evaluate the lecture (scholar and professional).
- Keep yourself up to date not only with the subject of the lecture but also with the techniques of lecturing and new approaches, such as methods of engaging the students (professional).

More information on lecture techniques and preparing for and delivering a lecture is widely available. See, for example, reports by Harden and Laidlaw (2017), Jeffries et al. (2017) and Brown and Manogue (2001).

The flipped classroom has been introduced as an alternative to the traditional lecture; this approach is described in Chapter 3.

Small group work

Small group activities can take many different forms, and the way in which students engage in group work will vary. The approaches can be placed on the continuum from student-centred to teacher-centred, and your role as a teacher will vary accordingly. At the teacher-centred end of the spectrum, the small group session consists of a seminar or tutorial or bedside teaching, with the teacher in the role of the information provider. There is likely, however, to be more student interaction than is found in a lecture situation. At the student-centred end of the spectrum, the teacher's role is one of facilitating the group. The group may even be student-led. Facilitating a small group is one of the most skilled tasks you can undertake as a teacher. You need to guide the work of the group and encourage the learners to interact. At the same time, you must guard against dominating the group.

Your role in relation to the small group can fall into one or more of the following categories:

- Chairperson – eliciting information and opinions from the group and managing the group process
- Consultant – providing information or specialist knowledge in an area
- Devil's advocate – confronting and challenging the group
- Counsellor – releasing tensions in the group when members feel threatened or some students dominate or do not participate in the discussions
- Assessor – assessing the students' performance

There has been much discussion, particularly in the context of PBL, as to whether the group facilitator should be a content expert or a person who has the facilitating skills but not necessarily the content expertise. In most situations, content expertise is seen as a valuable asset for the teacher. This is particularly so in bedside teaching, where the teacher serves as a role model. Content expertise on its own, however, is insufficient, and skills in group facilitation are essential.

Clinical teaching

The role of the clinical teacher is challenging:

- Consideration for the patient is paramount, and teaching students in the clinical context requires the permission of the patient. The well-being of the patient must be taken into account.
- Students will have different levels of prior experience and expertise. For some, this may be an early experience, and others may be on the point of graduating as a doctor. The approach to be adopted will vary accordingly.
- Tensions may exist between the time you have available for teaching and the time spent on clinical care of patients.
- Providing a holistic view of the patient's care may require collaboration with other healthcare professionals.

The clinical teacher requires:

- Expertise in the area of medical practice
- An understanding of how he or she can facilitate student learning
- Awareness of the local curriculum and expected learning outcomes
- An understanding of the students' progress and stage in the curriculum

The required knowledge and teaching skills are too often taken for granted, and it is assumed that if doctors are good practitioners, they are also good teachers. Unfortunately, this is often not so, and deficiencies and poor practice in clinical teaching are found. Problems most commonly identified include a lack of planning, inappropriate student supervision, lack of feedback to the learner and failure to appreciate basic educational principles about how students can learn most effectively and efficiently.

As well as in the hospital, in ambulatory care and in the community, clinical teaching can also be provided in a clinical skills centre, where students and trainees can develop and perfect their clinical skills with simulated patients or simulators. In the early years of the course, students can be introduced to communication skills using simulated patients, and the use of simulated task trainers allows them to practise procedures such as venesection or cardiopulmonary resuscitation. Simulators can also be used to demonstrate principles of physiology and clinical relevance using, for example, the Harvey cardiac simulator. A simulated experience may involve the use of:

- Simulated patients
- Simulators, both high fidelity and low fidelity
- Computer-based scenarios and virtual patients

Simulations should be used to complement, not replace, clinical experiences with patients.

Independent learning

Students now have greater access to learning resources, and your role as a teacher may be very different from the role of the teacher when you were a student. There is a switch in emphasis from the teacher as an information provider to the teacher as a facilitator of the student's learning. The role of facilitator is a more demanding one and requires an appreciation of the needs of the learners and the potential problems that students may encounter when working on their own. With the wider availability of learning resource material online, as well as in print, your responsibility as a teacher is to provide the student with the key to open the door to the rapidly expanding amount of information available. As we describe in Chapter 3, you act as an information coach rather than as an information conduit or transmitter. Students may need to be given guidance on how to access and evaluate sources of information online and on the use of tools such as Wikipedia, YouTube and Google (Friedman et al., 2016). As a teacher, you are responsible for:

- Creating a supportive learning environment for students that encourages independent learning, self-confidence, curiosity and the desire to continue to learn. Independent learning will be fostered by a climate that is flexible and responsive to the learner's needs.
- Briefing students on the role of independent learning in the curriculum and, if students are relatively inexperienced, providing counselling and advice on the skills.
- Working with students to help them develop their own learning plan.
- Communicating the core learning outcomes that it is expected students will address in their learning.
- Assisting students to identify appropriate learning resources and providing advice on how they can best be used.
- Advising and assisting students to monitor their progress and assess their mastery of the subject.
- Responding to problems that may arise and being available, perhaps at a specified time and place, to advise students.

Digital technologies are now omnipresent in medical education and, as a teacher, you need to be proficient in selecting and using the technologies (Ellaway, 2017). They can feature in a curriculum to different extents. Ten levels of digital application of e-learning in the teaching programme are noted in Table 5.6. The widespread use of digital media has blurred the boundaries between professional and personal lives.

Table 5.6 Ten Levels of incorporating digital applications into an education programme

Level	Description
0	Students do not use computers in formal or informal learning
1	E-learning is not part of the formal education programme but students use the Internet
2	A virtual learning environment is used to communicate, such as timetables or handouts
3	E-learning resources are identified and used to supplement existing teaching but this is not part of the formal timetable
4	E-learning resources are used with a specific intent distinct from the main existing teaching programme (e.g. for remedial students or self-assessment)
5	E-resources are used to fill gaps in the teaching programme where these exist
6	E-learning is incorporated into aspects of the teaching programme (e.g. problem-based learning groups)
7	E-learning replaces and serves as a substitute for some teaching (e.g. one or more lectures)
8	E-learning is used to introduce new dimensions or activities (e.g. collaborative learning)
9	Fully blended learning is introduced across the curriculum, combining e-learning with traditional approaches
10	E-learning replaces the face-to-face teaching

Students should be prepared for practice in a digital world and know how to acquire the necessary digital professionalism (Ellaway et al., 2015).

A blended curriculum

There is a growing trend for a blended learning environment, where the best of e-learning is combined with the best of face-to-face instruction (Khogali et al., 2011). We are seeing a convergence between the two learning environments, and this is an important trend in higher education today. Your challenge as a teacher or trainer is to plan a curriculum that embraces both approaches. A good example is the flipped classroom, where the teacher has to identify or create resource materials for the student to study before their participation in the whole-class session. There the teacher encourages the students' engagement with the topic and facilitates their learning through problem-solving exercises, discussions or a consideration of areas of difficulty.

Planning a blended approach may mean reconceptualising the role of lectures and placing a greater emphasis on independent learning. It gives you, as a teacher, the opportunity to provide students with learning experiences that might not otherwise be accessible to them and to offer a more student-centred approach to learning. The curriculum can provide more personalised adaptive learning geared to students' individual needs. Opportunities can also be scheduled for collaborative learning, with students working together locally and internationally.

Development of e-learning resources

The development of resources that combine pedagogy and technology appropriately is not an easy task. It requires a range of specialised skills that few teachers possess; a team approach is usually necessary, involving a content expert, an instructional designer, an educationist and a technologist. Most teachers will not wish or have the time to engage in the development of an e-learning programme from scratch. Resources can be created, however, in the form of podcasts or recorded lectures. Although this approach has limitations and may not incorporate the best educational strategies, in practice, it has been found to serve a useful purpose. Another option is for teachers to use material that has already been developed and, if copyright permits, incorporate all or part of it into their own teaching programme. This was described in Chapter 4.

Repositories such as YouTube, MedEdPORTAL (www.mededportal.org) and MedEdWorld (www.mededworld.org) offer a variety of content including video clips, images and self-assessment exercises. Value can be added if the material is annotated by the teacher and put in the perspective of the local context. Information about recommended resources, with the annotations, can be incorporated into a student's study guide.

If you are more ambitious, and with the author's permission, published material can be used as a starting point to build your own resources. A number of authoring systems are available that can help teachers who lack the necessary technical expertise create their own e-learning programme.

You may work with colleagues in the development and delivery of a massive open online course (MOOC). MOOCs are open access courses often based in higher education institutions and they have already attracted thousands of learners. They usually include a series of short videos, recommended reading and discussion forums, alongside automated assessment. In a Medical Teacher Twelve Tips feature, Pickering and colleagues (2017) have provided practice advice on developing and delivering a MOOC.

Integrating assessment and the curriculum

Having determined what it is expected that your students will learn (the learning outcomes), and having decided the most appropriate educational strategies and teaching methods to achieve this, it is essential that you give the same consideration to determining how you and your students will assess that they have achieved these outcomes.

In *Essential Skills for a Medical Teacher* (Harden and Laidlaw, 2017), we considered the six questions that as a teacher or examiner you should ask with regard to assessment. As a teacher, you should address these questions, regardless of your level of responsibility for assessment:

- **What** should be assessed? The assessment should clearly match the learning outcomes (Shumway and Harden, 2003).
- **How** should the student be assessed? The method should be fair, give consistent results (reliable), measure what you seek to measure (valid), be feasible and have a positive impact on the students and on the curriculum.
- **Why** are you assessing the student? The assessment can inform you whether the students have reached the learning outcomes expected at that stage of their education. Assessment also serves to motivate students and provides them with feedback to facilitate their further learning.
- **Who** should undertake the assessment? Responsibility may be with a national accrediting body or with the individual school. Self-assessment by students should also be encouraged as an important generic competence for lifelong learning. Peer assessment can also make a useful contribution, particularly in the assessment of professionalism and attitudes.
- **When** should assessment be undertaken? This should be both during and at the end of a course. An assessment of the student at the beginning of a course may also be informative for the student and the teacher.
- **Where** should the assessment be undertaken? This can be on the job in the clinical context as well as in the classroom (Norcini and Burch, 2007).

Your role as an assessor is discussed in more detail in Chapter 6.

Communicating information about the curriculum

Information about the curriculum should be readily available to all the stakeholders, including the students, the teachers, the accreditors or regulators and the future employers. This applies to the school's mission, the learning outcomes, the content included and the sequence in which it is covered, the educational strategies, the teaching and learning methods and the assessment. Traditionally, information was made available in the form of a syllabus which listed the courses, the classes, the lectures and the clinical clerkships. Some courses provided additional information about the content covered and recommended a reading list of books.

What is expected of the student and the education programme has now been made more explicit. Contributing to this is a statement of learning outcomes and milestones, what it is expected that the student will have achieved by each stage of the curriculum.

A description of Entrustable Professional Activities (EPAs) can also help illuminate what is expected of the student (ten Cate et al., 2015).

Curriculum map

A curriculum map is a useful communication tool. It provides an overview of the curriculum and shows the relationships between:

- The learning outcome
- The content
- The available learning opportunities and learning resources
- The assessment
- The scheduled courses

The concept of a curriculum map was introduced in chapter 4 and earlier in this chapter. A curriculum map allows you to answer questions such as:

- Where in the curriculum do students learn information handling skills? (The learning outcome node "information handling" is linked to the courses and learning opportunities where the topic is addressed.)
- When do students learn to measure blood pressure? (The practical skill "blood pressure measurement" is linked to the learning opportunities in the curriculum early or later, when the skill is covered.)
- Is the students' understanding of diabetes and their management of patients with the condition formally assessed? ("Diabetes" is linked on the map to the written and clinical assessments, where the students' competence relating to patients with diabetes is assessed.)
- What are the expected learning outcomes in relation to the cardiovascular system course? (The learning outcomes expected of students for the cardiovascular system and for individual lectures and sessions in the clinical skills centre are shown.)

With greater cooperation between curriculum developers, content experts and educational technologists, we will see the production of more sophisticated and illuminating maps of the curriculum on which you can map your own teaching and your students' learning progress.

Fostering an appropriate educational environment or climate

Insufficient thought is often given in a medical school to the educational environment. It is rarely mentioned or referred to when the curriculum is discussed, yet it plays a major part in students' learning and behaviour. There is, however, growing concern about the impact of the educational environment on the learner's performance (Gruppen et al., 2017). In a farming analogy, crops will grow from seeds sown only if the conditions, including the soil and the weather, are supportive. In an inhospitable environment, plants will not thrive. To a measure, the same is true of medical students who will not reach their true potential if the educational environment is not supportive.

The educational environment is affected by all the issues relating to the curriculum that we refer to in this chapter:

- If the mission of the medical school includes a social responsibility for the local community, is this perceived in the school as being encouraged and supported in terms of resources and curriculum activities?
- If the learning outcomes include team skills, does the climate in the school support collaboration or competition between students?
- Does the content covered and what is assessed create an atmosphere in which the emphasis is on the acquisition of facts or the ability to ask the right question and find an answer?
- Does what happens in the early years of the curriculum suggest that what is valued is medical science and research or clinical practice?
- Do staff–student relationships and how the curriculum process is managed encourage a student-friendly climate?

It is the educational environment that demonstrates what is valued in a school. A school that wishes to promote community-based medical practice must create an environment where experiences in the community and general practice are valued and where this is reflected in the learning opportunities provided and in the assessment. A school where student engagement is part of the mission should have an environment in which the student voice is encouraged in curricular committees and in the teaching activities through, for example, peer teaching.

Little attention has been paid to the educational environment in part because, as described by Genn and Harden (1986) and Genn (2001), it is a somewhat nebulous concept and is difficult to measure. You can inspect a curriculum timetable, a teaching method or an examination but you cannot touch the educational environment in the same way (Genn and Harden, 1986):

> Climate could easily be judged as a somewhat vague and ethereal concept. The climate of an educational environment, like the concept itself, is rather intangible, unreal and insubstantial, yet climate, in its effects, is pervasive, substantial and very real and influential. The establishing of this climate is almost certainly the most important single task of the medical teacher. As Stern (1970) rather poetically observed, the climate is indeed like a mist, and you can't stay long in the mist before becoming thoroughly soaked. (p. 112)

Various tools have now been described to measure the educational environment, and this has focused attention on the importance of the environment as part of a curriculum (Roff et al., 1997). As a teacher, you have a responsibility to contribute to and help shape the educational environment. You can influence the educational environment in your school through your input to curriculum planning and through your personal behaviour as a teacher. In one school, I (RMH) visited a lecture that was given before noon each day by a senior, internationally recognised, hospital-based clinician. A community-based attachment was scheduled one afternoon each week. However, its value was reduced by disparaging remarks from the lecturer about community-based practice and the afternoon assignment.

The use of space can also affect the educational environment, and this can have important consequences in the attitudes, behaviours and achievements of students. As a simple example, chairs arranged in a room in rows theatre style do not encourage discussion and contributions compared with when the chairs are arranged in a circle. Nordquist et al. (2016) have explored how the physical environment in a medical school affects how students behave and learn and the need for staff to engage with the use made of the physical space:

> ... technology has widened the range of spaces and places in which learning happens as well as enabling new styles of learning ... the involvement of relevant academic stakeholders who can identify the strategic direction and purpose for the design of the learning environments in relation to the emerging demands of the curriculum. (p. 755)

Your curriculum role as a manager and leader

It will be obvious from the description of the curriculum that its planning and implementation is a complex process. Curriculum developments, including integration, interprofessional education, team-based learning, PBL and OBE all add to the management challenges. The development and implementation of a curriculum is a dynamic process and, as a teacher, you have a managerial and leadership role to play, not only with regard to your own personal teaching responsibilities, but also to the curriculum overall. As we suggest in Chapter 8, you cannot simply delegate the management responsibilities to others.

Approaches to curriculum planning

We have identified in this chapter ten questions that you need to ask and what is expected of you as a curriculum planner in relation to these questions. Curriculum planning can be looked at from different perspectives. All of these elements are important and need to be taken into consideration, but particular attention is sometimes paid to one aspect (Harden, 1986):

- **An architect's approach.** Just as in architecture, work starts in curriculum planning, with a full specification of what is to be produced. The focus for curriculum planning is on a detailed statement about the graduates of the school and the expected learning outcomes.
- **A cookbook approach.** As in a cookbook, recipes comprise lists and the quantities of the ingredients, and a detailed list is made of all the contents

that have to go into the curriculum and how much time is allocated to each.

- **A railway approach.** The railway timetable comprises the routes and times when trains arrive at and depart from different stations. In the railway approach to the curriculum, the emphasis is on the students' timetable and their activities and venues at each hour of the day.
- **A mechanic's approach.** The car mechanic is concerned with the type of engine rather than the direction in which the car has to travel. From this perspective, the focus for the curriculum planning is on the physical facilities, the teaching approaches and the learning opportunities created.
- **A religious approach.** Just as in religion, where there is a principle or system of tenets held with devotion, so those responsible for planning the curriculum hold some value or curriculum strategy, such as PBL, to be of supreme importance.
- **A detective's approach.** Just as the detective has to assess the evidence and diagnose a problem at the scene of a crime, the emphasis in this perspective is on identifying problems in relation to the existing curriculum, with a view to producing a revised version.
- **A bureaucrat's approach.** Here the major concern is with the rules and regulations, sometimes imposed from outside, that govern an institution or school and its curriculum.
- **A magician's approach.** In this approach, a curriculum appears, just like a magician produces a rabbit out of a hat (Fig. 5.7). It is not clear how the curriculum has been derived or who has been responsible for its production.

Although these hopefully represent caricatures of curriculum planning. they occasionally represent what happens in practice. Today, in both undergraduate and postgraduate education, we should be far removed from a magician's approach to curriculum planning and should combine the other approaches, all of which have some merit when considered together.

The teacher as a curriculum developer, expert and master

The teacher as a curriculum developer

The teacher is familiar with the curriculum in the school, including the expected learning outcomes, the courses scheduled, the educational approaches in place and the assessment procedures. Teachers know how their own teaching responsibilities and course relate to the overall curriculum.

An expert curriculum developer

The expert curriculum developer has a more in-depth understanding of different approaches to curriculum planning in medical education and how the curriculum in his or her institution relates to these. They are actively involved in planning and

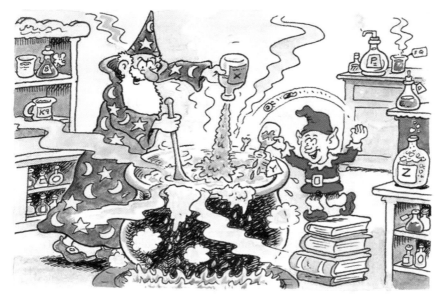

Figure 5.7 The magician's approach to developing a curriculum

implementing the curriculum in their own school and are likely to serve on the curriculum committee.

A master curriculum developer

The master curriculum developer has special expertise and experience in curriculum planning and is likely to have led or taken part in curriculum development in one or more schools. They will be recognised for their work and publications in the area nationally and internationally.

Take-home messages

1. All teachers have an important role to play in relation to curriculum planning in their school.
2. Teachers should have an overview of and be familiar with the school's vision, the expected learning outcomes, the educational strategies adopted, the teaching and learning methods used, the assessment approaches and the educational climate or environment.
3. Teachers will have a more in-depth commitment with regard to the curriculum as it relates to the course or element of the course for which they have a responsibility.
4. In some respects, teachers can be seen as pioneers supporting change in medical education and as the gatekeepers of reform in the curriculum.

Consider

- What is your role in the curriculum in your school?
- Are you familiar with the school's mission statement, with the learning outcomes it is expected the student will achieve, with the educational approaches and teaching methods adopted and with the assessment procedures? How do these relate to your own teaching?
- What sort of educational environment is present in your school? Has this been measured?
- When planning your education programme, think about giving students 1 hour each week to devote to what they want to learn.

Explore further

Brown, G., Manogue, M., 2001. Refreshing lecturing: A guide for lectures. AMEE Medical Education Guide No. 22. Med. Teach. 23, 231–244.

Callahan, D., 1998. Medical education and the goals of medicine. Med. Teach. 20 (2), 85–86.

Care, E., Luo, R., 2016. Assessment of Transversal Competencies. United Nations Educational, Scientific and Cultural Organization, Paris.

Cianciolo, A., Klamen, D., Beason, A., et al., 2017. ASPIRE-ing to Excellence at SIUSOM. https://www.mededpublish.org/manuscripts/983/v1.

Commission on Medical Education, 1932. Final report of the Commission on Medical Education. JAMA 99 (24), 2035–2036.

Couros, G., 2017. Accountability and action toward a shared vision. The principal of change. https://georgecouros.ca/blog/archives/7578.

Davis, M.H., Friedman Ben-David, M., Harden, R.M., et al., 2001. Portfolio assessment in medical students' final examinations. Med. Teach. 23 (4), 357–366.

Davis, M.H., Harden, R.M., 2003. Planning and implementing an undergraduate medical curriculum: The lessons learned. Med. Teach. 25 (6), 596–608.

Dornan, T., Littlewood, S., Margolis, S.A., et al., 2006. How can experience in clinical and community settings contribute to early medical education? A BEME systematic review. BEME Guide No. 6. Med. Teach. 28 (1), 3–18.

Dunn, W.R., Hamilton, D.D., Harden, R.M., 1985. Techniques of identifying competencies needed of doctors. Med. Teach. 7 (1), 15–25.

Ellaway, R.H., 2017. Using digital technologies. In: Dent, J.A., Harden, R.M., Hunt, D. (Eds.), A Practical Guide for Medical Teachers. Elsevier, London, pp. 1521–1561.

Ellaway, R.H., Coral, J., Topps, D., et al., 2015. Exploring digital professionalism. Med. Teach. 37 (9), 844–849.

Friedman, C.P., Donaldson, K.M., Vantsevich, A.V., 2016. Educating medical students in the era of ubiquitous information. Med. Teach. 38 (5), 504–509.

General Medical Council, 1993. Tomorrow's Doctors. GMC, London.

General Medical Council, 2009. Tomorrow's Doctors. GMC, London.

Genn, J.M., 2001. Curriculum, environment, climate, quality and change in medical education—a unifying perspective. AMEE Medical Education Guide No. 23. Med. Teach. 23, 445–454.

Genn, J.M., Harden, R.M., 1986. What is medical education here really like? Suggestions for action research studies of climates of medical education environments. Med. Teach. 8 (2), 111–124.

Gruppen, L.D., Rytting, M.E., Marti, K.C., 2017. The educational environment. In: Dent, J.A., Harden, R.M., Hunt, D. (Eds.), A Practical Guide for Medical Teachers. Elsevier, London, pp. 376–383.

Hafferty, F.W., Castellani, B., 2009. A sociological framing of medicine's modern-day professionalism movement. Med. Educ. 43 (9), 826–868.

Hafferty, F.W., Gaufberg, E.H., 2017. The Hidden Curriculum. In: Dent, J.A., Harden, R.M., Hunt, D. (Eds.), A Practical Guide for Medical Teachers. Elsevier, London, pp. 15–41.

Harden, R.M., 1986. Approaches to curriculum planning. Med. Educ. 20, 458–466.

Harden, R.M., 1998. Effective multiprofessional education: A three-dimensional perspective. Med. Teach. 20 (5), 402–408.

Harden, R.M., 2000. The integration ladder: A tool for curriculum planning and evaluation. Med. Educ. 34, 551–557.

Harden, R.M., 2001. Curriculum mapping: A tool for transparent and authentic teaching and learning. AMEE Guide No. 21. Med. Teach. 23 (2), 123–137.

Harden, R.M., 2007. Learning outcomes as a tool to assess progression. Med. Teach. 29 (7), 678–682.

Harden, R.M., 2016. Curriculum planning in the 21st century. In: Bin Abdulrahman, K.A., Mennin, S., Harden, R.M., et al. (Eds.), Routledge International Handbook of Medical Education. Routledge, London.

Harden, R.M., Crosby, J.R., Davis, M.H., et al., 2000. Task-based learning: The answer to integration and problem-based learning in the clinical years. Med. Educ. 34 (5), 391–397.

Harden, R.M., Davis, M., 2001. Med. Teach. 23 (2), 231–244.

Harden, R.M., Davis, M.H., 1998. The continuum of problem-based learning. Med. Teach. 20 (4), 317–322.

Harden, R.M., Laidlaw, J.M., 2017. Essential Skills for a Medical Teacher, second ed. Elsevier, London.

Harden, R.M., Laidlaw, J.M., Ker, J.S., et al., 1998. Task-Based Learning: An Educational Strategy for Undergraduate, Postgraduate and Continuing Medical Education. AMEE Medical Education Guide No. 7. AMEE, Dundee, Scotland.

Harden, R.M., Sowden, S., Dunn, W.R., 1984. Some educational strategies in curriculum development: The SPICES model. ASME Medical Education Booklet No. 18. Med. Educ. 18, 284–297.

Harden, R.M., Stamper, N., 1999. What is a spiral curriculum? Med. Teach. 21, 141–143.

Hunter, I., Murphy, B., McEwan, J., et al., 2002. Experience with a free-text pilot progress test for undergraduate medical students. Presented at the 10th Annual Ottawa Conference, Ottawa, Ontario, Canada, July 2002.

Jeffries, W.B., Huggett, K.N., Szarek, J.L., 2017. Lectures. In: Dent, J.A., Harden, R.M., Hunt, D. (Eds.), A Practical Guide for Medical Teachers. Elsevier, London, pp. 44–51.

Khogali, S.E.O., Davies, D.A., Donnan, P.T., et al., 2011. Integration of e-learning resources into a medical school curriculum. Med. Teach. 33 (4), 311–318.

Mandin, H., Harasym, P., Eagle, C., et al., 1995. Developing a "clinical presentation" curriculum at the University of Calgary. Acad. Med. 70 (3), 186–193.

Nikendei, C., Ben-David, M.F., Mennin, S., et al., 2016. Medical educators: How they define themselves – results of an international web survey. Med. Teach. 38 (7), 715–723.

Norcini, J., Burch, V., 2007. Workplace-based assessment as an educational tool: AMEE Guide No. 31. Med. Teach. 29 (9), 855–871.

Nordquist, J., Sundberg, K., Laing, A., 2016. Aligning physical learning spaces with the curriculum: AMEE Guide No. 107. Med. Teach. 38 (8), 755–768.

Pickering, J.D., Henningsohn, L., DeRuiter, M.C., et al., 2017. Twelve tips for developing and delivering a massive open online course in medical education. Med. Teach. 39 (7), 691–696.

Race, P., 2000. Task-based learning. Med. Educ. 34, 335–336.

Reeves, S., Fletcher, S., Barr, H., et al., 2016. A BEME systematic review of the effects of interprofessional education: BEME Guide No. 39. Med. Teach. 38 (7), 656–668.

Roff, S., McAleer, S., Harden, R.M., et al., 1997. Development and validation of Dundee Ready Education Environment Measure (DREEM). Med. Teach. 19, 295–299.

Shumway, J.M., Harden, R.M., 2003. The assessment of learning outcomes for the competent and reflective physicians. AMEE Medical Education Guide No. 25. Med. Teach. 25, 569–584.

Simpson, J.G., Furnace, J., Crosby, J., et al., 2002. The Scottish doctor – learning outcomes for the medical undergraduate in Scotland: A foundation for competent and reflective practitioners. Med. Teach. 24 (2), 136–143.

Spady, W.G., 1988. Organising for results: The basis of authentic restructuring and reform. Educ. Lead. October, 4–8.

Spady, W.G., 1993. Outcome-Based Education. ACSA Report No 5. Australian Curriculum Studies Association, Australia.

Stern, G.G., 1970. People in Context. Wiley, New York.

Taylor, D., Miflin, B., 2010. Problem-based learning: Where are we now? AMEE Medical Education Guide No 36. AMEE, Dundee, Scotland.

ten Cate, O., Chen, H.C., Hoff, R.G., et al., 2015. Curriculum development for the workplace using Entrustable Professional Activities (EPAs). AMEE Guide No. 99. Med. Teach. 37 (11), 1–20.

Tong, A.S.Y., Adamson, B., 2008. Curriculum change and the pioneering teacher. Curric. Pers. 28 (1), 45–54.

Toohey, S., 1999. Designing Courses for Higher Education. Open University Press, p. 4.

Chapter 6

The teacher as an assessor and diagnostician

In one way or another, most practising physicians are involved in assessing the competence of trainees, peers, and other health professionals.

Ronald M. Epstein, 2007

Your role as an assessor is one of your most important responsibilities.

- The importance of assessment
- Your role as assessor
- Your assessment responsibilities
- Assessment as a challenge
- A school's *Assessment PROFILE*
- **P**rogramme-focused assessment
- Assessment and the **R**eal world
- **O**utcome-based and competency-based assessment
- *For* learning, with feedback

- **I**mpact of assessment on the student and the curriculum
- **L**earners' engagement with assessment
- **E**valuation of the assessment
- The teacher as an assessor, the expert assessor, the master assessor
- Take-home messages
- Consider
- Explore further

The importance of assessment

As a teacher, you are an assessor and diagnostician (Fig. 6.1).

The assessment of students' achievements and whether they have the competencies and capabilities to pass on to the next phase of the curriculum, to graduate as doctors or to complete their training as specialists, is arguably the most important decision made in the education programme. But assessment is an area where, even among experts, there is often disagreement:

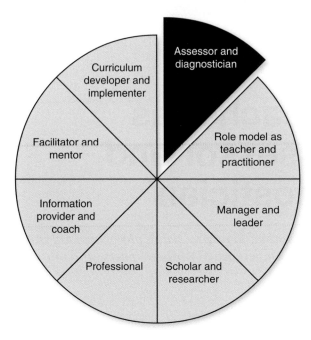

Figure 6.1 The teacher as an assessor and diagnostician

- What is the best standard setting procedure?
- Should we have national examinations or should each school be charged with implementing an assessment process embedded in the school's curriculum with external quality control?
- Should we use multiple-choice questions (MCQs) as a written examination or constructed response questions more related to clinical practice?
- In the objective structured clinical examination (OSCE), should we use global rating scales or checklists, and how do we come to a decision as to a student's overall performance?
- How valid is the situational judgement test?
- What is the role of peer assessment and the patient in assessment decisions?

It could be argued that if the teaching and learning programmes are working well, assessment is less important. However, this cannot be guaranteed, and there is a need to reassure all the stakeholders that the learner has achieved the required competencies. It is also important to provide feedback to students and to you, the teacher, about a student's progress – your role as a diagnostician.

Assessment of the learner is important for the student, for the public, for the school, for accreditation bodies, for researchers and innovators and for you, the teacher:

- From the perspective of the learner, the assessment determines whether he or she progresses to the next phase of the education programme or, at the end of the course, graduates as a doctor or specialist. Are there gaps or deficiencies in her or his mastery of the learning outcomes which need to be corrected?

- The assessment reassures the public that the doctor has the necessary knowledge, skills and attitudes to serve the patients for whom they will be responsible.
- The assessment provides the medical school or postgraduate training programme with an indicator of the quality of the education programme it provides and may suggest areas where improvement is necessary.
- For an accrediting body, the assessment process provides an indication as to whether the programme is reaching the standard expected by the accreditors.
- The assessment results can provide information about a new approach in the curriculum for a researcher or innovator and contribute to a judgement of its value.
- Decisions about the assessment can clarify the goals and desired outcomes of learning.
- Assessment can also be seen as a process that communicates to the student what is valued in the curriculum.

There is a need for a greater level of understanding and assessment literacy in a medical school at all levels, from a teacher to the head of school or programme director, including administrators and those concerned with providing educational support. We discuss in this chapter how an understanding of assessment methodology is important for you as a teacher and your role. However, more than any other role, that of assessor is particularly challenging, and it is likely that many schools will employ a psychometrician to support faculty in this highly complex area.

Your role as assessor

You may have a major role as an assessor in your school, with responsibility for aspects of the assessment process. If your main responsibilities lie elsewhere, you still have an important role to play with regard to assessment. In one way or another, most practising physicians are involved in assessing the competence of trainees, peers and other health professionals (Epstein, 2007). As a teacher, your responsibilities as an assessor are described below:

- Examinations are important for your students. As a teacher, you should be familiar with the school's arrangements with regard to assessment of students – the timing and the format, the areas assessed and the implications for students of their performance in an examination.
- The assessment of the students' mastery of the aspects of the course for which you are responsible provides valuable feedback as to how well you have done your job as a teacher. Do your students achieve the required

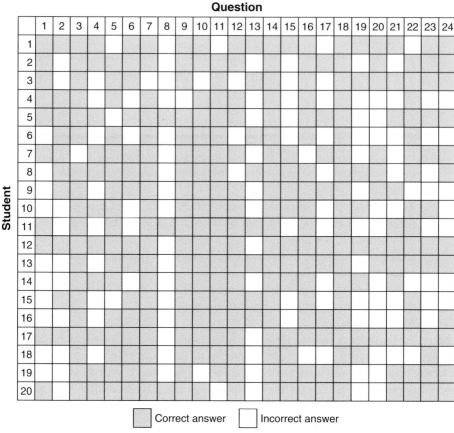

Figure 6.2 Performance of 20 students in 24 questions in an endocrinology multiple-choice question examination

pass mark? Do some students excel? Are some students struggling? The examinations may identify unexpected deficiencies. Fig. 6.2 shows student performance in 24 MCQ questions on endocrinology in an end-of-course examination. What do you conclude, looking at the results? Some students performed better than others, but most students answered most of the questions correctly. The results for question 8, however, stand out. Almost no student got the correct answer. It was not a poorly worded question, and it was on a topic that the students were expected to know. On examining the recording of the relevant lecture and the lecture handout, it was found that the teacher had provided the students with misleading information.

- It is important that the teaching and assessment are aligned. Does your teaching match what is covered in the examination? If not, is there a problem with the examination or with your teaching?
- You should provide learners with feedback about their successes and failures, and guidance should be given about their future studies.

Assessment is not only a measure of the students' achievements to date and their past learning, but should serve also as a guide for their future learning.

- You may be expected to participate as an examiner in the planning and delivery of a written paper assessment, an OSCE, a portfolio assessment or a work-based assessment. You may be asked to serve as an examiner at a station in an OSCE or to mark a written answer.
- As a teacher and a stakeholder in the curriculum. you have a broader responsibility for the assessment process. You can influence the school's approach to assessment indirectly or directly through membership in an assessment or curriculum committee. The school's approach to assessment is discussed below in terms of its "Assessment PROFILE". The issues discussed are of relevance to all teachers in the school, not just to a small group charged with the assessment policies and arrangements.

Your assessment responsibilities

You have important responsibilities as an assessor, as shown in Fig. 6.3. The different steps with regard to assessment in your institution are outlined in Table 6.1. You may be involved in one or more of these steps.

Decisions about the school's or institution's overall approach to assessment, including the scheduling of the assessment (Steps 1 and 2) – As a teacher, you may be a member of an assessment committee, with overall responsibility for the assessment processes in the medical school or postgraduate institution. If you are

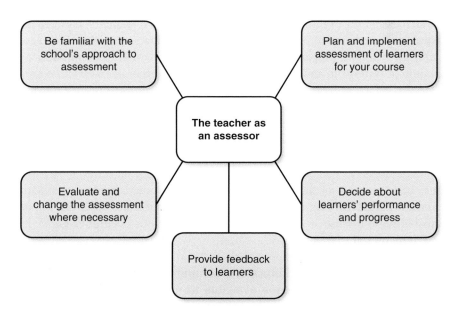

Figure 6.3 The teacher's responsibilities as an assessor

Table 6.1 Ten steps in a school's or institution's assessment programme

1. Decisions are made about the institution's overall approach to assessment in relation to the issues identified in the school's *Assessment PROFILE*.
2. The overall timing and form of examinations, the learning outcomes assessed, the tools to be used and the staff responsible are determined.
3. Individual assessments such as an Objective Structured Clinical Examination (OSCE) or written examination are developed, and the learning outcomes assessed are specified.
4. The students are briefed about the examination, including its form, areas covered and the implications for their progress.
5. The resources for the examination are prepared. This will vary depending on whether it is paper-based, computer-based or clinical.
6. The examination is implemented, and evidence about the students' performance is collected.
7. Based on the evidence obtained from this and other assessments, decisions are made about the individual student as to whether they have reached the standard required.
8. Feedback is provided to students about their performance in the examination.
9. Feedback is also provided to examiners and teachers.
10. The examination process is reviewed.

in this position or wish to have an impact on education decisions in your school, you should have an understanding of the key issues relating to assessment, as described later in this chapter.

Planning and implementing the assessment of students in line with the school's agreed approach to assessment (Steps 3, 4, 5 and 6) – You may be responsible for an element of an examination designed to assess the students' competence in the aspect of the education programme for which you are responsible. For example, this may involve the preparation of questions for a written examination paper, preparation of stations in an OSCE or serving as an examiner in an OSCE. A surgeon may serve as an examiner at a station in an OSCE where the examinee has to take a history from a patient with abdominal pain. At another station, a physician may assess how a student advises a patient on discharge from hospital following a myocardial infarction. As a teacher, you may have overall responsibility as lead or coordinator for an examination. This requires management skills, an understanding of the basic principles of assessment and an understanding of the learning outcomes to be assessed. You may be responsible for the blueprint for the examination that relates the examination to the expected learning outcomes. The lead examiner in an OSCE has important responsibilities and these are discussed in more detail in the *Definitive Guide to the OSCE* (Harden et al., 2016).

Decisions about an individual student's competence or capability in the area assessed, based on the evidence available from this and other assessments (Step 7) – You may be involved in setting the standards or pass mark for an examination. This may require you to work with a member of staff who has experience with different approaches to the standard setting and the necessary statistical proficiency.

In the case of an OSCE, you may be asked to contribute to decisions about the required overall pass mark using the borderline regression or other method. However, psychometrics is just one aspect of standard setting. In decisions about whether a student should pass an examination, you should have a view on issues, such as the extent to which students should be able to compensate for deficiencies in one aspect of their performance with their performance in other areas. In the Dundee final examination, students were required to demonstrate in their portfolios a minimum standard in all twelve learning outcome domains. Poor performance in one domain could not be compensated for by good performance in another domain. In an OSCE, decisions are required about whether it is necessary for students to achieve a minimum standard in each of a specified number of stations or whether a pass mark is set for the examination based on their overall performance. Should there be aspects of competence, such as communication skills, where a minimum level of competence is required?

Provision of feedback to students about their performance and to the teachers about the performance of their students (Steps 8 and 9) – Providing the learner with feedback following an examination is an important responsibility. Lack of attention to the provision of appropriate feedback to students about their performance following an examination is one of the most frequent complaints from students. In Chapter 4, we highlighted the value of feedback in facilitating students' learning and this is discussed further later in the chapter.

Whether or not you are directly involved with an examination, you should receive feedback about the performance of students for whom you have had teaching responsibilities. A poor performance in an examination or an element of it might indicate an area where improvements in your teaching programme are indicated. Poor performance of students in an examination implies a problem with the examination or with the teaching.

An evaluation of the examination (Step 10) as part of quality assurance of the educational programme – Postexamination analysis of examination data can improve the examination cycle, as described by Tavakol and Dennick (2012).

Different levels of expertise in assessment and the assessment tools and in the areas to be assessed are required, depending on the role expected of you.

Assessment as a challenge

Your role as assessor is important but it is also challenging.

Assessment is an area in medical education where there have been many developments. For example, there has been a move from paper-based to computer-based assessment

Changes are taking place in the use of the OSCE with the adoption of technology and the assessment of competencies such as those related to teamwork, interprofessional collaboration, patient safety, and cultural competence (Harden et al., 2016). New

Table 6.2 Some newer features or approaches to assessment

Assessment tool	Description
Computer-based problems, including virtual patients	The decisions taken by the learner managing a patient presented virtually online are assessed.
Direct observation of procedural skills (DOPS)	The DOPS is a variation of the Mini-CEX. The learner is watched and scored carrying out a procedure on a real patient.
Mini-clinical evaluation exercise (Mini-CEX)	In a Mini-CEX, the student is engaged in an authentic, workplace-based patient encounter. The examiner watches and scores the student taking a focused history, performing a relevant physical examination and providing a diagnosis and management plan.
Multiple-mini interview (MMI)	The MMI usually consists of a series of 5–8 minute stations designed to assess whether a student has the attributes for admission to medical school.
Multisource feedback (360 degrees)	Evidence is collected systematically from a number of individuals who are in a legitimate position to make a judgement about the learner's performance.
Portfolios	Evidence is collected by learners about their achievement of the learning outcomes and presented in a portfolio.
Programmatic/ Programme-focused assessment	Decisions are based on multiple data points collected over time, with separation of the assessment moment and decision moment.
Progress testing	Students in all years of school sit the same examination, which samples all the subjects covered in the curriculum.
Script concordance test	In a script concordance test, students are given a brief evolving patient scenario and asked to make judgements regarding diagnostic or management options. The learner is assessed on the amount of agreement or concordance between his or her response and that of a panel of experts.
Situation judgement tests	Situational judgement tests are designed to assess judgement or knowledge of appropriate behaviour in work-related situations. The answers are usually in MCQ format.

approaches have been developed to work-based assessment. Fundamentally different approaches are being adopted about how students are assessed for admission to medical studies. Some newer approaches to assessment in addition to the traditional essay, MCQ or OSCE now in use are given in Table 6.2.

It is not uncommon to find a lack of agreement or differences of opinion among experts on approaches to implementing assessment in practice

This may relate to the use of an assessment tool such as the situation judgement test, the use of constructed response versus MCQs, the need to correct for guessing

Table 6.3 Consensus statements and recommendations for assessment in the healthcare professions

Source	Theme
Amin et al., 2011[a]	Technology-enabled assessment.
Boursicot et al., 2011[a]	Performance assessment.
Hodges et al., 2011[a]	Assessment of professionalism.
Norcini et al., 2011[a]	Criteria for good assessment.
Prideaux et al., 2011[a]	Assessment for selection for the healthcare professions and specialty training.
Schuwirth et al., 2011[a]	Research in assessment.
Rogers et al., 2017	Assessment of interprofessional learning outcomes.

[a]From the Ottawa 2010 Conference.

in a written examination, the merits of checklists versus global rating scales in an OSCE and the advantages and disadvantages of a national licensing examination. These differences have been highlighted at the Ottawa Conferences on the Assessment of Competence in Medicine and the Healthcare Professions, and an attempt has been made to reach consensus in a number of areas in the form of published consensus statements, as set out in Table 6.3.

There are regional and national differences in approaches to assessment

A greater emphasis has been placed on psychometrics in the USA and more on examiner judgement in Europe. Standardised or simulated patients are used in OSCEs in the USA, whereas real patients, along with simulated patients, have an important role to play in other countries.

There may be differences of opinion about the approach to arriving at pass/fail decisions

The setting of standards to inform pass/fail decisions requires a theoretical understanding of the approach to the standard setting adopted and a grasp of statistics. Perhaps the most widely used method for written assessments has been the Angoff approach, with the borderline regression method used in the OSCE (Norcini and McKinley, 2017). However, the choice of the standard setting approach is only one aspect of pass/fail decisions (Harden et al., 2016). Important decisions need to be taken, as described above, on issues such as the extent to which students can compensate for poor performance in one part of an examination with better performance in another part. Rather than a decision made on an aggregate score, there are arguments that students should be expected to achieve a minimum standard in each outcome domain assessed.

In coming to a decision as to whether a learner has achieved a required competence, a challenge relates to whether evidence from different sources over a period of time should be considered, as described below for programmatic assessment

There is debate as to whether the length of the examination should be standard for all students or whether it should be adjusted, with borderline students requiring a longer examination to assess reliably whether they have or have not achieved the standard expected

Such "sequential testing" has been attracting more attention. It allows more assessment effort to be directed to students when this is necessary.

Decisions need to be taken about the student who "fails" the examination, with regard to remedial work required and the support provided

When should students be allowed to sit a repeat examination, and on how many occasions? When should students who fail examinations be encouraged to leave the course, or is there a responsibility to support them in achieving the standard required?

Assessment may involve ethical decisions about issues such as cheating (Bandaranayake, 2011)

Recently, at one school, an OSCE for 270 students had to be repeated and the results for the first examination set aside when it was found that a few students had cheated by providing colleagues with information about stations in the examination.

Traditionally, the teacher is the examiner, and the student is the person who is assessed. The value of peer assessment is now recognised

In many ways, students are in a better position than the teacher to make decisions about outcomes relating to the behaviour and attitudes of their colleagues (Box 6.1).

Box 6.1 The value of peer assessment of attitudes and professionalism[a]

A doctor in the UK was found to have behaved unethically and was convicted in court for the death of a number of his patients. At medical school, he had passed all the required examinations and indeed in some he was in the top 10% of students. I had the opportunity to speak with a colleague who had been in the same year at medical school as the doctor concerned. He said that he was not surprised about the subsequent behaviour of the doctor as while he was a medical student the other students in the class were aware of his inappropriate attitude to his studies, to medicine and to patients. However, this was not assessed in the examinations. Peer assessment might have revealed the problem.

[a]*Ronald M. Harden, General Secretary, AMEE, Professor of Medical Education (Emeritus), University of Dundee, Dundee, UK.*

A school's *Assessment PROFILE*

In this section, we return to the key decisions to be made by a school or postgraduate body with regard to its assessment practice. As we have argued, every teacher should be familiar with where their institution stands on the issues and should have a voice relating to their institution's position.

The SPICES curriculum model (Harden et al., 1984; Harden and Laidlaw, 2017) has been widely used and has proved to be a useful tool in planning and evaluating a curriculum. As described in Chapter 5, it offers six dimensions with regard to a curriculum on which the school and the teacher should have a position. The *Assessment PROFILE* offers a similar tool to describe a school's assessment strategy. Seven dimensions are described, each with a more traditional perspective of assessment as an anchor at one end and a trend or direction in which assessment is moving at the other end of the continuum. The position on each of the dimensions should not be considered as polarised, with schools placed on the extreme left or the extreme right on each dimension. Rather, each of the seven dimensions, as with the SPICES model for the curriculum, represents a continuum. A school's position on each continuum will vary, with the school being perhaps more to the left on some dimensions and more to the right on others. Teachers can reflect where they believe the school currently stands on each dimension on the continuum and where they would like it to be. This can be compared with students' perceptions of the school's position. Assessment is often a fiercely contested terrain. An analysis and discussion of the different perceptions can contribute to the formation of a consensus policy regarding assessment in the institution.

A summary of the seven *Assessment PROFILE* dimensions is given in Table 6.4 and Fig. 6.4, with the end anchor points identified in each dimension.

The trend	Traditional
Programme-focused	Compartmentalised
Real world	Ivory tower
Outcome/competency-based	Content and time-based
For learning (with feedback)	*Of* learning (no feedback)
Impact	No impact
Learner engagement	No learner engagement
Evaluation of assessment	No evaluation

Figure 6.4 The school's *Assessment PROFILE*

THE TEACHER AS AN ASSESSOR AND DIAGNOSTICIAN

Table 6.4 The school's *Assessment PROFILE*

The trend	The traditional
Programme-focused	**Compartmentalised**
Assessment decisions about a learner based on an aggregation and analysis of evidence from different sources over time	The more traditional reductionist approach to assessment
Longitudinal assessment with triangulation of assessment evidence	Assessment fragmented with decisions taken based on isolated events and single examinations at one point in time
Real world	**Ivory tower**
Valid and authentic assessment in the real world of learning outcomes related to the learner's capability to function as a practising health professional	An assessment programme reflecting a curriculum with a theoretical emphasis rather than an emphasis on the knowledge, skills and attitudes necessary for medical practice
Assessment for capability	
Outcome-based or competency-based	**Content and time-based**
Assessment mapped on a blueprint to the expected learning outcomes or competencies. The standard expected of the learner is fixed, and the time required to reach the standard is variable	The time required to complete a course of study is fixed and the standard learners achieve is variable. The emphasis is on assessing content areas
For **learning (with feedback)**	*Of* **learning (no feedback)**
Assessment *for* learning	Assessment *of* learning
Feedback based on the learner's performance provided to guide the learner's further studies	Judgements made on the learner's competence to progress or fitness to practice
Test-enhanced learning	
Impact	**No impact**
Impact of assessment on the learners and on their learning	No impact of assessment on the learner's approach to learning
Impact of results of assessment on teacher and curriculum decisions	No impact of the assessment results on the teacher or curriculum decisions
Assessment-led innovation	
Learner engagement	**No learner engagement**
Learners engaged with planning and decisions relating to the assessment process	Learners not engaged with planning or decisions relating to the assessment process
Learners contribute to examination preparation activities	Learners do not contribute to examination preparation activities
Peer assessment	Self-assessment not encouraged
Assessment of learners' own competence – self-assessment	
Evaluation of the assessment	**Assessment process not evaluated**
Quality control of the assessment process including whether it is fair, acceptable, valid, reliable and has a positive impact on the learner and on the curriculum	No quality control of the assessment process, including whether it is fair, acceptable, valid, and reliable and has an impact on the learner and on the curriculum

Programme-focused assessment

Programme-focused assessment (PFA) is the assessment of student learning specifically designed to address key programme learning outcomes. It switches the emphasis away from the assessment at the individual course or module level. McDowell has asked (2012, p. 1): "Do your students experience their programme as a whole or do they see it as 'ticking off' modules and the marks attained?" McDowell (2012) has described PFA as:

> assessment of student learning specifically designed to address key programme (course of study such as a Bachelor's or Master's degree) learning outcomes ... PFA shifts the balance away from assessment at the module, unit or component level which is where much attention and effort is currently focused. PFA is integrative in nature, assessing the knowledge, understanding and skills that represent key programme aims. (p. 1)

An individual examination or assessment is useful and gives a student and the teacher feedback about the student's progress. However, it is only one data point and has limited utility. Van der Vleuten et al. (2017) have argued that pass/fail decisions should be based on many data points and that evidence from different sources over time should be used to make a final high-stakes decision about a student's competence in an area. They have termed this *programmatic assessment*. Programmatic assessment, or PFA, requires aggregation or combination of the information about the student's competence across assessment methods. Van der Vleuten et al. (2017) have likened assessment data points to the pixels in a photograph. An individual pixel may not tell you much, and many pixels are needed to understand the image. In a traditional approach to assessment, the aggregation occurs across the different elements of a single examination – the different questions in a written examination and the different stations in an OSCE.

In *Twelve Tips for Programmatic Assessment*, van der Vleuten et al. (2015) noted that a feature of programmatic assessment is:

> There is a decoupling of assessment moment and decision moment. Intermediate and high-stakes decisions are based on multiple data points after a meaningful aggregation of information and supported by rigorous organisational procedures to ensure their dependability. (p. 641)

It is more meaningful in the assessment of the learner's performance and also in the provision of feedback to the learner to aggregate only elements relating to the same outcome domain, such as communication skills. In the case of an OSCE, as described by Harden et al. (2016), you can look at a learner's profile across the different domains. In programmatic assessment, the OSCE evidence relating to each domain is combined with other evidence about the student's competence relating to the same domain. Judgement of the student's competence should be based on this broader assessment of the evidence relating to the student's competencies. Decisions about a student's communication skills should not be based on a single

OSCE performance but should take into account evidence from a number of sources, such as portfolios, problem-based learning tutor ratings, multisource feedback from clinical attachments and peer assessment (Fig. 6.5). Van der Vleuten et al. (2015) have suggested:

> *The basic tenet of programmatic assessment is to capitalise on the complementarity of different assessment methods by seeking to achieve their most fruitful constellation, rather than pursuing perfection – in terms of fulfilment of all possible quality criteria – in each of these methods individually. (p. 295)*

The UK General Medical Council (2011, p. 8), in their advice to medical schools on assessment, has recommended that "the consideration of performance in various assessments throughout the course may make it easier to reach sound decisions about individuals' fitness to practise and preparedness."

The principles of programme-focused assessment are compatible with the principle of longitudinal and repetitive assessment as found in the progress test. This can be part of a comprehensive programme of assessment which has an educational impact (Heeneman et al., 2016).

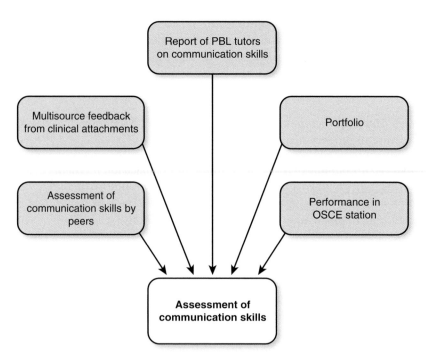

Figure 6.5 Sources of evidence to inform decisions about a student's communication skills

Increasing interest has been shown in the use of portfolios as a powerful assessment tool, capturing the student's achievements over a period of time rather than providing a snapshot at one specific time (Friedman Ben-David et al., 2001; van Tartwijk et al., 2009). These provide a multidimensional view of the student's achievements and offer a valuable tool which can contribute to a programme-focused approach to assessment. The portfolio has been likened to a family photograph album put together over time, with some high-resolution photographs and others of lower resolution but nonetheless contributing to the album.

Implementing programme-focused assessment presents a challenge particularly in a traditional medical school. McDowell (2012) suggested the following:

> Many implementations of PFA do not cover the whole programme at all stages. If the approach to PFA is new to the programme team and new within their department or university, it might be better to start small, with PFA at one level or within a few programme components....Launching a new programme or making major revisions to an established programme may offer a good opportunity to introduce a substantial implementation of PFA. (p. 4)

Assessment and the Real world

Those in medical schools have been accused of working in ivory towers, out of touch with the needs of society and the community they serve (Harden, 2016). As described in Chapter 5, there has been a move to locate the curriculum to a greater extent in the real world, with a recognition of the importance of the relevance of what is taught and learned. This has been reflected in more clinical and basic science integration, in the use of education strategies such as problem-based learning and in a greater use made of clinical experiences in the community. Paralleling these changes in approaches to teaching and learning has been a move to greater relevance and authenticity in assessment. To be maximally effective as an educational tool, any system of assessment should model the realities of practice as closely as possible.

The concept of an authentic assessment has been embraced enthusiastically by the stakeholders and is recognised as a desirable feature of an assessment (Cumming and Maxwell, 1997):

> Of course, it is as difficult to be against authentic assessment as to be against apple pie and motherhood. It is obviously a 'good thing'. The alternative presumably would be inauthentic assessment and nobody would want that. Authentic assessment is clearly 'the way to go.' (p. 2)

"Authenticity is achieved," suggested Eva et al. (2016), "when assessment protocols accurately reflect the domain of practice such that 'studying to the test' or learning to 'game the system' equates with learning to practice well." (p. 905)

Examples where assessment is related to the real world include:

- The use of MCQs, with clinical scenarios as the stem replacing MCQs with a highly theoretical focus
- The use of a portfolio where students demonstrate their achievement of the expected learning outcomes, including the application of the basic sciences, health promotion and ethics, to the patients they document (Friedman Ben-David et al., 2001)
- A greater emphasis on performance assessment with the use of instruments such as the OSCE (Harden et al., 2016). In their article, Wei et al. (2015) defined performance assessment as "tasks that ask students to produce work or demonstrate their knowledge, understandings, and skills in ways that are authentic to the discipline and/or the real world."
- Work-based assessment using instruments such as the mini clinical evaluation exercise (mini-CEX) (Norcini and Burch, 2007)
- The assessment of competencies as they relate to medical practice, including professionalism, team-working skills and patient safety and error management
- The use of assessment relating to whole tasks (van der Vleuten et al., 2015)
- The use, as described below, of outcome- or competency-based assessment

The move in Miller's pyramid from "knows" to "does" (Fig. 6.6) represents a move to greater authenticity, with the learner assessed in more professionally authentic tasks (Miller, 1990). At New Lanark in the UK in the 18th century, the silent monitor

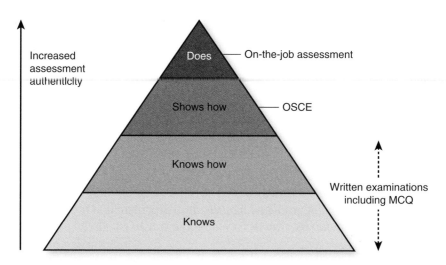

Figure 6.6 Miller's pyramid (1990) and increased assessment authenticity as one moves higher up the pyramid

was an early example of on-the-job assessment. In Robert Owen's textile mills, a small block of wood hung over the employee's workspace, with the front colour indicating the foreman's assessment of the previous day's conduct, from white for good through black for bad (Donnachie and Hewitt, 1993).

This move to more authentic assessment in the real world can be referred to as "assessment for capability." The assessment programme can incorporate different levels of authenticity, and this will change as the student progresses through the curriculum. It is important from the outset, however, to have an element of authenticity; the assessment instrument should in some way reflect the real world of medical practice. Look at the assessment record of three young doctors described in Box 6.2. To whom would you refer your mother as a patient? On the basis of the information provided, many would choose Dr Taylor because portfolio assessment was probably the most authentic and relevant assessment, and the MCQ performance was probably the least authentic.

Outcome-based and competency-based assessment

The move to outcome-based and competency-based education has been a major trend in medical education. It represents a move of emphasis from process and how students learn through methods such as lectures and problem-based learning to product and what students learn (Harden and Laidlaw, 2017). Learning outcomes have been specified using a range of frameworks by bodies such as the Accreditation

---

Box 6.2 To which doctor would you refer your mother?

Margaret Williams as a trainee passed a series of multiple-choice question (MCQ) examination papers covering the basic and clinical medical sciences and the practice of medicine. These included questions on clinical skills, therapeutics and ethics, and legal responsibilities. The questions had been vetted by a panel of senior examiners and an appropriate pass mark had been set along with criteria for "distinction." Margaret was awarded distinction marks in two papers.

Bob McGregor not only achieved a clear overall pass mark in a series of objective structured clinical examinations (OSCEs) but passed in every station in each postgraduate examination. Stations tested among other things – history taking, communication skills, physical examination of the patient, practical procedures, and problem solving.

David Taylor had prepared a portfolio which comprised evidence collected by him that he had achieved the required learning outcomes. This included a record of the patients he had seen, the procedures he had carried out, his competence in these and his analysis of what he had learned. The portfolio also included assessments of his clinical competence by his clinical supervisors against each of the learning outcomes and reports from nurses in the wards where he had been working and from patients he had seen. Four senior doctors who reviewed the portfolio judged that he had achieved all of the learning outcomes and was competent to practise medicine.

Council for Graduate Medical Education (ACGME), the Royal College of Physicians and Surgeons of Canada and the Scottish Medical Schools. They include domains such as communication skills, physical examination, practical procedures and generic competencies such as empathy, culture competence, teamwork skills and information-handling skills, as described in Chapter 3. Doctors need to know how to ask the right questions, where to look for the answers and how to evaluate the answers received. These learning outcomes should be addressed in the design of an assessment.

Tomorrow's Doctors (General Medical Council, 2009), requires that: "All the outcomes for graduates will be assessed at appropriate points during the curriculum, ensuring that only students who meet these outcomes are permitted to graduate." Your responsibility as an assessor in an outcome-based curriculum includes:

Identifying the learning outcomes to be assessed, both in respect of generic competencies relating to the curriculum overall and also relating to the course for which you are responsible

This is discussed in Chapter 5, and Table 5.3 describes some of these generic competencies.

Work with patients and other members of the healthcare team in creating the assessment tool. Patients can help construct stations in an OSCE or provide a valuable input into developing an entrustable professional activity (EPA). El-Haddad and colleagues (2016) in Austria worked with patients in developing an EPA relating to the management of low back pain that aligned best clinical practice with patient expectations.

Selecting a range of instruments to be used in the assessment of the specified learning outcomes

The assessment tools should assess not just the learner's theoretical knowledge but the application of the knowledge to practice and the appropriate skills and attitudes.

Preparing a blueprint relating the assessment to the specified learning outcomes

This should match the learning outcomes to the different assessment instruments used and the different elements within each instrument, such as the stations in an OSCE.

Taking responsibility that learners achieve the expected learning outcomes or competencies

This includes the provision of appropriate feedback and the necessary support, as described below. The commitment of the teacher to the student's success is an often ignored feature of outcome-based education, as described by Spady (1994).

Table 6.5 Key differences between traditional and outcome-based approaches

Approach	Fixed	Variable
Traditional	Time to complete	Standard achieved
Outcome-based, competency-based	Standard achieved	Time to complete

Moving from a time-based approach, where what is fixed is the time of study, with the standards achieved by the students variable, to an outcome-based approach, where what is fixed are the standards achieved and what is variable is the time required by the learner to achieve the standards (Table 6.5)

This is probably the most challenging feature of outcome-based assessment. It can be applied more easily to elements within a course than to a whole course. In the Biochemistry Learning Laboratory in Dundee, students were able to work at their own pace. On completion of a module, they were assessed on their mastery of the module and, if they had achieved the expected learning outcomes, they then moved on to the next module (MacQueen et al., 1976).

For learning, with feedback

There has been a reconceptualisation of assessment from assessment *of* learning to assessment *for* learning (Schuwirth and van der Vleuten, 2011). Traditionally, assessment has been seen as separate from the learning process. Students completed a course of study and were then assessed on their mastery of it. On the basis of this, decisions were taken about whether students should progress to the next phase of their studies or, in the final year, whether they were fit to graduate and practise as a medical practitioner. In assessment *for* learning, assessment is embedded within the learning process and helps guide the student's learning. Students in Dundee rated the OSCE and the feedback provided to them on their performance as one of the most powerful and rich learning experiences.

As a teacher, you have as a major responsibility monitoring your students' progress, identifying areas where required standards have been reached and where there are gaps or deficiencies and providing your students with appropriate feedback. This is why we coupled in this role of assessor your responsibility as a diagnostician. You should help students find the difference between their current status and their desired goals.

As described in Chapter 4, however, how feedback is provided to the learner is critical. Feedback to students with regard to their performance—their strengths and weaknesses—is often done badly or not at all, and lack of appropriate feedback is one of the most common complaints of learners in undergraduate, postgraduate and continuing education. Feedback needs to be timely, specific and related to the expected learning outcome and non-judgemental. Importantly, the learner should be given guidance and support about how they might remedy any difficulties identified. Feedback should be part of a dialogue between the student and the teacher, with the aim of students working to improve their mastery of the learning outcomes.

Assessment can be viewed as part of the learning process. Studies have demonstrated that time spent by students assessing their competence may be more rewarding than simply spending the equivalent time in further study of the subject. This has been termed *test-enhanced learning* (Lafleur and Côté, 2016; Larsen and Butler, 2013). Students, by testing themselves, increase their long-term retention and their understanding of what is being examined.

Assessment of a student's performance during a course, with feedback provided, has been described as formative assessment. The distinction previously made between formative and summative assessments, however, is now less clear-cut. A holistic view on assessment is emerging in which formative and summative assessment strategies are combined (van der Vleuten et al., 2017). Feedback to students about their mastery of the learning outcomes may contribute to a portfolio of evidence about students' progress and achievement of the learning outcomes. A summative end-of-course assessment need not be confined to the decision about the student's progression. It can also identify the student's strengths and weaknesses. The examination should not be seen as marking the end point of the student's learning on completion of a course. No student is perfect. Although achievements should be celebrated and rewarded, any deficiencies should be identified and constructively communicated to the student and to those responsible for the next stage of the learner's education.

Schuwirth and van der Vleuten (2011) have written about assessment *for* learning: "Behind this rather inconspicuous terminology hides nothing short of a revolution in the conceptual framework of assessment." A medical school or postgraduate training body that does not recognise this can be deemed to be irresponsible.

Impact of assessment on the student and the curriculum

The assessment, in terms of its content, format, timing and feedback provided, can have a major impact on the behaviour of students, and it is well recognised that assessment drives learning (Newble, 2016; van der Vleuten, 1996). In Dundee, the inclusion of a station on otolaryngology in the final OSCE had more impact on the student's view of the importance of the subject than other changes made in the curriculum and teaching of the subject. Peter Dieter, a leading expert in medical education in Germany, recognises that assessment drives learning (Box 6.3).

The results of an examination should be taken seriously by the teacher. To some extent, the results provide evidence about the degree of success or failure

Box 6.3 Assessment drives learning – make the most of it[a]

I teach biochemistry in a preclinical curriculum (lectures, 250 students; seminars, 20–24 students; laboratory courses), in which all faculty exams are fact-based, multiple-choice questions and in which the students have to pass a national state exam consisting half of fact-based multiple-choice questions and half of an oral examination. Students are particularly interested in teaching that allows them to pass the exams and helps them to answer the fact-based multiple-choice questions, but are less interested in the understanding of the biochemical processes. To achieve both learning how to answer fact-based multiple-choice questions and also understanding of the biochemical processes, I have made a deal with the students: introduction of interactive PBL lectures and seminars. In lectures I often ask comprehension questions and the first student to give the correct answer is rewarded with Haribo Gold Bears ("Haribo Lectures"). In seminars the students first have to answer five multiple-choice questions (taken from former state exams) and afterwards I discuss the questions and answers with respect to the underlying biochemical principles and clinical context. This initiative gave me the nickname "Professor Haribo".

[a]Peter Dieter, Professor, Carl Gustav Carrus Medical School, Dresden University of Technology, Dresden, Germany.

of the teaching. There are no bad students, only bad teachers. The cause of poor student performance should be analysed; this may be a result of a problem with the teaching and learning programme or may reflect a problem with the examination.

The assessment can also have an impact on the teacher and on curriculum development, which may not be for the good. Teaching to the test is a fact of life. National licensing examinations, although ensuring the maintenance of minimum standards, may also influence a school's approach to curriculum design and implementation and discourage curriculum innovation.

Learners' engagement with assessment

The importance of the students' voice and the engagement of students with the curriculum is now recognised, as discussed in Chapter 4. Student engagement with a curriculum and the medical school is one of the indices of excellence in education in a medical, dental or veterinary school, as assessed in the ASPIRE initiative (www.ASPIRE-to-excellence.org). Students are perceived not simply as customers or clients but as active partners in curriculum decisions and the learning process. This applies also to assessment:

- Students can be members of an assessment committee and share responsibility for the assessment process. They would normally be excluded, however, from decisions relating to an individual student's performance.

- Students can help formulate policy with regard to assessment issues such as honesty, cheating and plagiarism.
- Peer assessment, particularly relating to issues of attitudes and professionalism, can be part of the assessment process (see Box 6.1).
- Students can take responsibility for the development of practice examinations designed to prepare the student for the formal assessment.
- Students can be given some responsibility for assessing their own progress.

Self-assessment may be done badly, with poorer students often overestimating their own performance. The skill of self-assessment is, however, an important one for students to acquire as an essential skill for their continuing education and lifelong learning after graduation from medical school. The importance of self-assessment has been highlighted by Costa and Kallick (1992):

We must constantly remind ourselves that the ultimate purpose of evaluation is to have students become self-evaluating. If students graduate from our schools still dependent upon others to tell them when they are adequate, good or excellent, then we've missed the whole point of what education is about.

Evaluation of the assessment

Because of its importance and the associated complexities, quality control and evaluation of the assessment process are critical. The assessment process should be judged in terms of:

- Validity – is it measuring what should be measured – the specified learning outcomes?
- Reliability – is it reliable, providing consistent results and avoiding examiner and other biases?
- Fairness – is it fair, including how students with disabilities or cultural differences are assessed?
- Acceptability – is it accepted by staff and students as an approach to assessment?
- Feasibility – can it be implemented with the resources available, and are sufficient resources made available?
- Impact – does it have a positive impact on the students, on the curriculum and the teachers?

On the basis of these criteria, it can be decided whether the examination is fit for purpose or what changes are needed in relation to the assessment tools adopted and how they are used. The ASPIRE-to-Excellence initiative (www.ASPIRE-to-Excellence. org) describes best practice in the field of assessment and what represents excellence in a school's assessment programme.

The teacher as an assessor, the expert assessor, the master assessor

The teacher as an assessor

Teachers should be familiar with the assessment programme in the school, including what is assessed, when and how. They should understand some basic principles relating to assessment, as set out in the *Assessment PROFILE*.

An expert assessor

The expert teacher will be actively involved in the assessment programme and will take the lead in one or more initiatives. He or she will have particular responsibility for one or more elements in the assessment programme. Although some general principles apply, expertise in assessment is not a generic capability. The teacher may be an expert in running OSCEs but not in portfolio assessment.

A master assessor

The master assessor will be recognised for his or her experience and expertise in one or more aspects of assessment and is likely to have innovated in the area. He or she will have published and communicated nationally and internationally in the field of assessment.

Take-home messages

1. As a teacher, you have an important role to play in assessment. The extent of your commitment to assessment of students on your own course and in the curriculum as a whole will vary. You should be familiar with the school's assessment process and its impact with regard to the part of the teaching programme for which you are responsible.
2. Assessment is a complex and changing subject. An understanding of the principles and trends, as outlined in the *Assessment PROFILE*, is important when decisions are made about assessment.
3. Decisions about what to include in an examination, the format of the examination and the final decisions about whether the student has reached the standard required to progress or graduate is dependent on your judgement as an examiner. Even the so-called objective MCQ is subjective in terms of what has been chosen to assess, how the question is worded and the standard expected of the student.

Consider

- What is your current role as an assessor?
- What would you like your role as an assessor to be?

- Where do you stand on the seven continua described in the *Assessment PROFILE*?
- In the previous chapter, we suggested that you ask six questions about assessment: What? How? Why? When? By whom? Where? These are discussed in more detail in *Essential Skills for a Medical Teacher* (Harden and Laidlaw, 2017).

Explore further

Amin, Z., Boulet, J.R., Cook, D.A., et al., 2011. Technology-enabled assessment of health professions education: consensus statement and recommendations from the Ottawa 2010 conference. Med. Teach. 33 (5), 364–369.

Bandaranayake, R.C., 2011. The ethics of student assessment. Med. Teach. 33 (6), 435–456.

Boursicot, K., Etheridge, L., Setna, Z., et al., 2011. Performance in assessment: Consensus statement and recommendations from the Ottawa Conference. Med. Teach. 33 (5), 370–383.

Costa, A.L., Kallick, B., 1992. Reassessing assessment. In: Costa, A.L., Bellanca, J.A., Fogarty, R. (Eds.), If Minds Matter: A Foreword to the Future, vol. 2. Hawker Brownlow Education, PA, USA. pp. 275–280.

Cumming, J.J., Maxwell, G.S., 1997. Contextualising authentic assessment. Assess. Educ. Princ. Pol. Pract. 6 (2), 177–194.

Donnachie, I., Hewitt, G., 1993. Historic New Lanark: The Dale and Owen Industrial Community since 1785. Edinburgh University Press, Edinburgh.

El-Haddad, C., Damodaran, A., McNeil, P., 2016. A patient-centered approach to developing entrustable professional activities. Acad. Med. 92 (6), 800–808.

Epstein, R.M., 2007. Assessment in medical education. N. Engl. J. Med. 356 (4), 387–396.

Eva, K.W., Bordage, G., Campbell, C., et al., 2016. Towards a program of assessment for health professionals: From training into practice. Adv. Health Sci. Educ. 21 (4), 897–913.

Friedman Ben-David, M., Davis, M.H., Harden, R.M., et al., 2001. Portfolios as a method of student assessment. AMEE Medical Education Guide No 24. Association for Medical Education in Europe, Dundee, Scotland.

General Medical Council, 2009. Tomorrow's Doctors. General Medical Council, London.

General Medical Council, 2011. Assessment in Undergraduate Medical Education: Advice Supplementary to Tomorrow's Doctors (2009). General Medical Council, London.

Harden, R.M., 2016. Curriculum planning in the 21st century. In: Bin Abdulrahman, K.A., Mennin, S., Harden, R.M., et al. (Eds.), Routledge International Handbook of Medical Education. Routledge, London, pp. 113–127.

Harden, R.M., Laidlaw, J.M., 2017. Essential Skills for a Medical Teacher. Elsevier, London.

Harden, R.M., Lilley, P.M., Patricio, M., 2016. The Definitive Guide to the OSCE. Elsevier, London.

Harden, R.M., Sowden, S., Dunn, W.R., 1984. Some educational strategies in curriculum development: the SPICES model. Med. Educ. 18 (4), 284–297.

Heeneman, S., Schut, S., Donkers, J., et al., 2016. Embedding of the progress test in an assessment program designed according to the principles of programmatic assessment. Med. Teach. 39 (1), 44–52.

Hodges, B.D., Ginsburg, S., Cruess, R., et al., 2011. Assessment of professionalism: Recommendations from the Ottawa 2010 Conference. Med. Teach. 33 (5), 354–563.

Lafleur, A., Côté, L., 2016. Programmes' and students' roles in test-enhanced learning. Med. Educ. 50 (7), 702–708.

Larsen, D.P., Butler, A.C., 2013. Test-enhanced learning. In: Walsh, K. (Ed.), Oxford Textbook of Medical Education. Oxford University Press, Oxford, UK (Chapter 38).

MacQueen, D., Chignall, D.A., Dutton, G.J., et al., 1976. Biochemistry for medical students: A flexible student-oriented approach. Med. Educ. 10 (5), 418–437.

McDowell, L., 2012. Programme-Focused Assessment. Programme Assessment Strategies. University of Bradford, Bradford, UK.

Miller, G.E., 1990. The assessment of clinical skills/competence/performance. Acad. Med. 63 (9), S63–S67.

Newble, D., 2016. Revisiting 'the effect of assessments and examinations on the learning of medical students'. Med. Educ. 50 (5), 498–501.

Norcini, J., Anderson, B., Bollela, V., et al., 2011. Criteria for good assessment: Consensus statement and recommendations from the Ottawa 2010 Conference. Med. Teach. 33 (3), 206–214.

Norcini, J., Burch, V., 2007. Workplace-based assessment as an educational tool: AMEE Guide No. 31. Med. Teach. 29 (9), 855–871.

Norcini, J., McKinley, D.W., 2017. Concepts in assessment including standard setting. In: Dent, J.A., Harden, R.M., Hunt, D. (Eds.), A Practical Guide for Medical Teachers. Elsevier, London, pp. 252–259.

Prideaux, D., Roberts, C., Eva, K., et al., 2011. Assessment for selection for the health care professions and specialty training: Consensus statement and recommendations from the Ottawa 2010 Conference. Med. Teach. 33 (3), 215–223.

Rogers, G.D., Thistlethwaite, J.E., Anderson, E.S., et al., 2017. International consensus statement on the assessment of interprofessional learning outcomes. Med. Teach. 39 (4), 347–359.

Schuwirth, L., Colliver, J., Gruppen, L., et al., 2011. Research in assessment: consensus statement and recommendations from the Ottawa 2010 Conference. Med. Teach. 33 (3), 224–233.

Schuwirth, L.W.T., van der Vleuten, C.P.M., 2011. Programmatic assessment: From assessment of learning to assessment for learning. Med. Teach. 33 (6), 478–485.

Spady, W.G., 1994. Outcome-Based Education: Critical Issues and Answers. American Association of School Administrators, Arlington, VA.

Tavakol, M., Dennick, R., 2012. Post-examination interpretation of objective test data: Monitoring and improving the quality of high-stakes examinations: AMEE Guide No. 66. Med. Teach. 34 (3), e161–e175.

van der Vleuten, C.P.M., 1996. The assessment of professional competence: Developments, research and practical implications. Adv. Health Sci. Educ. 1 (1), 41–67.

van der Vleuten, C.P.M., Heeneman, S., Schuwirth, L.W.T., 2017. Programmatic assessment. In: Dent, J.A., Harden, R.M., Hunt, D. (Eds.), A Practical Guide for Medical Teachers. Elsevier, London, pp. 295–303.

van der Vleuten, C.P.M., Schuwirth, L.W.T., Driessen, E.W., et al., 2015. Twelve tips for programmatic assessment. Med. Teach. 37 (7), 641–646.

van Tartwijk, J., Driessen, E.W., 2009. Portfolios for assessment and learning. AMEE Guide No. 45. Med. Teach. 31 (9), 790–801.

Wei, R.C., Pecheone, R.L., Wilczak, K.L., 2015. Measuring what really matters. Kappan. 97 (1), 8–13.

Chapter 7

The teacher as a role model

As a general rule, teachers teach more by what they are than by what they say.

Unknown

Example isn't another way to teach. It is the only way to teach.

Albert Einstein

More attention should be paid to the impact, both positive and negative, of the teacher as a role model.

What is a role model?

In earlier chapters, we looked at your actions and at what you do as a teacher. You inform students through lectures and other means, as described in Chapter 3. You facilitate their learning through small group work and the provision of learning resources and opportunities, as described in Chapter 4. You plan and deliver a curriculum, as described in Chapter 5, and you assess whether students have achieved the expected learning outcomes, as described in Chapter 6. In contrast, as a role model, you are identified less by what you do as a teacher and more by who you are and your personal behaviour in the classroom and clinical contexts. Despite its importance, of the eight roles of the teacher described in this book, the teacher as a role model has attracted least attention. Indeed, you may not have thought much about your importance as a role model for your students (Fig. 7.1). As noted by Subha Ramani, a general physician and medical education specialist, and by Liz Mossop, head of teaching and learning at a veterinary school, teachers may not be consciously aware of this role and its potential impact on students (Boxes 7.1 and 7.2). There is a lack of understanding of the complex phenomenon of role modelling (Passi et al., 2013).

Although it was only in the second half of the 20th century that the term *role model* came into the vocabulary, the concept was rooted in tradition. The first Native American physician, Charles Alexander Eastman (1991), described the role model in the education of a Native American child: "We watched the men of our people and acted like them in our play, then learned to emulate them in our lives." (p. 20)

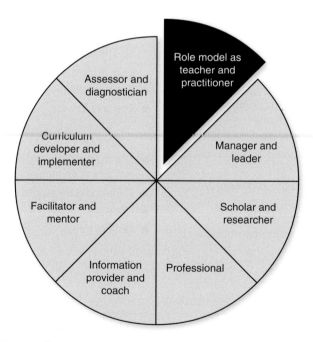

Figure 7.1 The teacher as a role model

Box 7.1 My role as a role model[a]

Role modelling is an intrinsic aspect of my role as a clinical teacher, more often implicit than explicit. As I mature as a professional educator, I increasingly believe that clinical teachers should be consciously aware of this role and its potential impact on learners' career choices; practise good clinical habits always, and debrief with learners about the "softer" side of medicine. Learners rate qualities such as enthusiasm and humanism higher than medical expertise as indicative of excellent clinical teachers. Thus, it is important for institutions to engage in faculty development initiatives that discuss this vital educational strategy, that of role modelling.

[a]Subha Ramani, Director of Education Innovations and Scholarship, Internal Medicine Residency Program, Brigham and Women's Hospital, Assistant Professor of Medicine, Harvard Medical School, Boston, Massachusetts, USA.

Box 7.2 The importance of role modelling[a]

During my transition from practitioner to clinical teacher there was one element that I was very unaware of and did not appreciate until much later – that of being a role model. Whilst my responsibilities as a clinician were of crucial importance to the health and well-being of my patients and clients, suddenly as an educator I became aware of a new responsibility to my students. My influence as part of the hidden curriculum of my institution on the professional identity formation of our students was something of a threshold competency in my development as a teacher – once I'd worked this out, my teaching skills improved immensely. In veterinary education, a key element of this is our role modelling of attitudes towards animal welfare, a constant struggle in veterinary professionalism when there are clients, society and the business side of practice to consider. I try to be openly reflective about these challenges with my students and encourage them to actively consider the behaviours they see around them and reject inappropriate role models. Role modelling is now almost the first thing I discuss with new teachers in our faculty, and hopefully their development is a little easier because of this.

[a]Liz Mossop, Professor of Veterinary Education, School of Veterinary Medicine and Science, University of Nottingham, UK.

Prior to the 21st century, the education model in medicine was one of an apprenticeship. The doctor to whom the learner was attached was the role model for the learner and demonstrated the practice of medicine through work as a physician, with the student learning from his or her actions and thought processes. The aim of the learners was to mirror the teachers in their own behaviour. Tim Dornan (2005) argued that an apprenticeship in medicine is as powerful a learning model today as it was a century ago, and that although the goals of education must be defined rather than be left to chance, "tacit knowledge and attitudes must be given due recognition and allowed to pass from teacher to learner by role modelling." In this chapter, we explore the teacher as a model for the student in a 21st century curriculum.

But, what is a role model? There are a variety of definitions from which to choose:

- The *Oxford English Dictionary* defines a role model as "a person looked to by others as an example to be imitated" (http://www.askoxford.com).
- Dake and Taylor (1994) have defined role modelling as "teaching by example and learning by imitation."
- Bandura (1977) has described role modelling as "a process that allows students to learn new behaviours without the trial and error of doing things for themselves."
- A role model, according to *Stedman's Medical Dictionary*, is "a person who serves as a model in a particular behavioural or social role for another person to emulate."
- Role models, suggested Paice et al. (2002), are people we can identify with who have the qualities we would like to have and are in a position we would like to reach.

Which definition do you prefer? All have their own message, but we prefer Dake and Taylor's definition, because it highlights role modelling from the perspective of the teacher and the student.

The importance of the teacher as a role model

The importance of the teacher as a role model is well documented. Role modelling affects what students learn and is an integral and important component of medical education (Wright et al., 1998; Paice et al., 2002). A systematic review of the literature by Passi et al. (2013), based on 39 published studies, highlighted role modelling as an important process for the professional development of learners. Dan Tosteson (1979), Dean of Harvard Medical School, has highlighted the importance of the teacher as a role model:

We must acknowledge…that the most important, indeed, the only, thing we have to offer our students is ourselves. Everything else they can read in a book…Relations with other persons drive our feelings and thus our actions.

David Irby (1986) has also emphasised the importance of the teacher as a role model:

Faculty members demonstrate clinical skills, model and articulate expert thought processes, and manifest positive professional characteristics. Through this modelling process student knowledge, skills and attitudes can be changed profoundly. (p. 40)

In the UK, the General Medical Council (2002) has recommended:

Every doctor who comes into contact with medical students should recognise the importance of role models in developing appropriate attitudes and behaviour towards patients and colleagues. (p. A13)

Very much to the point were comments by two emergency medicine physicians, Hazan and Haber (2017), when they highlighted the importance of the role model:

> *It may be overwhelming to you, the teacher, to realize that everything you say is being ingrained in some young student-doctor's brain, that what you say and do will forever affect the way the person in front of you practices medicine, and beyond that, will in some way influence the lives of thousands of patients and their family members. We should not shy away from this responsibility. We need to acknowledge that our words and actions have influence beyond the four walls of the emergency department, and we must take this responsibility seriously…Wouldn't you rather be remembered for the rest of a medical student's or resident's career as the person who showed empathy, respect, love, and consideration rather than the one who was jaded, disrespectful, and unkind toward someone who sought your help in the ED? (p. 2–3)*

Attention to the perceived deficiencies in graduates, such as poor communication skills, lack of empathy and other characteristics of the good practitioner, have been the focus for many changes in medical education. These reforms, however, have not usually featured the roles and responsibilities of the teacher and doctor as a role model, despite the fact that these elements are best acquired by role modelling, where repeated negative learning experiences may adversely affect the development of professionalism in medical students and residents.

Six reasons why role models are important

Your responsibilities as a role model are important for a number of reasons. We describe six of these, as shown in Fig. 7.2.

Career choice

As a teacher, you can have a significant impact on your students' choice of career, both positive and negative (Campos-Outcalt et al., 1995). Brock and Harper (2016) have noted:

> *As final year students, we are often asked about potential career choices and many of us have excluded specialties based on experiences we have had during our clinical attachments. (p. 960)*

Exposure to role models in a particular clinical field was found by Wright et al. (1997) to be strongly associated with medical students' choice of clinical field for residency training. The role model has a significant effect on a student's self-confidence in pursuing a career in a certain area. A lack of surgical role models is one reason why more female students do not choose this specialty. Heidi Chumley, an experienced clinical teacher, sees her role as a woman as being helpful to students (Box 7.3).

The impact of doctor role modelling was examined by Passi and Johnson (2016b) using interviews with consultants and focus groups with medical students. The

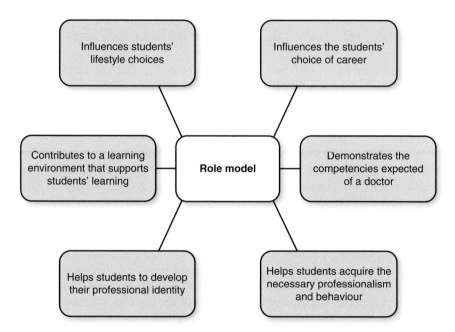

Figure 7.2 Six reasons why the role model is important

Box 7.3 My role as a woman[a]

Being a role model is particularly fulfilling. As students' professional identity formation accelerates in the clinical years, they look around for people like them. Seeing people like them who are successful gives them confidence that they can be successful as well. In addition to being a doctor, I was also a wife and a mother. I found the medical students who were women wanted to hear about my personal life and to talk about theirs as they were trying to understand how they would balance a career as a physician and a life with children. At these times, these students didn't need to see me as Superwoman – they needed to see me as a normal woman, like them. I enjoyed normalizing the role of doctor/wife/mom.

[a]Heidi Chumley, Executive Dean, American University of the Caribbean School of Medicine, Cupecoy, St. Maarten.

consultants described as "vital" the influence of role models on their choice of career:

Role models are vital, vital...You do things that you find very good as a student...I became a urologist because I was taught extremely well within the urology departments...Great teachers...For me no other reason...I think that role models are very important.

I was influenced by one person...I was doing cardiology at the time...he opened my eyes to the possibilities and made it sound exciting and so yes, definitely influenced my career."

The students also highlighted the influence of role models on their choice of career:

> *Even though I know how hard surgery is…I am really interested in it… because all the surgeons have such high job satisfaction and love the job.*

> *We do talk a lot about what we think of different consultants…some people, everyone likes them and those people are held in high esteem…it does influence what speciality we choose.*

The finding that medical students who work with the best internal medicine attending physicians and residents in their internal medicine clerkship are more likely to choose an internal medicine residency (Griffith et al., 2000) is further evidence that role models can affect a student's or trainee's career choice.

Good role models are particularly important in the community and rural settings (Amalba et al., 2017):

> *When medical students observe and are mentored by doctors working as health care physicians in the rural communities, this may have an influence on their choice of specialty and practice location through the role modelling they either passively or actively received. (p. 178)*

The importance of the doctor as a role model in the community was illustrated by students' comments following a community-based attachment in Ghana (Amalba et al., 2017):

> *A pleasant attitude put up by a role model towards the trainees would make them develop a favourable attitude to working in the rural community.*

> *If role models have a positive attitude toward work in the rural area it could encourage trainees to also work in rural areas.*

> *Dedication to work in spite of non-availability of certain facilities/amenities and the ability to improve the lives of community members by a role model can help others adapt to the situation and learn to work in rural communities.*

Understanding the competencies expected of a doctor

In addition to influencing career choice, role modelling also allows the learner to develop a more general understanding of the competencies expected of a doctor. The role model provides the student with first-hand experiences of the competencies that they need to acquire as a healthcare professional.

Statements of the expected learning outcomes, as described in Chapter 4, set out the abilities that a student should have on graduation as a doctor. The doctor as a role model illustrates this in practice. In medicine, learning outcomes, such as communication skills, empathy, teamwork and decision-making, become more meaningful for the student and come alive when they are seen in practice rather than on a theoretical list on paper or described in a lecture. When you review the expected learning outcomes for the course with students, you can invite them to illustrate the learning outcomes with examples from observation in practice of the doctor with whom they are working. This can help clarify any misunderstandings and reinforce what is expected of them.

Helping students acquire the appropriate professionalism and behaviour

The values, attitudes and behaviours required of a healthcare professional are most likely to be acquired by students through observation of the teachers and doctors with whom they work and aspire to emulate. As noted by Shapiro (2002), role modelling is the most effective way of teaching empathy to students. Angela Fan, a teacher in Taiwan, describes how she tries to serve as a good role model to foster students' compassion (Box 7.4). Role modelling is an efficient model of teaching and learning as the student learns while working with the doctor as he or she manages patients in day-to-day work. Brock and Harper (2016) have described the acquisition of professionalism from a student perspective:

We have had various lectures and workshops surrounding the topic of professionalism. Although these sessions provide us with a framework, the moulding into professionals is predominantly a result of the environment we encounter on placement. Furthermore, observing doctors breaking bad

---

Box 7.4 Compassion, commitment and humanity[a]

The faculty is the foundation for an academic institution. In this information age, students can learn knowledge through many sources and self-learning techniques. The duties of medical teachers extend far beyond the mere imparting of theories or clinical skills. We shall expect ourselves to convey and decode the humanistic value and ethics into the minds of future physicians and to cultivate them to form a core set of morals in their profession.

Today's doctor is as much a humanist as a scientist. As a medical teacher, I hope to strengthen our students' understanding of the human experience and human suffering in the different layers of human lives. However, I hope to cultivate their critical thinking capabilities and help them develop their own humanistic judgement and value. At the same time, I expect myself to serve as a good role model and provide the environment and learning experiences to foster their compassion and commitment to human beings and humanity.

Medicine is the essence of both a society's humanity and its prosperity, while the medical teacher carries the burden of shaping the future of medicine.

[a]*Angela Pei-Chen Fan, Associate Professor of Psychiatry, Internal Medicine, Faculty of Medicine, National Yang-Ming University, Taipei, Taiwan.*

*news, consulting families, and handling difficult consultations is a continual
learning process for students throughout their training. (p. 960)*

Without doubt, role modelling is one of the most powerful means of transmitting
values, attitudes and patterns of thoughts and behaviour to students (Bandura, 1986).
Students learn by observing and imitating the clinical teachers who they respect.
Students learn not just from what their teachers say, but also from what they do in
their clinical practice and the knowledge, skills and attitudes they exhibit. McAllister
et al. (1997, p. 53) have suggested that "being a role model is widely recognised as
critical in shaping, teaching, coaching and assisting future clinicians as it is the most
powerful teaching strategy available to clinical educators."

Role modelling can have a greater impact on the student than other teaching methods.
Falvo et al. (1991) have found role modelling to be educationally more effective in
enhancing the students' ability to communicate with patients about immunodeficiency
compared with lecture and discussion sessions. Douglas (1999) has described vividly
her experience of terminal care as a trainee and the lessons learned from her trainer:

> *Jimmy [her trainer] was an inspirational doctor and man, and I miss him
> terribly. His legacy to me, as a trainer myself now, is to remind me of the
> importance of teaching by example, which matters as much as, if not more
> than, anything that happens in a tutorial. (p. 889)*

The importance of the role model was also emphasized by Sir Donald Irvine (1999),
President of the General Medical Council in the UK. He has suggested that "the
model of practice provided by clinical teachers is essential because students learn
best by good example."

Passi and Johnston (2016b) have also identified the importance of role modelling in the development of professionalism, as illustrated by quotes from survey
participants:

> *Role modelling is really important…we develop our professional role with
> patients, colleagues…We learn how to behave.*
>
> *Role modelling is important in professionalism…as issues such as integrity
> are difficult to teach, you cannot push/you just have to let it come out…
> You cannot give a lecture on professionalism and hope they become
> professional.*

In programmed learning, an education approach that attracted a lot of attention in
the 1960s, two learning strategies were described, the *rul-eg* and the *eg-rul* approaches.
In the *rul-eg* approach, students first learned the principles and theory and then
studied applications of these in practice. In the *eg-rul* approach, the student first
worked on practical examples and, from these, identified and subsequently mastered
the principles and theory.

We have suggested elsewhere that this is a key principle in problem-based learning (Harden and Davis, 1998). This *eg-rul* strategy is relevant in terms of the teacher as a role model. The student first sees the doctor as an example of what is expected of them and then proceeds to learn the competencies necessary to perform as a physician. An example is the relatively new Hofstra University Zucker School of Medicine in New York. Students spend the first 6 weeks of their medical programme working with paramedics and serving as members of a team in an ambulance responding to emergency calls. Talking with students there, two things struck me (RMH). The first was their high level of motivation and enthusiasm for the medical course that followed. Secondly, I was impressed by the fact that they were already learning not just the knowledge and skills expected of a health professional, but also the necessary attitudes and professionalism.

Development of a professional identity

Attention has been paid in recent years to the development in students and trainees of their identity as a doctor. This can occur from an early stage in their training, and role models are critically important in the transformation of the student to a doctor. In a systematic review of the value of clinical experience early in the curriculum, Dornan et al. (2006) have found that "early experience helps medical students socialise to their chosen profession. It helps them acquire a range of subject matter and makes their learning more real and relevant."

The students' experiences and the teachers to whom they are attached have an important part to play in the establishment of the students' identity. Passi and Johnston (2016a) have suggested that "the development of professional identity is a complex, often subconscious, process that effectively takes place through positive role modelling throughout the curriculum."

They found that both consultants and students described the nurturing impact of role modelling as "moulding," with students describing the process as "moulding of our professional identity" and consultants describing it as "groomed from day one as we know what the public expect." One consultant noted that "there was a consultant who really made me into consultant material...it was his personality...He moulded me into consultant material." Participants reported that they developed an idea of what type of doctor they would want to be through role modelling.

Professional identity can be developed if clinicians serving as role models provide authentic learning experiences that allow the student, under supervised conditions, to assume aspects of a doctor's work. As noted by Birden et al. (2016):

> *A supportive environment where students are allowed to assume some of the decision making and clinical aspects of the doctor's role under supervised conditions can provide authentic learning experiences, treating medical students as junior colleagues, producing junior doctors who are likely to fare better in developing their professional identity. (p. 946–947)*

Contributing to a learning environment that supports students' learning

The learning environment or climate plays a key part in the student's learning, as described in Chapter 5. It is the learning environment that sets the stage for effective teaching and learning. The desired education strategy may be unsuccessful if the environment fights against it; to paraphrase Peter Drucker, "the climate eats strategy for breakfast." Creating an appropriate educational environment, however, is not easy. Good role models can make a significant contribution, as described by Teh Kailin, a postgraduate trainer in Singapore (Box 7.5). Through role models, the learning environment can encourage students to evaluate their own competence and to search for information to keep themselves up to date. Writing about the role of the teacher in the clinical environment, Ramani and Leinster (2008) argued that "modelling life-long learning requires that the teacher is willing to admit ignorance and prepared to learn from students."

The learning style of the teacher contributes to the learning style adopted by the student. This has been demonstrated by Shein and Chiou (2011). The students' learning style was assessed before and after the course and related to the teacher's learning style. They found that after a semester, the learning style of students became associated with that of their role model.

An educational environment in which the delivery of cost-conscious healthcare is valued should be encouraged as the learning environment where role modelling is a key element that influences the learners' future practice patterns. Cost-conscious medical care is on today's agenda, and appropriate role models can help prepare future doctors to address health care costs. Students, however, may encounter conflicting doctor role modelling behaviour. Leep Hunderfund et al. (2017) have found that while some observed cost-conscious behaviours, others observed "wasteful behaviours

---

Box 7.5 A role model in postgraduate education[a]

When medical officers first start their rotation in the polyclinic, they are given time to sit in with me and their supervisors to observe how we manage patients and communicate with them. Throughout the 6-month posting, I also help them to deal with challenging patients and, whenever they encounter difficulties, to meet their expectations and demands. Through these opportunities to observe their seniors, medical officers can develop and enhance their clinical and communication skills.

By my personal example I demonstrate the need to keep up to date as a teacher. I attend meetings, workshops and conferences relevant to medical teaching, e.g. the Asia-Pacific Medical Education Conference, bimonthly Train-the-Trainer sessions and Medical Forums conducted by NHGP, to keep myself abreast with advances in medical knowledge and new approaches to postgraduate medical training.

[a]Teh Kailin, Family Physician, National Healthcare Group Polyclinician (NHGP), Singapore.

such as excessive use of diagnostic tests and unnecessary referrals which may erode values taught in more formal settings and adversely affect students' intended and actual behaviours."

Lifestyle choices

A role model is important not only from professional perspectives, as described above. The teacher as a role model can also influence the students' lifestyle choices. For example, the teacher as role model is more effective in discouraging students from smoking than lectures or other forms of teaching on the topic.

A doctor, teacher and person as a role model

The teacher serves as a role model from three different perspectives (Cruess et al., 2008):

- The teacher as a doctor or scientist
- The teacher as a teacher
- The teacher as a person

The doctor as a role model

The doctor has an impact on the student as a role model, as highlighted by Samy Azer, an experienced teacher (Box 7.6).

Box 7.6 The teacher as role model[a]

I still remember my first exposure to bedside learning when I was a medical student: an elderly patient with neurological changes and a professor in internal medicine teaching us and eliciting clinical signs. At the end of the session, I saw him on his knees near the patient's bed, delicately placing her socks back on the feet while talking to her. It struck a chord within me.

To me, this reflected care, support, love, and humbleness of the teacher. When the teachers are role models and their actions are the standardization of excellence, they inspire their students and colleagues around them. The impact on learners could be lifelong. Now nearly 30 years later and having been working in several different countries overseas, I totally believe that teaching professionalism is not about a set of lectures on professional values, it is rather what we say and what we do as clinicians and as teachers in day-to-day practice. If you want your students to become professionals, let them watch, observe, experience, and reflect on their own feelings. It is always small things we do or say that usually leave the greatest imprint on a learner.

However, a small percentage of students may have totally different views about role models and may show no changes, even after a period of socialization with a role model.

---

[a]Samy Azer, Professor of Medical Education, Chair of Curriculum Development and Research Unit, College of Medicine, King Saud University, Saudi Arabia.

But what are students and trainees looking for in a doctor as a role model? The features identified include (Althouse et al., 1999; Wright, 1996):

- A good relationship with the patient
- Compassion for and dedication to the patients
- A holistic approach to the patient
- Enthusiasm for and dedication to their specialty
- Demonstration of excellent clinical reasoning skills
- Integrity

A more comprehensive list of features of a good model prepared by de Sousa (2004) is given in Box 7.7. I (RMH), as a house surgeon in the Western Infirmary, Glasgow,

---

Box 7.7 A Good Role Model[a]

Shows an attitude of compassion, openness and integrity

Is punctual, has a pleasing look, is friendly

Is well organized, gives clear instructions

Has a balanced personality

Looks after himself or herself

Masters knowledge in his or her field of expertise

Has sound clinical reasoning

Speaks clearly, with precision and in a language understandable to the patient

Assures continuity of care

Remains up-to-date and cultivates intellectual curiosity

Establishes a confident relationship with patients and their families

Possesses a good sense of professional responsibility

Plans the investigation (choice of tests, cost–benefit and risks) and interprets the results

Treats the patient and carries on the follow-up

Knows and respects his or her limits

Demonstrates good technical skills

Conducts the interview with patience and gentleness; is sensitive to the patient's reactions

Shows empathy

Considers the patient's point of view during the interview, particularly during decision-making

Emphasizes a biopsychosocial approach

Demonstrates intellectual exactness and critical judgement

Demonstrates good control of a medical interview

Respects the patient as a person

[a]As described by Jaime Correia de Sousa (2004).

learned from Sir Charles Illingworth that the most important person in the ward was the patient. If he was concerned about a patient, he not uncommonly came into the ward on a Sunday morning to see the patient. He noted that some patients developed a deep vein thrombosis in the leg and, in an attempt to prevent this, developed a leg support for the patients. What also had an impact on me was his enthusiasm for his subject and for his staff, many of whom went on to become distinguished professors of surgery and deans of medical schools.

With the greater emphasis on work-based training and on-the-job learning, and with curriculum developments, such as the early introduction of clinical experiences and the longitudinal integrated clinical clerkships, the importance of the doctor as a role model has become even more important. This responsibility does not rest only with senior doctors. The move to have students shadow a junior doctor as a formal part of their training programme places the junior doctor in an important position where his or her behaviour and attitudes are likely to influence the student.

The teacher as a role model

Teachers serve as powerful role models for students, regardless of whether they are a clinician or a basic scientist. Whether the teacher is perceived as having a passion for her or his subject and for teaching students and as being honest and trustworthy has an impact on the students. The quality of time is more important than the amount of time spent by students with their teacher. Althouse et al. (1999) examined how clinical instructors, designated by their medical students as influential role models, described their teaching and their relationships with students. They reported:

> *Medical students and their models did not generally spend large amounts of time together. Often they met only briefly after patient encounters to discuss care of a specific patient. This finding indicated that the quantity of time physicians spent with their students was not nearly as important as the quality of the time. Regardless of the amount of time spent together, students chose models who were more than just a good instructor or clinically competent. Students chose models who demonstrated a dedication to their speciality and patients, a love of teaching, and a caring personality, which fostered an environment of mutual respect. The role models were genuinely interested in facilitating the growth of the students, which manifested in being selected by students as a model. (p. 120)*

The recognised attributes of the teacher as a good role model include:

- Enthusiasm and passion for teaching and for student learning
- Engagement and effective communication with students
- Priority given to teaching, with time spent with students
- Teaching directed to meet the learner's needs and feedback provided to the learner

> **Box 7.8** Hall of Mirrors[a]
>
> One of the valuable lessons I have learned is that effective teaching is very dependent on the quality of the relationship that you are able to establish with the student or resident, whether it is in the clinic, the small group or the large classroom. I attribute any success I have had to interacting with my students, patients and co-workers as though they are guests in my home. Picture all of the relationships you have in your life as a giant Hall of Mirrors. Every relationship you have and the quality of that relationship should ideally be variations of mirror images of each other. I think of this often when I am with my patients and students are observing. To be authentic, we need to be able to mirror the caring and evidence-based culture that is embedded in our care of patients, in our relationship with our students and in all of our professional relationships. Shedding light on your personal Hall of Mirrors, and being mindful of the reflections, can enable you to be consistently responsive to the ever-changing needs and challenges of teaching and learning.
>
> [a]*Ivan Silver, Psychiatrist, Toronto, Canada.*

- Compassion
- Trustworthiness
- Sense of humour
- Integrity

If they relate appropriately to the student, teachers have the ability to share the importance of the subject and to kindle in the student a curiosity and quest for a better understanding of the topic than it is possible to derive from a handout or online resource. Regrettably, however, teachers may serve as poor role models. Beaudoin et al. (1998) found that most students in a Canadian medical school considered their teachers to be insensitive to their anxieties as students. Ivan Silver, a psychiatrist in Toronto, highlights in Box 7.8 that teachers need to be able to mirror in their relationships with students the caring that is embedded in the care of patients.

The students of today are not only the doctors, but also the teachers of tomorrow. Their experience as students and the teacher role models that they encounter will influence their future practice as a teacher.

The teacher as a personal role model

The teacher, in addition to serving as a role model from both a medical and teaching perspective, influences the student through his or her personal behaviour. We described above, for example, how smoking is less frequent in students if the teacher does not smoke. This personal aspect of a role model has received less attention but it is nonetheless important. Professor Sir Charles Illingworth, a keen hill walker and climber, invited his staff to join him on expeditions. As a result, some developed their own enthusiasm for exploring the Scottish hills and even climbing the Munros (the name given to the 277 Scottish mountains of at least 3,000 feet [914 m] in height). Peter Forsey, a consultant cardiologist, competed successfully in *Robot Wars*, in which radio-controlled machines go into battle; the robot that he had built was powered by two hospital trolley motors. We have no evidence, but we would be surprised if this did not create an interest in his staff and students in the use of technology.

Professor Sir Edward Wayne, professor of medicine at the University of Glasgow, was a good role model. On his retirement from medicine, he devoted himself to other activities and founded a retired professional men's group and a photographic club and became the governor of a local school. In these activities, he demonstrated the same attributes of leadership and an active, searching mind as he had as a teacher in medicine.

As a junior member of staff in the department of medicine at the Western Infirmary in Glasgow, I (RMH) remember the discussions over coffee in the ward sister's room following the morning ward round and in the once-monthly evening journal club held in the houses of members of staff. Although these occasions focussed on medical issues, they also provided opportunities to get to know the senior members of staff as individuals. Sadly, such informal meetings with colleagues are now less common. We mention these anecdotes to illustrate that the teacher serves as a role model, not just as a doctor or a teacher but as an individual whose behaviour can have an influence on the students and junior staff.

We recently ran Essential Skills in Medical Education courses in Uruguay and Argentina and were impressed with the engagement and enthusiasm shown by the staff. One reason was that the dean and vice chancellor of the universities were excellent role models and attended and took part enthusiastically throughout the course.

The bad role model

We have described the value of the teacher as a role model, with students emulating their behaviour. This, however, can be negative as well as positive. Tensions may arise when the student observes discordance between the behaviour and attitude of the teacher when communicating with patients and what they have been taught about relationships with patients in lectures. It is also too easy for students to assume that what they see in practice, although it contradicts what they have been taught, represents the real world of medical practice and is what they should emulate. A concern is that students who observe cases of unprofessional behaviour in a bad role model are more likely to participate in such behaviours themselves, and once a student has engaged in such unprofessional behaviour he or she is more likely to do it again. Franco et al. (2017) have described how students who observe unprofessional behaviour may reflect this later in their own behaviour:

> …the student who observed or participated in unprofessional behaviour
> seemed to enter into a vicious circle: once the student had observed,

*participated in or misjudged a certain form of unprofessional behaviour, the
likelihood that he/she would do so again in the future increased. (p. 217)*

Problems can arise if the doctor as a role model does not meet in their own behaviour
the ethical standards expected (Bloch, 2003):

*If a series of teachers fail as ethical role models, students may well
become disillusioned with their chosen profession. Instead of having an
eager, energetic approach to medical life, they may become cynical and
embittered. If insufficient good role models are available, students may miss
the opportunity, at a formative period in their development, to enhance
their own ethical capabilities. (p. 168)*

The dissonance between the ethical behaviour of doctors as observed by students
and the ethical behaviour they have been taught to expect may cause confusion and
even distress on the part of the student. There is a need to provide an opportunity
for students to discuss in a safe environment the everyday ethical dilemmas as they
are encountered (Paice et al., 2002).

In a conversation I (RMH) had with a group of medical teachers about problems
identified relating to the teaching programme, concern was expressed about the
number of students who arrived late for lectures, and the question was raised about
whether the door of the lecture theatre should be locked to prevent the late arrivals
from joining the lecture. On talking with the students, however, it emerged that the
lecturers themselves had set a bad example with regard to timekeeping by often
arriving late or cancelling a lecture at short notice.

Students tend to be drawn to and emulate senior doctors who have responsibility
and status but who may emphasise the biomedical model of care and are less interested
in their patients' social, psychological and cultural problems. One result is that the
students' empathy decreases.

Bad role models are a not uncommon problem. Tagawa (2016) asked final-year
medical students whether they observed good and desirable or undesirable role models
who made them feel "I should not behave like that." Of the 115 students, 113
observed desirable role models, with only two students encountering only undesirable
role models; 85 students also observed undesirable role models, particularly in terms
of their relationships with patients, other people and teaching, rather than clinical
competence.

It is important that you recognise the importance of positive and negative role models
to students' development. Role models are not usually discussed with students.
However, you should encourage students not to imitate their role models blindly but
to be critical and selectively adopt the behaviours and attitudes of different role
models. This is an example of the value of reflection by the student as part of the
learning programme.

The way forward

We have discussed the problem of the bad role model. How do you become a good role model? What action is required in your school or institution to promote good role models? Developing this role is different from developing the other roles described in this text. When it comes to how to deliver better lectures, develop strategies to facilitate learning, assess a student's competence, serve as a manager or leader or undertake research, you can read about it, attend courses or even learn from experience, hopefully with useful feedback from peers and students. Learning to be a "good" role model is different. However, there are things that can be done to enhance your value as a role model:

- The first step is to recognise that role modelling is an important feature of the education programme. Squires (1999) has noted:

  It is important to identify modelling as a distinct function and heading in order to draw attention to what is a pervasive but sometimes unconscious, and even denied process in education. Teachers may not see themselves as models, and may even regard the very idea as pretentious and paternalistic. (p. 47)

- The impact of the teacher as a role model should be emphasised as it relates to what the teacher does as a medical practitioner, as a teacher and in relation to personal attitudes and behaviours. The teacher should be aware of the impact of what they are modelling, positive or negative.

- The school should acknowledge the importance of role modelling by recognising and rewarding in some way teachers who are good role models. Faculty members who model and perpetuate poor behaviour should not be allowed to interact with students (Schwartzstein, 2015):

  ....we can ensure that the clinical faculty who supervise our students are selected for, and trained to enhance, their ability to support rather than undermine these values; faculty members who model and perpetuate poor behaviour ought not be allowed to interact with students. We can make it clear that teaching students is a privilege and that we have high expectations for those chosen for this task. (p. 1587)

- Role modelling should be included in faculty development activities – it is often not addressed. Many of the attributes associated with being an excellent role model are related to skills that can be acquired and to modifiable behaviour (Wright et al., 1998). Lublin (1992) has noted:

  ...all teachers are always role models for students. So there may be need for developmental activities for teachers which deal not just with the mediation of medical knowledge and skills, but which also

sensitize teachers to the effect they have on students' acquisition of attitudes and values towards the medical role and the teaching role.

- All teachers should be encouraged to reflect on their responsibilities as role models and the important effect that this can have on student learning and their attitudes and behaviours. They should be aware that any action observed by a learner constitutes role modelling. All their actions affect students. As suggested by Cruess et al. (2008), they should make a conscious effort to articulate what they are modelling and to make the implicit explicit.
- Students should be encouraged to think about their learning from role models and how they can pick an amalgam of different role models (Shuval and Adler, 1980). Time should be available to facilitate debriefing because of the potential danger of inappropriate role models. Students should be encouraged to reflect on and assess their teachers professional behaviour so that they can discern those that are worth emulating (Benbassat, 2014).

Role models should reflect education change

We have seen and will continue to see developments in medical practice and health care delivery. These developments include a greater involvement of patients in their management, a greater emphasis on collaboration and teamwork and a greater use of technology. Meg Gaines, a distinguished Clinical Professor of Law, at a meeting of the American Medical Association's Accelerating Change in Medical Education consortium discussing the physician of the future, highlighted the importance of role modelling with regard to a greater role of patients in the education process: "Students do what they see us do, not what we tell them. So we need to co-create curriculum with patients, families and communities. We have to walk our talk. There's no way around it." (Smith, 2016)

In education, we have seen significant changes in the curriculum, including outcome-based education, vertical and horizontal integration, interprofessional education, student-centred learning and the use of new technologies, including simulation and e-learning and, as described in this text, there have also been changes in the roles of the teacher. One recently recognised change is the need for students, when seeking information, to master the skills of asking the right question, to know where to seek information and to know how to evaluate the answers they obtain. The teacher as a role model needs to show by example the use of the Internet to ask the right question in response to a clinical query, to look for the answer on the Internet and to know how to evaluate the responses they have found and recognise when they have sufficient information without further searches. The problem is that some teachers may themselves not have these skills.

Marshall McLuhan (McLuhan and Fiore, 2008) stated that "we look at the present through a rear-view mirror. We march backwards into the future." The role model that students see may have represented good practice in the past, but things may have changed. The senior teacher may be more at home with the role of information provider than facilitator and may need to come to terms with this if he or she is to be a valuable role model in a situation in which there is greater engagement of students in the education programme. We need to ensure that students are not constrained by role models emphasising the past and that they are encouraged to reflect on this and consider the changes that are now taking place in medical practice.

The teacher as a role model, an expert role model and a master role model

The teacher as a role model

The teacher serves as a good role model whose behaviour and actions should be emulated by the students.

The teacher as an expert role model

The teacher has looked at the importance of role models and how this contributes to the students' learning experience and has contributed to enhancing the value of role models in the school.

The teacher as a master role model

The teacher is not only a good role model, but also has studied the value of role models in the curriculum and different approaches to role modelling and is recognised nationally and internationally as an authority in that area.

Take-home messages

1. Although less obvious and visible than the other roles we have described, the teacher's responsibility as a role model is as, if not more, important. The role is often underestimated. The teacher as a role model is not the icing on the cake. It is the cake itself. The teacher as a role model has a powerful influence on students' career choice, on their understanding of what is required to become a doctor and the development of their professional identities, on the acquisition of appropriate professional behaviours, including learning skills, and on the creation of an educational environment conducive to learning.
2. As far as possible, the curriculum should be arranged so that students spend more time with teachers who are good role models. In practice, this may be difficult to organise.
3. Students should be taught how and when to learn from and emulate a role model, selecting traits from different role models as appropriate. They should identify bad role models as exhibiting behaviours to be avoided.

Consider

- Think of the different ways a role model may influence a student, as illustrated in Fig. 7.2.
- To what extent are you a "good" role model for your students?
- Are your students briefed on how to respond to "bad" role models? Are they helped to recognise learning from role models as a skill that needs developing?

Explore further

Althouse, L.A., Stritter, F.T., Sterner, B.D., 1999. Attitudes and approaches of influential role models in clinical education. Adv. Health Sci. Educ. Theory Pract. 4 (2), 111–122.

Amalba, A., Abantanga, F.A., Scherpbier, A.J.J.A., et al., 2017. Community-based education: The influence of role modeling on career choice and practice location. Med. Teach. 39 (2), 174–180.

Bandura, A., 1977. Self-efficacy: Toward a unifying theory of behavioural change. Psych. Rev. 84 (2), 191–215.

Bandura, A., 1986. Social Foundations of Thought and Action. Prentice Hall, Upper Saddle River, NJ.

Beaudoin, C., Maheux, B., Cote, L., et al., 1998. Clinical teachers as humanistic care-givers and educators: Perceptions of senior clerks and second-year residents. CMAJ 159 (7), 765–769.

Benbassat, J., 2014. Role modeling in medical education: The importance of reflective imitation. Acad. Med. 89 (4), 550–554.

Birden, H., Barker, J., Wilson, I., 2016. Effectiveness of a rural longitudinal integrated clerkship in preparing medical students for internship. Med. Teach. 38 (9), 946–956.

Bloch, S., 2003. Medical students and clinical ethics. Med. J. Aust. 178 (4), 167–169.

Brock, S., Harper, L., 2016. Incentives for role models; our most invaluable resource. Med. Teach. 38 (9), 960–961.

Campos-Outcalt, D., Senf, J., Watkins, A.J., et al., 1995. The effects of medical school curricula, faculty role models and biomedical research support on choice of generalist physician careers: A review and quality assessment of the literature. Acad. Med. 70 (7), 611–619.

Cruess, S.R., Cruess, R.L., Steinert, Y., 2008. Role modelling – making the most of a powerful teaching strategy. BMJ 336 (7646), 718–721.

Dake, S.B., Taylor, J.A., 1994. Do as I do: The importance of the clinical instructor as role model. J. Extra Corpor. Technol. 26 (3), 140–142.

Davis, M.H., Harden, R.M., 1999. AMEE Medical Education Guide No. 15: Problem-based learning: A practical guide. Med. Teach. 21 (2), 130–140.

de Sousa, J.C., 2004. Being a role model for students in your practice. http://studylib.net/doc/8030858/being-a-role-model-for-students-in-your-practice.

Dornan, T., 2005. Osler, Flexner, apprenticeship and "the new medical education". J. R. Soc. Med. 98 (3), 91–95.

Dornan, T., Littlewood, S., Margolis, S.A., et al., 2006. How can experience in clinical and community settings contribute to early medical education? A BEME systematic review. Med. Teach. 28 (1), 3–18.

Douglas, A., 1999. A lesson learnt, an inspirational teacher. BMJ 319, Oct. 2. 889.

Eastman, C.E., 1991. The ways of learning. In: Nerburn, K., Mengelkoch, L. (Eds.), Native American Wisdom. New World Library, San Raphael, CA, p. 20, (Chapter 3).

Falvo, D.R., Smaga, S., Brenner, J.S., et al., 1991. Lecture versus role modelling: A comparison of educational programs to enhance residents' ability to communicate with patients about HIV. Teach. Learn. Med. 3 (4), 227–231.

Feudtner, C., Christakis, D.A., Christakis, N.A., 1994. Do clinical clerks suffer ethical erosion? Students' perceptions of their ethical environment and personal development. Acad. Med. 69 (8), 670–679.

Franco, R.S., Franco, C.A.G., Kusma, S.Z., et al., 2017. To participate or not participate in unprofessional behaviour—is that the question? Med. Teach. 39 (2), 212–219.

General Medical Council, 2002. Tomorrow's Doctors: Recommendations on undergraduate medical education. http://www.gmc-uk.org/static/documents/content/Outcomes_for_graduates _Jul_15.pdf.

Glicken, A.D., Merenstein, G.B., 2007. Addressing the hidden curriculum: Understanding educator professionalism. Med. Teach. 29 (1), 54–57.

Griffith, C.H., Georgensen, J.C., Wilson, J.F., 2000. Speciality choices of students who actually have choices: The influence of excellent clinical teachers. Acad. Med. 75 (3), 278–282.

Harden, R.M., Crosby, J., 2000. AMEE Guide No. 20: The good teacher is more than a lecturer – the twelve roles of the teacher. 22(4), 334–347.

Harden, R.M., Davis, M.H., 1998. The continuum of problem-based learning. Med. Teach. 20, 317–322.

Hazan, A., Haber, J., 2017. Mindful EM: The impact factor of the hidden curriculum. Emerg. Med. News 39 (4), 22.

Irby, D.M., 1986. Clinical teaching and the clinical teacher. J. Med. Educ. 61, 35–45.

Irvine, D., 1999. The performance of doctors: The new professionalism. Lancet 353 (9159), 1174–1176.

Kenny, N.P., Mann, K.V., MacLeod, H., 2003. Role modelling in physicians' professional formation: Reconsidering an essential but untapped educational strategy. Acad. Med. 78, 1203–1210.

Leep Hunderfund, A.N., Dyrbye, L.N., Starr, S.R., et al., 2017. Role modelling and regional health care intensity: U.S. medical student attitudes towards experience with cost-conscious care. Acad. Med. 92 (5), 694–702.

Lublin, J.R., 1992. Role modelling: A case study in general practice. Med. Educ. 26 (2), 116–122.

McAllister, L., Lincoln, M., Maloney, D., McLeod, S., 1997. Facilitating Learning in Clinical Settings. Stanley Thornes, Cheltenham, UK.

McLuhan, M., Fiore, Q., 2008. The Medium is the Message: An Inventory of Effects. Penguin Modern Classics, London.

McMurray, J.E., Schwartz, M.D., Genero, N.P., et al., 1993. The attractiveness of internal medicine: A qualitative analysis of the experiences of female and male medical students. Ann. Intern. Med. 199 (8), 812–818.

Nelms, T.P., Jones, J.M., Gray, D.P., 1993. Role modelling: A method for teaching caring in nursing education. J. Nurs. Educ. 32 (1), 18–23.

Oxford English Dictionary, Role model. http://www.oed.com/view/Entry/275493?redirectedFro m=role+model#eid.

Paice, E., Heard, S., Moss, F., 2002. How important are role models in making good doctors? BMJ 325 (7366), 707–710.

Passi, V., Johnson, N., 2016a. The hidden process of positive doctor role modelling. Med. Teach. 38 (7), 700–707.

Passi, V., Johnson, N., 2016b. The impact of positive doctor role modelling. Med. Teach. 38 (11), 1139–1145.

Passi, V., Johnson, S., Peile, E., et al., 2013. Doctor role modelling in medical education: BEME Guide No. 27. Med. Teach. 35 (9), e1422–e1436.

Ramani, S., Leinster, S., 2008. AMEE Guide No. 34: Teaching in the clinical environment. Med. Teach. 30 (4), 347–364.

Schwartzstein, R.M., 2015. Getting the right medical students – nature versus nurture. N. Engl. J. Med. 372 (17), 1586–1587.

Shapiro, J., 2002. How do physicians teach empathy in the primary care setting? Acad. Med. 77 (4), 323–328.

Shein, P.P., Chiou, W.B., 2011. Teachers as role models for students' learning styles. Soc. Behav. Personal. 39 (8), 1097–1104.

Shuval, J., Adler, I., 1980. The role of models in professional socialization. Soc. Sci. Med. 14, 5–14.

Smith, T.M., 2016. The physician of the future: More like da Vinci. https://wire.ama-assn.org/education/physician-future-more-da-vinci.

Squires, G., 1999. Teaching as a Professional Discipline. Falmer Press, London.

Tagawa, M., 2016. Effects of undergraduate medical students' individual attributes on perceptions of encounters with positive and negative role models. BMC Med. Educ. 16, 164.

Tosteson, D.C., 1979. Learning medicine. N. Engl. J. Med. 301 (13), 690–694.

Walton, H., 1985. Overview of themes in medical education. In: Goodlad, S. (Ed.), Education for the Professions. Society for Research into Higher Education and NFER-Nelson, Windsor, UK, pp. 49–51.

Wright, S., 1996. Examining what residents look for in their role models. Acad. Med. 71 (3), 290–292.

Wright, S.M., Kern, D.E., Kolodner, K., et al., 1998. Attributes of excellent attending-physician role models. N. Engl. J. Med. 339 (27), 1986–1993.

Wright, S., Wong, A., Newill, C., 1997. The impact of role models on medical students. J. Gen. Intern. Med. 12 (1), 53–56.

THE TEACHER AS A ROLE MODEL

Chapter 8

The teacher as a manager and leader

Teachers who choose the path of teacher leadership...become owners and investors in their schools, rather than mere tenants.

Roland Barth (2001)

Every teacher has a management and leadership role.

- The manager and leader role is important
- The teacher's management responsibilities
- The teacher as a leader
- The management cycle
- Management and leadership strategies
- Collaboration
- Negotiation and conflict
- Organising and participating in meetings
- Adaptive leadership

- Student engagement
- Change in medical education as a management and leadership challenge
- Innovation in medical education
- Cost of medical education
- Teacher manager/leader, expert or master?
- Take-home messages
- Consider
- Explore further

The manager and leader role is important

Management and leadership are very much on today's agenda in medicine. It is now accepted that doctors as part of their medical practice have a management and leadership role. Expertise in management and leadership is important, not only for the healthcare professional's work in clinical practice, but also for his or her role as a teacher.

When we described the different roles of the teacher (Harden and Crosby, 2000), the role as manager was not included. We assumed that this was addressed by the other educational roles described. Since then, the role of the teacher as a manager has become more important for a number of reasons and merits separate consideration as a distinct role for the teacher (Fig. 8.1). Teachers must be capable of taking

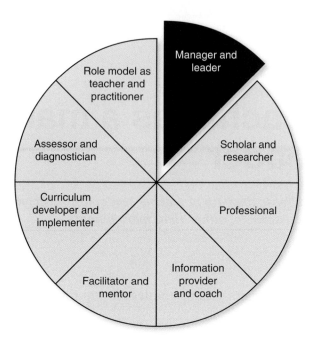

Figure 8.1 The teacher as a manager

responsibility for difficult decisions in situations of complexity and uncertainty in their day-to-day work with curriculum development, teaching and learning and assessment of students' competence. Some teachers may think that taking on formal management or leadership responsibilities as a teacher is an abdication and abandonment of their primary responsibilities as a teacher. We argue, however, that management and leadership are important roles alongside and contributing to the other seven roles for the teacher we describe. Judy McKimm, a senior medical educator and manager and former Dean of Medical Education at Swansea University Medical School, highlights in Box 8.1 the importance of the teacher as leader.

Reasons for the increasing importance attached to the teacher as a manager and leader include:

- Medical education has become more complex with a move to integrated teaching and horizontal and vertical integration in the curriculum, the concept of a flipped classroom, problem-based learning as a learning strategy and outcome or competency-based education. No longer is it reasonable for a teacher to address his or her subject in the curriculum in isolation. Planning, collaboration and negotiation with colleagues are required.
- There are increasing pressures on the teacher to be accountable for the education programme to the profession, including accrediting bodies, to

Box 8.1 The importance of leadership[a]

I've been teaching since 1986 when I started working in further education. With a teaching load of 25 hours a week, working with adult learners and disaffected 16–19 year olds, I learned my 'classroom craft' over eight years. I also learned that I loved developing curricula and the importance of good leadership and management for high quality learning. An MA in Education and an MBA, plus working in different education sectors gave me confidence to move into my first 'big' medical education job at Imperial College. Taking a leadership role in developing a new curriculum and medical school is a huge challenge, opportunity and privilege. Good curriculum design needs the art of good leadership and knowledge of the 'industry' (expert leadership) and a flair for 'what works' and why. If it is not practical and sustainable then it's hallucinatory: this is where management skills come in. Experience gained from these two jobs has stood me in good stead over the nearly 30 years I've been working in education around the world on educational projects and programmes. Learning about education in different contexts and how to lead and manage pragmatically and with agility is essential for teachers wanting to deliver the best quality education.

[a]*Judy McKimm, Director of Strategic Educational Development and Programme Director, MSc in Leadership for the Health Professions, Swansea University Medical School, Swansea, UK.*

the public, including students and their parents, and to the government that contributes funding. Quality control and related management issues are now a requirement.

- Students are now more actively engaged in the curriculum with a student voice. They are considered as partners in the process rather than simply consumers. This provides important opportunities but also comes with tensions and related management issues.
- At a time of financial constraints, cost-effectiveness (Walsh, 2014) has to be taken into consideration, particularly with more sophisticated education resources available, including online learning, virtual reality and hi-fidelity simulators. We argue that decisions need to be taken about how the resources can be used most effectively and efficiently. Should every hospital, for example, have a clinical skills laboratory?
- There has been an expansion in the number of students admitted to medical studies, including students from diverse backgrounds, often without matching funding. This brings its own management problems.
- Distributed learning is now relatively common, with students based at a number of different sites for their education programme (Bates et al., 2011). This too presents its own management challenges.
- "Education without borders" (Wass and Southgate, 2017) is also on today's agenda, with greater educational collaboration between schools nationally and internationally and between the different healthcare professions.

- Finally, and importantly, as we discuss later, this is a time of change. Transformation in medical education in the 21st century is on today's agenda. Catalysts include changes in healthcare delivery systems, advances in medicine and developments in education such as the move to outcome-based education. Strategies are required if we are to bring about educational change.

The teacher's management responsibilities

For these different reasons, you will be required to take a management and leadership role in implementing the education programme and, in particular, facilitating change in the part of the course where you have an impact. Teachers will vary in their management responsibilities, and the same teacher will vary in her or his responsibilities at different times. A few may have overall responsibility for managing their medical school or speciality training programme and, for them, this may be their main contribution to the education programme, demanding much if not all of their time. Others may be responsible for a course or part of the educational programme. Every teacher, however, has some management responsibility if their teaching is to be delivered effectively and efficiently as part of the undergraduate or postgraduate education programme. The management and leadership issues described in this chapter are relevant, therefore, to all teachers. What we are talking about is a wide spread of responsibility for management in the medical school or education institution, even when on the surface the management structure appears hierarchical, and decisions appear to rest with the dean and a few senior staff.

You can view your role as a teacher manager at three levels (Fig. 8.2):

- *Institutional level* – this involves participating in the process of managing the overall medical school or education institution, including the curriculum, as a stakeholder in the success of your school.
- *Course level* – this involves managing interactions with others in collective decision making relating to that part of the education programme for which you are responsible.
- *Personal level* – this involves self-management and the application of management principles to your day-to-day life and to your work as a teacher, including setting objectives, planning how these will be achieved, implementing the plan, monitoring the progress and responding to feedback.

The teacher as a leader

With increasing complexity in medical education, the distinction between management and leadership has become blurred, with the manager assuming leadership skills

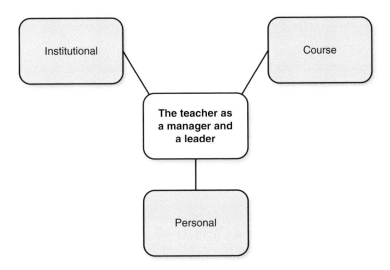

Figure 8.2 The teacher may be a manager and leader at different times

whilst leadership per se embraces being a manager (Bin Abdulrahman and Gibbs, 2016; McKimm and Lieff, 2013). Effective leaders require management skills, and vice versa. As a teacher, you are not only a manager but also a leader, with responsibility for innovating and bringing about change in your teaching where required. We discuss your role as a change agent and innovator later in this chapter.

Highlighting the importance in schools of teachers as leaders, Hess (2015) wrote:

> *Frustrated by schools and systems that consume their time and passion, teachers can find it all too easy to retreat to their classrooms. But doing so leaves them trapped in a classroom cage, stuck with systems and policies that they find frustrating or incoherent. Cage-busting teachers reach out in ways that identify the problems and surface workable solutions. (p. 59)*

Alex MacQueen, an anatomist in Dundee in the 1970s, was not content to sit back and continue to teach anatomy with a traditional approach. He reached out and, working with Bob Pringle, a surgeon, introduced a "living anatomy" approach, in which students learned their anatomy as it related to outpatients and patients in the hospital ward. Management, according to Kotter (1990), is about the production of predictability and order, whereas leadership is about change and the creation and implementation of new visions relating to change in an institution. The living anatomy course is an example.

On occasion, there may be a teaching leadership vacuum in a medical school resulting in a failure to introduce required new approaches in the curriculum. Teachers can respond to this challenge formally and informally. Like Alex MacQueen, you can demonstrate leadership skills and bring about change without holding a formal leadership position (Bin Abdulrahman and Gibbs, 2016).

Most teachers are not born leaders and have to learn leadership skills. The list of new books purporting to offer indispensable but varying advice to would-be leaders is endless. Maddux (2002) has concluded that:

> *The popular and academic literature is marked by so much confusion, disarray, shoddy thinking, and charlatanism, that the serious reader might be tempted to dismiss the concept of leadership as unworthy of serious consideration. (p. 42)*

In thinking about leadership, we should move away from the concept of leadership as described by Rear Admiral Chester Ward. Lynch and Kordis (1988) quoted Chester Ward: "(The) great leader is one for whom his men will CHEERFULLY give up their lives. That is the real test of leadership." Admiral Rickover responded:

> *I have not been able to find a single person in my organization who would die for me, much less CHEERFULLY die for me. This definitely shows I am not a leader in accordance with Admiral Ward's definition. Incidentally, when Admiral Ward's article came out I telephoned him and asked him how many in his office had volunteered cheerfully to die for him, whereupon he hung up on me.*

It is recognised that interpersonal skills and appropriate personal attributes are important for leadership (Davis and Harden, 2002). Openness, concern and the capacity to work effectively with others are needed. The good leader is not narcissistic, egocentric, hypercritical, isolated or abrasive under pressure. Good leaders show concern for the people they work with, make their expectations clear and follow through on issues. The concept of emotional intelligence is also important in leadership and, the more complex the job, the more emotional intelligence matters (Goleman, 1998). Goleman has defined five components of emotional intelligence:

- Self-awareness: The ability to recognise and understand one's own moods, emotions and drives and their effect on others.
- Self-regulation: The ability to control impulses and moods and to think before acting.
- Motivation: A passion to work that goes beyond financial reward or status.
- Empathy: The ability to understand the emotional makeup of others and to treat people according to their emotional reactions.
- Social skill: The ability to manage relationships and build networks.

Leadership can be said to be the ability to combine emotions and cognition. The leader needs both academic ability and a high level of competence at work, but the leader also needs wisdom, courage, justice and love in going about his or her work. It is the emotional intelligence that creates the difference between the average practitioner and the star performer or leader. Can emotional intelligence be learned? Goleman (2004) believes that it can:

> It is fortunate, then, that emotional intelligence can be learned. The process is not easy. It takes time and, most of all, commitment. But the benefits that come from having a well-developed emotional intelligence, both for the individual and for the organization, make it worth the effort. (p. 10)

Doctors must be capable of regularly taking responsibility for difficult decisions in situations of clinical complexity and uncertainty (General Medical Council, 2009). They are expected to offer leadership and to work with others to change systems when it is necessary for the benefit of patients. The same is true for the teacher who, to be an effective leader, needs to learn to adapt to the ever-changing world of education. This concept of adaptive leadership is discussed further below.

Geurin (2016), in his blog, has argued that to be successful as a teacher you must be both a manager and a leader. He accepts the importance of the teacher as a manager, but argues that the teacher as a leader is more important than a teacher as a manager:

- Leaders create a vision for learning. They communicate why the learning is important.
- Leaders build strong relationships with students and establish a positive learning culture.
- Leaders are inspiring and energizing. They have passion for what they are doing and it's contagious. For a manager, efficiency is more important than passion.
- A leader is careful to ensure that students don't feel disrespected, overlooked or misunderstood. When things go wrong, leaders help shoulder the blame.
- Leaders have honest and clear communication with students, including delivering hard truths when necessary.
- Leaders lead by example. They model the types of behaviours and mindsets that they want to see in others. Managers don't feel the need to set an example.
- An effective leader anticipates any needs and works to stay in front of problems. Managers react. Leaders prevent. Managers think about today; leaders think about tomorrow.

The management cycle

Views about management and leadership have developed. The concept of a management cycle, however, remains relevant. Think about this management cycle only as a guide to assist you in the different education tasks in which you may be engaged (Fig. 8.3).

Plan the teaching activity

What are the objectives? These may be, for example, to enhance the students' learning experience through the introduction of simulators, encourage students' teamwork skills through interprofessional education (IPE) or support students in difficulty through the provision of feedback.

Organise the activity

Consider who should be involved and how their collaboration can be ensured, the resources that are necessary and any associated cost. What time scale is envisioned? What problems may arise, and how can they be managed?

Implement the activity

Put the plan into action and provide the necessary leadership. It is likely that success will depend on good communication, appropriate delegation and effective teamwork.

Monitor the activity

Evaluate the results as part of a curriculum or course evaluation. This may lead to further modification of the activity and is also necessary for quality assurance.

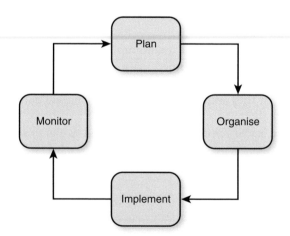

Figure 8.3 The management cycle

Management and leadership strategies

A range of models has been described for management and leadership in practice (McKimm and Lieff, 2013). Quinn et al. (1996) have described a management format based on the different roles of the manager (Fig. 8.4), defining eight managerial leadership roles and identifying three key competencies for each role.

Mentor role

- Understanding self and others
- Communicating effectively
- Developing subordinates

Facilitator role

- Building teams
- Using participative decision making
- Managing conflict

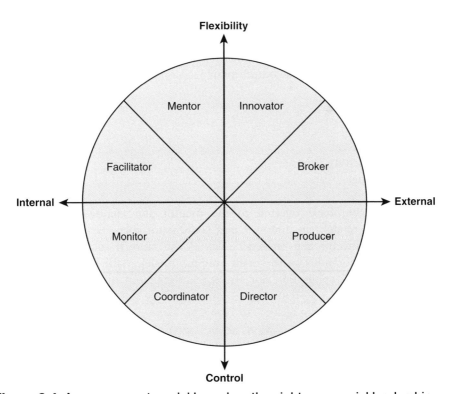

Figure 8.4 A management model based on the eight managerial leadership roles

(Quinn et al., 1996)

Monitor role

- Monitoring individual performance
- Managing collective performance
- Managing organisational performance

Co-ordinator role

- Managing projects
- Designing work
- Managing across functions

Director role

- Visioning, planning and goal setting
- Designing and organising
- Delegating effectively

Producer role

- Working productively
- Fostering a productive work environment
- Managing time and stress

Broker role

- Building and maintaining a power base
- Negotiating agreement and commitment
- Presenting ideas

Innovator role

- Living with change
- Thinking creatively
- Creating change

Quinn et al. (1996) have referred to the mentor and facilitator roles as the human relations model, the monitor and coordinator roles as the internal process model, the director and producer roles as the rational goal model, and the broker and innovator roles as the open systems model. With little modification, the Quinn model is appropriate for the teacher-manager and leader in medical education.

You can reach some general conclusions about how, as a teacher, you should approach your role as a manager or leader. The approach you adopt, however, should vary and be related to a specific context or situation at a particular point in time. Here are some guidelines:

- Make sure that there is a shared vision that is explicit and feasible for the education programme or approach under consideration. To be a successful teacher-manager or teacher-leader, you need a powerful and clear vision of what is to be achieved. This applies whether it is a medical school programme, an element of the programme such as special study modules (electives) or a single lecture.

- You may sometimes need to be authoritative and directive when exerting your authority, particularly if you are head of a school, a lead for a course or a chair of a committee, whereas at other times you may need to share the decision making and be supportive to those working with you and delegate work to them.
- As an effective manager or leader, you should emphasise the building of a consensus, listen carefully to the different views expressed and recognise the value of emotional congruence and harmony within the institution.
- Take steps to value your colleagues and their aspirations. This is particularly important in IPE, in which the culture of different professions can vary significantly.
- Collaboration with other teachers is of value and is essential in an integrated curriculum. Collaboration may be with individuals in your own department or speciality or with individuals from other departments. The ability to communicate and think together with others is important and allows you to take their wisdom and experience into consideration. Collaboration as an essential management skill is discussed further later.
- Like collaboration, how you negotiate and deal with conflict is an important management skill. As described below, dealing with conflict can have a positive as well as a negative aspect.
- Try to create a supportive environment within your department or medical school that encourages the achievement of the vision and objectives of the school.
- Serve as a role model for others by demonstrating personal values and a passion for the work while at the same time showing humility. Build trust and a commitment to others.
- As a teacher-manager or leader, be resilient. Inevitably there will be failures as well as successes. It is important to avoid personal burnout. This is discussed further in Chapter 10, the teacher as a professional.

Collaboration

Because of the great importance of collaboration as a management strategy, we explore this approach in more depth, including the factors that can lead to successful collaboration. There are many stakeholders in the education programme, as highlighted in Fig. 8.5. Effective collaboration between the stakeholders and working with them as a team is essential for the delivery of a successful education programme. Collaboration between subject experts, technologists and educationalists is important in the development of new teaching initiatives, as described in an evaluation of the UK and Teaching and Learning Technology Programme (Coopers and Lybrand, 1996):

> *Where we saw inspirational materials, we found that they had often emerged from a synthesis of computing, subject discipline and educational expertise. The presence of these three elements seemed to be a precondition for the production of materials that we could recognise as excellent.*

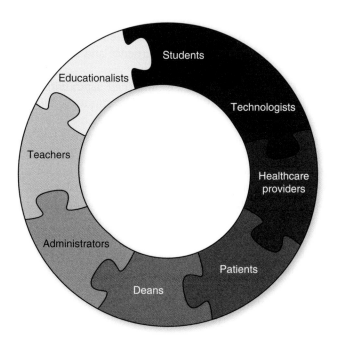

Figure 8.5 Collaboration and the stakeholders in medical education

If an integrated curriculum is to be delivered, collaboration is necessary and involves:

- Teachers responsible for other topics in the same phase of the curriculum. This is necessary for the implementation of the integrated programme in practice.
- Teachers responsible for other phases. Medical scientists and clinicians need to work together in the design and delivery of the education programme.
- Other healthcare professionals. IPE is on today's agenda in medical education and requires cooperation between the different healthcare professions.
- Recent graduates. They can provide a useful perspective on the education programme and where change may be desirable.

- Patients. They can have a useful input to planning the curriculum and can contribute to the teaching and learning programme.
- Students. As we describe later in the chapter, students should be engaged and have a voice in matters relating to the curriculum.

Collaboration may be difficult, particularly between teachers of different seniority and with different levels of power. As Woody Allen (1983) said in this context: "and the lion and the lamb shall lie down together, but the lamb won't get much sleep." Backer and Norman (1998) have suggested:

> ...collaboration has been defined as an unnatural act between non-consenting adults. We all say we want to collaborate, but what we really mean is that we want to continue doing things as we have always done them while others change to fit what we are doing. (p. 7)

The benefits of collaboration, however, are great. The poet Mattie Stepanek said, "Unity is strength ... when there is teamwork and collaboration, wonderful things can be achieved." Collaboration can lead to a more effective teaching and learning programme. It can also enhance your motivation and self-satisfaction as a teacher and provide additional recognition of your achievements. It can have other benefits too. In Dundee, we found that healthcare professionals who had not previously worked together professionally in clinical practice or research, after collaboration in the development of an educational programme on the cardiovascular system, went on to undertake productive joint research work.

Given the importance of collaboration for the teacher-manager, we will explore what works and what does not work. A report on collaboration and what makes it work by Mattessich et al. (2001) has reviewed and summarised the existing research literature on factors that influence the success of collaboration:

The success of a collaboration can be determined by the following equation:

Collaboration = (Vision × sharing strategies × learning experience)/(negative mindset)

Factors related to the **vision** that influence the success of a collaboration include:

- A vision with concrete collaborative goals
- An agreed and shared vision
- A unique purpose that can be achieved through the collaboration

According to Kotter (1996, p. 72), a good change vision should be "imaginable, flexible, feasible, desirable, focused and communicable."

In the development of a **sharing strategy**, communication using a common vocabulary is important. The move to outcome-based education with clearly defined learning outcomes provides such a vocabulary for education initiatives. Determination of the learning outcomes required for entrustable professional activities (EPAs) also provides a focus (see Chapter 5).

An examination of the curriculum maps for the different healthcare professions, such as medicine and nursing, can identify areas of overlap and is a good starting point for IPE. Concept maps can be used in the same way to support IPE (Daley et al., 2016).

If a collaboration is to be successful it is important that it has as its aim the creation of **meaningful learning experiences**. These need to be meaningful for all the collaborators.

A **negative mindset** with regard to possible collaboration may need to be overcome. Leonard and Leonard (2003) have referred to "… persisting negative mindsets about the actual desirability of shared work and the resistance to moving beyond the traditional models of teacher relationships."

Arguments against collaboration that need to be countered are that collaboration takes too much time, collaboration destroys individual characteristics and collaboration removes our competitiveness. Fragmented visions with socially embedded knowledge structure and framework constraints also need to be addressed. There may also be a concern about personality conflicts, with a wide diversity of opinion. However, such differences and diversity of opinion can be an advantage. John-Steiner (2006) has suggested that "collaboration thrives on diversity of perspectives and on constructive dialogue between individuals negotiating their differences while creating their shared voice and vision."

If you are to deliver an excellent education programme, your challenge is to develop meaningful new collaborations that supersede the traditional silos in which education in healthcare professions operate. These silos currently operate in the different healthcare professions (e.g. medicine, nursing, dentistry and pharmacy), in the different phases of medical education (e.g. undergraduate, postgraduate and continuing), and within medicine itself across the different disciplines (including the basic science/clinical divide). Collaborations crossing these divides, facilitated by the teacher as a manager-leader, can result in a richer, more effective education programme and may even address education challenges not yet overcome.

Negotiation and conflict

Negotiation is another important management strategy that merits particular consideration. Increasing demands placed on teachers from teaching, research, clinical work and administrative activities can be stressful and may result in tensions and conflicts. There may be a clash of opposing ideas, disagreements or differences of views between members of staff. This may result from staff defending their own subject when asked to change the focus of their teaching in line with redefined learning outcomes or from requests to reduce the input of their subject to the curriculum. Conflicts may also result from staff in the same department or teaching unit having different education philosophies and opposing ideas about the education strategies to be adopted from the curricular options, as described in Chapter 5.

Conflict is not necessarily bad. As we have suggested, managed appropriately, it can lead to a constructive sharing of different views, with an improved outcome for the educational programme. Improved ideas can develop through active debate and argument with problems in the system identified. Unfortunately, however, this may not happen, and the results may be antagonism and hostility.

The best resolution to a conflict is one where both parties appear to win and the problems responsible for the conflict are solved. This is not easy to achieve, however, and short-term solutions may need to be adopted. Two longer-term solutions with win-win positions for those concerned are described below:

Agree on a common goal for the education programme rather than pursue individual interests

It may be possible to persuade all concerned to work together and to rise above the problem to create a more authentic curriculum, where the objective is to qualify doctors who have the capabilities necessary to meet the needs of the patients they will serve. An example of such a win-win situation was seen in the Dundee curriculum in the 1970s. There was understandable and not unexpected opposition by some teachers to the proposal to replace some lectures with self-learning resources to be made available in a newly established learning resource centre. At the same time, there was a recognition that the increased number of students admitted to the medical school could not all be accommodated for their clinical training at the Ninewells Teaching Hospital. Excellent clinical facilities were available at hospitals in Perth and Stracathro, about twenty miles away to the east and west of Dundee. Although all teachers believed it was desirable, it was not possible for students in the third year of a 5-year curriculum to take advantage of these opportunities while at the same time attending lectures in Dundee. The answer, to which everyone agreed, was to replace some of the lectures with independent learning resources. An agreed common goal for all concerned was to make possible additional clinical placements out of Dundee, and this was feasible only with the replacement of some lectures in Dundee with other learning resources – a win-win situation.

Identify a solution that meets the different aspirations of all concerned

The number of hours allocated to the learning of anatomy in the early years of the course in Dundee medical school was significantly reduced. The anatomists, who cared for their subject and its future, raised serious objections. A major concern was that students with a possible interest in the subject would have insufficient time to develop this interest and would be less likely to take up a career later as an anatomist.

The situation was resolved by creating special study modules in anatomy in the curriculum, which proved attractive and allowed some students to spend an extended period studying the subject. At the same time, the core anatomy that all students were expected to master was identified and, with the spiral curriculum, students revisited the subject in the later years. This vertical integration was ensured through a portfolio assessment in the final examination, in which basic scientists as well as clinicians served as examiners. The result of these initiatives was that the anatomists no longer opposed the reduction of hours in the early years because their key aspirations for the subject were met. Some students with a particular interest in the subject had an opportunity to study anatomy in more depth, and other students were required to master a core extending into the later years of the course. The aspirations of other teachers and the curriculum developers were also met.

Organising and participating in meetings

Meetings are a common management tool, and almost certainly some of your time will be spent attending meetings. These may be curriculum or course committees, assessment committees, selection committees, appointment committees or committees responsible for an aspect of the school's programme, such as a fitness to practice committee. A committee may be set up with a limited life span to tackle a specific problem such as cheating by students or to prepare for a special event such as a school's anniversary.

If properly run, a committee can successfully achieve its objectives and serve as a useful means of communication and decision making for the education programme. If poorly run, it can be frustrating and a waste of time.

If you are a member of a committee, here are some suggestions:

- Prepare for the meeting, and read the relevant papers.
- Arrive on time.
- Minimise the chance of interruptions from phone calls or emails during the meeting.
- Present your own views on the topic succinctly, and be constructive.
- Allow others to present their view without interrupting.
- Accept the chairperson's authority and decisions.
- Note any actions that you have been asked to undertake, and complete these within the allocated time frame.
- Check the meeting minutes when circulated, and let the chair or secretary know if you disagree with any points.

If you are chairing a committee meeting, here are some guidelines:

- Consider what you wish the meeting to achieve and, if necessary, contact individual members of the committee in advance to prepare yourself.
- Ensure that all members are briefed in advance with an agenda and appropriate background papers.

- Ensure that the key persons will be present at the meeting.
- Check that appropriate audiovisual facilities are available, if required.
- If the meeting is to be recorded, ensure that participants are aware of this.
- Establish the meeting protocol at the outset, such as whether questions will be taken at any time or at the end of an item.
- Manage time, and ensure that priority is given to areas where key decisions are required.
- Give all members of the committee an opportunity to speak, and listen to their views and concerns.
- At the end of the meeting, summarise the views expressed, the decisions taken and any follow-up actions.
- Produce a record of the meeting, highlighting the agreed decisions, actions to be taken, by whom and by what date.

Increasingly, meetings are held online using web conferencing or Skype. This may present additional challenges for the chair and the participants, especially if several countries and time zones are involved. Increased concentration may be needed, particularly if the Internet connection is less than ideal or if a participant is difficult to hear; it is advisable to limit the length of the meeting to no more than 1 hour unless a break is scheduled. Although there are obvious advantages in terms of cost and convenience, online meetings may be less suitable than face-to-face meetings for in-depth discussions on a topic. In addition to the suggestions noted for face-to-face meetings, the following are important considerations for online meetings:

- When selecting a time for the meeting, take account of the time zone(s) of participants and select one that suits the majority, or the least indispensable participant(s).
- Ensure that participants receive the link to join the meeting in good time and that it is clear in which time zone the meeting will take place. Send the link again a few hours before the meeting is due to start as a gentle reminder. Suggesting some basic instructions on how to use the platform is also helpful.
- Don't leave it to the last minute to log in to your meeting platform. Overnight updates to software may cause access delays, raising stress levels.
- Ask participants to log in a few minutes before the allotted start time to minimise potential delays.
- A welcome slide and some music may reassure participants that their video and audio are working.
- Run through the essentials for those who might be new to use of the platform, such as muting microphones to avoid feedback, the potential advantage of using a head set, using the chat box if one exists and clicking the raised hand icon to ask a question.
- Remind participants that if they have a webcam, they are on view throughout the meeting, and warn them if you intend to record the session.

Adaptive leadership

Earlier we suggested that the changing emphasis on leadership embraces the concept of the adaptive leader. A key ability of a leader is to be able to respond to a complex and, in some cases, intractable challenge facing education (Mennin, 2013; Mennin et al., 2016). Traditionally, the leader was seen as the expert in change, like the orchestra conductor or the general in the army, with everyone else looking to the leader for direction. In today's environment in medical education, leadership and your role as a teacher-leader is taken out into the real and complex world of implementing the curriculum when the position changes. As noted by Mennin et al. (2016):

> *Because you are working in complex environments, with many demands and tight constraints, you have to integrate your teaching and leadership into your day-to-day work, just as your students and staff do. When your teaching takes place out of the classroom and into the community or institutions where care is delivered, you immediately encounter uncertainty. When your organization or community goes through a significant change, you lose your ability to set and meet expectations. Performance in authentic learning settings becomes much more emergent – more flexible, sensitive, and responsive leadership and teaching is necessary, as rigid approaches are less likely to succeed. (p. 15)*

In the AMEE Essential Skills in Medical Education course, Mennin et al. (2016) described the following:

- The need for a teacher leader to recognise that only some issues can be solved with existing resources and knowhow.
- The need to recognise more complex issues that cannot be easily solved and require adaptive action (as defined below).
- The importance of collaborating across disciplines, organisations and social boundaries and how to negotiate conflict to achieve shared interests.
- The importance of maintaining flexibility and making continual adjustments as necessary.
- Recognition of results that are "excellent enough".

Mennin et al. (2016) have suggested that the adaptive leader will change disagreement into shared exploration, defensiveness into self-reflection, assumptions into questions and judgement into curiosity.

In their book *Adaptive Action: Leveraging Uncertainty in Your Organization*, Eoyang and Holladay (2013) have defined adaptive action as "an elegant and powerful method for engaging with dynamical change in an ever-emerging, always self-organizing world" (p. 30) and suggested that we should ask ourselves the following questions:

- *What?* What do we see when looking around our environment? What has changed, and what has remained the same? What are the trends and emerging patterns? What can we learn from past experiences?
- *So what?* What surprises you about your observations, and what do they mean to you and to other stakeholders? Are there opportunities or a desire to change existing patterns and to create new ones?
- *Now what?* What actions should we take, individually and collectively? What outcomes might we expect? What data should we collect to evaluate the outcomes in this iterative process?

The single biggest failure of leadership is to treat adaptive challenges like technical problems (Heifetz and Linsky, 2002). Technical problems are easy to identify, often lend themselves to quick and easy (cut and dried) solutions and often can be solved by an authority or expert. Examples of technical problems in medical education are the redesign of an objective structured clinical examination (OSCE) to include an assessment of skills in prescribing, scheduling time in the programme to discuss with students issues relating to career choice and the requirement to assess students' work in an elective or student-selected component in the curriculum. The required change in a "technical problem" can usually be clearly defined and specified and a solution proposed which will be generally acceptable and can be implemented fairly quickly.

In contrast, adaptive challenges are difficult to identify and easy to deny, require changes in values, beliefs, roles, relationships and approaches to work and require change not just in one area but across the organisation. Examples of adaptive challenges are attempts to introduce IPE with collaboration between different healthcare professionals, the adoption of an outcome-based model of education with a move away from a time-based to a standard-based approach and a change from an emphasis on students' acquisition of knowledge to their knowing how to access sources of knowledge and evaluate them. There may be reluctance in acknowledging these adaptive challenges, and solutions may require new approaches to the curriculum and may take some time to implement.

Student engagement

In many schools, students are increasingly engaged with matters relating to the curriculum. Students are considered not just as consumers but as partners in the learning process. In the ASPIRE-to-Excellence initiative (www.aspire-to-excellence.org), schools are recognised for excellence in their education programme, and student engagement is one of the categories in which schools can elect to be assessed. Students may be engaged in different ways, each with different management and leadership implications. These include:

- Students are involved in governance decisions and have representation on key committees.
- Students are involved in decisions about staff appointments and promotions.

- Peer assessment contributes to the assessment programme.
- Students contribute to the teaching programme through peer-to-peer learning.
- Students have an impact on the curriculum through membership on curriculum committees.
- Students are engaged in planning their own learning.

Student engagement is discussed further in Chapter 4.

Change in medical education as a management and leadership challenge

Effective management is essential if schools are to cope with and respond to change, whether the change arises from internal rearrangements in the medical school or institution or from external factors. Debra Klamen, an educator deeply involved in improving medical education at the Southern Illinois University School of Medicine, highlights in Box 8.2 the importance of the teacher as a change agent.

Change is now an integral function of organisational life and education (Olver, 1996). Olver has suggested that "Rather than viewing equilibrium as the norm, change and transition are more typical of contemporary life." Change is more likely to be maintained as a characteristic of education than stability.

The need for change in medical education was identified in the *Lancet* report, "*Health professionals for a new century: Transforming education to strengthen health systems in an interdependent world*" (Frenk et al., 2010): "Professional education has not kept pace with these challenges, largely because of fragmented, outdated, and static curricula that produce ill-equipped graduates."

Box 8.2 The teacher as a change agent[a]

If I had to sum it up, I would describe my teaching role in medical education to be that of a change agent. My job as a curricular dean and chair of a department of medical education automatically puts me in more usual teaching roles, such as curriculum planner and developer, assessor, and mentor/role model. However I believe all of these can be summed up in the same manner. What I do is see *potential* and then develop it, whether that be in curricula, assessments, or individual students and faculty. Seeing students bloom into their best possible versions of themselves, and knowing I had a part of that, really makes my job a labor of love. Seeing young faculty members new to medical education come into the school and thrive is a thrill. The same is true of watching new and innovative assessment tools and methodology, or even whole curricula, come into being, often after many hours of hard work and negotiation, and make the gray hairs all worthwhile. I can think of no position which would be more valuable and fulfilling to me than that in which I have been honored to take part.

---

[a]*Debra Klamen, Senior Associate Dean for Education and Curriculum, Professor and Chair, Department of Medical Education, Southern Illinois University School of Medicine, Springfield, Illinois, USA.*

Change in medical education is difficult. Indeed, it has been suggested that it is easier to move a cemetery than to change a curriculum. Change was recognised to be difficult in the report *Australian Medical Education and Workforce into the 21ˢᵗ Century* (Committee of Inquiry into Medical Education and Medical Workforce, 1988):

> *The Committee recognises that, if it were given the task of designing a medical education system for Australia de novo, it might well choose to take quite different approaches. It would certainly wish to remove some of the discontinuities in the system. It accepts, with some regret, that to redesign the entire system is not feasible for many reasons, historical, financial and political.*

With regard to change in medical education, there is a need to think out of the box, as described by Hess (2010):

> *...repeated attempts to improve a fundamentally outdated outmoded structure. Rather than explore and develop new structures, reformers pour their faith and resources into making the existing structure more effective. They tend to color safely within the lines—largely because those lines are so taken for granted that would-be reformers don't realise there is an alternative. (p. 10)*

As Henry Miller (1966), Dean of Medicine at the University of Newcastle, UK, has suggested, all teachers have a responsibility for change:

> *It is useful occasionally to take a fresh look at a situation which we who are busily occupied in its day-to-day activities are often inclined to regard as immutable. In fact, of course, the present situation presents nothing more than a stage in an untidy historical process to which each generation must make its contribution, and effective change depends on continuing examination and criticism.*

Good ideas for change in medical education may stagnate in a curriculum bureaucracy if this is committed to maintaining the status quo. What is seen as disruptive innovation is at best given only passing attention and at worst is ignored. Sclerotic bureaucracy, territorial warfare, incompetence and ignorance about the process have been enemies of change in education (Harden, 1998). Effective leadership is essential if the obstacles to change are to be overcome.

As a teacher, you should be a change maker and not simply a recipient of change. You should not be isolated from change in the medical education programme but should be part of it. Many of the 3,500 abstracts submitted for the AMEE 2017 Conference in Helsinki described innovations and changes in medical education brought about by practising teachers who were able to innovate and bring about change in their own institution. Your participation in the change process cannot

Table 8.1 Guidelines for managing change

1. Establish the need or benefit for the change. This must be shared by all on whom the change will have an impact.
2. Look at the sources of power to act or to move the change forward and the forces which might hinder it.
3. Design the innovation, taking into account its feasibility, the resources needed, appropriate time scale and those involved in the change.
4. Consult widely with all those affected by the change.
5. Publicize the change widely, taking feedback with a view to amending the proposal.
6. Agree on detailed plans to implement the change with those concerned.
7. Implement the proposals using an appropriate implementation.
8. Provide support in dealing with difficulties and maintaining the change.
9. Modify the plans, redesigning the system in the light of experience.
10. Evaluate the outcomes.

Adapted from Gale, R., Grant, J. 1997. Managing change in a medical context: Guidelines for action, AMEE Medical Education Guide No. 10. Med Teach. 19(4), 239–249.

only be effective in bringing about change, but can also be satisfying for you and can help prevent burnout.

Hodgins (2005) has challenged us to think of our role in bringing about change:

> This future is ours for the choosing if we can muster the courage to ignite the transformation from vision to reality by simply imagining that this bright future is now possible and begin shaping its design and implementation. The trick is that it will take all of us to imagine, design and build. If you can imagine this previously impossible dream now, you are already part of the solution. (p. 243–4)

Gale and Grant (1997) described in AMEE Guide No. 10 strategies that can help you cope with change (Table 8.1). These strategies have been thoroughly tested, are firmly rooted in practice and have been found to work in a broad range of contexts.

Innovation in medical education

As a manager and leader, the teacher is concerned with innovation. In Chapter 9, as an aspect of scholarship, we describe the teacher as a researcher and innovator. The teacher may personally set an example of innovation by introducing into the curriculum new approaches to teaching, learning and assessment. More importantly, however, the teacher as a manager and leader creates within the school a culture of innovation, in which teachers are empowered to innovate in pursuit of a better educational experience for their students. There is a push for **transformation and transformative change** in medical education (Frenk et al., 2010). A focus on **innovation** may be less threatening, as described by Walsh (2017), a middle school principal:

> A culture of innovation suggests to me a culture of continuous improvement. It's not the destination, but the journey...If I am in a good

"place", transforming makes me feel apprehensive....why transform? I am in good shape! However, if I am in a good place, innovating enlivens me! it challenges me to take something good and make it better! I add to some total universal value in innovating. In transforming, I feel called to move away from that "thing" that was seemingly effective. Now why would anyone want to do that?

Quinn (2017) has argued that "Innovation is about creating an environment where people can be exposed to different concepts, interact productively, experiment safely and be allowed time to reflect."

The innovation can address any aspect of the teacher's role – how we communicate information, how we facilitate learning, how we design and implement a curriculum, including the learning outcomes and the approaches to teaching, learning and assessment, and the approaches we adopt to role modelling. The aim may be to solve a problem, to provide a better experience for students, to be more productive and efficient or to lower cost.

As teachers, we have a number of roles in innovation, as described by Kelly and Littman (2008) in their book *The Ten Faces of Innovation*:

- An anthropologist – observes human behaviour and brings new insight.
- An experimenter – prototypes new ideas, learning by trial and error.
- A cross-pollinator – translates values from other fields.
- A hurdler – overcomes obstacles in path to innovation.
- A collaborator – brings collaborators together to work on solutions.
- A set designer – creates a stage on which innovation can happen.
- The caregiver – understands students' needs and looks after them.
- A storyteller – communicates the value of innovation.
- The experience architect – designs compelling experiences.
- A director – gathers together staff and sparks their creativity.

Which of these roles do you fulfil?

Medical education, perhaps more than any other professional education, is in a permanent state of change, in which innovation is the rule rather than the exception. All the roles of the teacher as described in this text have witnessed major changes since the late 1990s. Based on a literature review and an analysis of the factors leading to the successful adoption of the OSCE in South African medical schools, Lazarus and Harden (1985) have provided a checklist of factors facilitating the adoption of an innovation (Table 8.2). The attributes of a successful innovation were described by Schneider (2014) as:

- Perceived significance – the idea seems significant.
- Philosophical compatibility – the idea is reasonable and appropriate for use, not just the wish of outsiders.
- Occupational realism – the idea must be practical and easy to use.

Table 8.2 Checklist of factors facilitating the change process

Factor	Features
Attributes of the innovation	Relevance
	Compatibility
	Adaptability
	Advantageousness
	Simplicity
	Available resources
	"Triability"
	Observability
The environment	Active openness
	Freedom to innovate
	Information linkage
	Leadership
	Power
The potential user	Participation
	Social network
	Informal personal contact
	Reference group identification
	Ownership of innovation
	Opinion leader
Method of dissemination	Resources available
	Workshops and seminar
	Lectures
	Hands-on experience
	Informal discussions
	Committees
	User participation

Adapted from Lazarus, J., Harden, R.M. 1985. The innovative process in medical education. Med Teach. 7(314), 333–342.

- Transportability – simple principles can be easily implemented and can be adopted for different situations.

We have described how these contributed to the wide adoption of the OSCE (Harden et al., 2016). The bottleneck to change in medical education, it can be argued, is not a lack of innovative ideas but rather an understanding of the role of the innovative process and the factors that facilitate it (Lazarus and Harden, 1985).

Cost of medical education

Cost may be a factor in management and leadership decisions. Educational decisions are usually made on the basis of a desire to improve (or maintain) the quality of the education delivered. They may be made on the basis of personal experiences, on prejudices or on research as to what works and what does not work, on the students' examination performances or progress after qualification, and on student or staff satisfaction and acceptance decisions. Cost is seldom taken into consideration and there are few publications on the topic (Walsh, 2014). The cost associated with the education programme, however, is particularly important at a time of financial constraint, when more is expected of the teacher, with fewer resources. Return on investment must also be considered because medical education interventions have an impact on medical practice for decades to come.

Although questions regarding cost are appropriate, they are seldom asked with regard to education decisions, such as the replacement of lectures with the use of learning resource materials, the use of an OSCE as an assessment tool or a move from a model where students are admitted to medical school directly from school to one where there is graduate entry, students having completed another college degree. The graduate entry approach offers a significantly more expensive option, with a longer overall education programme and graduates who are older when they qualify, with fewer years to practise medicine before they retire. In discussions about a graduate versus direct from school entry to medicine, one seldom hears the question of cost discussed.

One reason that cost has been relatively ignored is that it is difficult to calculate or estimate in the educational context. This can be illustrated in the case of the OSCE, for which a number of studies have examined costs (Harden et al., 2016). The situation is complex, however, and the cost will vary considerably. It depends, for example, on whether real patients or simulated patients are used and, if simulated patients, whether they are trained volunteers claiming only travel expenses or professional simulated patients who are paid for contributing. The question also to be asked in relation to the cost of the OSCE is whether there is another, less expensive tool available that assesses the student's clinical competence equally well and identifies students who do not have the required clinical knowledge, skills and attitudes. Assessment of the cost is also difficult when it comes to taking into account the implications of wrong decisions – passing students who should fail and failing students who should pass. The situation is further complicated by the fact that the value of the OSCE approach lies not just as an assessment tool; its value as an aid to learning must also be factored into the cost estimate. With the move to assessment *for* learning, as described in Chapter 6, this is important.

Financial constraints and consideration of costs of medical education present a challenge but can, on occasion, even be helpful in forcing us to be more creative and to think about resources in different ways (Calvo and Miles, 2012).

Teacher manager/leader, expert or master?

Teacher manager/leader

The teacher reflects on her or his role as a manager and leader in particular as it relates to personal teaching responsibilities. The teacher looks at his or her day-to-day activities, such as attending meetings and collaborating with colleagues, and considers how these could be more effective and efficient.

Expert manager/leader

The expert manager/leader will have developed skills through reading and/or participation in courses on the subject. He or she is likely to have specified management or leadership responsibilities in her or his own institution and will have applied appropriate strategies in this context.

Master manager/leader

The master manager/leader is likely to have studied management and leadership in more depth and may have done research in this area. He or she is recognised nationally and perhaps internationally for his or her expertise in the area. He or she may have contributed to courses or publications on the topic.

Take-home messages

1. A good teacher is a skilled manager and leader. There are few things you can do successfully in medical education without management and leadership skills. You may not like to think of yourself as a manager or leader but, as a teacher, you have an important management and leadership role to play in your school's education programme. This responsibility can be an informal as well as a formal one.
2. Your role as teacher manager/leader is key at a time of significant change in medical education.
3. As a teacher, you need to be at the same time a leader and a follower, a dreamer and a doer.
4. The implementation of an education programme relies on collaboration and teachers working as members of an education team, negotiating and resolving any conflicts or differences of opinion as they occur.
5. The optimum management or leadership strategy will depend on the context in which you operate and will vary with time.

Consider

- Reflect on your own role as a manager or leader with regard to your own personal activities, the teaching programme for which you are responsible and the overall curriculum and medical school or institution.

- Where do you stand with regard to Quinn's roles of a manager (page 205)?
- Do you have the leadership skills as set out by Geurin (page 203)?
- Is there anything you would do differently or strategies that you would emphasise more relating to collaborating, negotiating, participating in meetings and engaging students?
- Are you an "adaptive" manager and leader (page 214)?

Explore further

Allen, W., 1983. Without Feathers. Ballantine Books, New York.
Backer, T.E., Norman, A., 1998. Best practices in multicultural coalitions: Phase 1 report to the California Endowment. Human Interaction Research Institute, Encino, California.
Barth, R.S., 2001. Teacher leader. Phi Delta Kappan. 82 (6).
Bates, J., Frost, H., Schrewe, B., et al., 2011. Distributed Education and Distance Learning in Postgraduate Medical Education. The Future of Medical Education in Canada. The Association of Faculties of Medicine of Canada (AFMC), Ottawa, Canada.
Bin Abdulrahman, K.A., Gibbs, T., 2016. Recognising leadership and management within the medical school. In: Bin Abdulrahman, K.A., Mennin, S., Harden, R.M., et al. (Eds.). Routledge International Handbook of Medical Education. Routledge, London, (Chapter 22).
Calvo, N., Miles, K.H., 2012. Turning crisis into opportunity. Educ. Lead. 69 (4), 19–23.
Committee of Inquiry into Medical Education and Medical Workforce, 1988. Australian Medical Education and Workforce into the 21st Century. Australian Government Publishing Service, Canberra, Australia.
Coopers & Lybrand, Institute of Education, Tavistock Institute, 1996. Evaluation of the teaching and learning technology programme (TLTP). Active Learning. 5, 60–63.
Daley, B.J., Durning, S.J., Torre, D.M. 2016. Using concept maps to create meaningful learning in medical education. MedEdPublish. 5 (1). Available at: https://www.mededpublish.org. https://doi.org/10.15694/mep.2016.000019
Davis, M.H., Harden, R.M., 2002. Leadership in education and the strategy of the dolphin. Med. Teach. 24 (6), 581–582.
Eoyang, G.H., Holladay, R.J., 2013. Adaptive Action: Leveraging Uncertainty in Your Organization. Stanford University Press, Redwood City, CA.
Frenk, J., Chen, L., Bhutta, Z.A., et al., 2010. Health professionals for a new century: Transforming education to strengthen health systems in an interdependent world. Lancet. 376 (9756), 1923–1958.
Gale, R., Grant, J., 1997. Managing change in a medical context: Guidelines for action, AMEE Medical Education Guide No. 10. Med. Teach. 19 (4), 239–249.
General Medical Council, 2009. Tomorrow's Doctors: Outcomes and standards for under graduate medical education. General Medical Council, London.
Geurin, D. 2016. 7 Reasons 'Classroom Leadership' Is Better Than 'Classroom Management.' http://www.davidgeurin.com/2016/12/7-reasons-classroom-leadership-is.html.
Goleman, D., 1998. Working with Emotional Intelligence. Bloomsbury, London, p. 185.
Goleman, D., 2004. What makes a leader? Harv. Bus. Rev. 1–11.
Harden, R.M., 1998. Change – building windmills not walls. Med. Teach. 20 (3), 189–191.
Harden, R.M., 2008. E-learning – caged bird or soaring eagle? Med. Teach. 30 (1), 1–4.
Harden, R.M., Crosby, J.R., 2000. The good teacher is more than a lecturer—the twelve roles of the teacher: Guide No 20. Med. Teach. 22 (4), 334–347.
Harden, R.M., Lilley, P.M., Patricio, M.F., 2016. The Definitive Guide to the OSCE. Elsevier, London.
Heifetz, R., Linsky, M., 2002. Leadership on the Line: Staying Alive Through the Dangers of Leading. Harvard Business Review Press, Boston.

Hess, F.M., 2010. The Same Thing Over and Over – How School Reformers Get Stuck in Yesterday's Ideas. Harvard University Press, Cambridge, MA.

Hess, F.M., 2015. Bursting out of the teacher's cage. Kappan. 96 (7), 58–63.

Hodgins, W., 2005. Into the Future of meLearning: Every one learning…imagine if the impossible isn't! In: Masie, E. (Ed.), Learning: Rants, Raves and Reflections. Pfeiffer, USA.

John-Steiner, V., 2006. Creative Collaboration. Oxford University Press, New York.

Kelley, T., Littman, J., 2008. The Ten Faces of Innovation. Profile Books, London.

Kotter, J.P., 1990. A Force for Change: How Leadership Differs from Management. Free Press, New York.

Kotter, J.P., 1996. Leading Change. Harvard Business Press, Cambridge, MA.

Lazarus, J., Harden, R.M., 1985. The innovative process in medical education. Med. Teach. 7 (314), 333–342.

Leonard, L., Leonard, P., 2003. The continuing trouble with collaboration: Teachers talk. Curr Issues Educ. 6 (15). Retrieved from http://cie.asu.edu/ojs/index.php/cieatasu/article/view/1615

Lynch, D., Kordis, P.L., 1988. Strategy of the Dolphin: Winning Elegantly by Coping Powerfully in a World of Turbulent Change. Hutchinson Business Books, London.

Maddux, C.D., 2002. Information technology in education: The critical lack of principled leadership. Educ. Tech. 42 (3), 41–50.

Mattessich, P.W., Murray-Close, M., Monsey, B.R., 2001. Collaboration: What Makes It Work, second ed. Turner Publishing, Nashville.

McKimm, J., Lieff, S.J., 2013. Medical education leadership. In: Dent, J.A., Harden, R.M. (Eds.), A Practical Guide for Medical Teachers, fourth ed. Elsevier, London, (Chapter 42).

Mennin, S., 2013. Health professions education: complexity, teaching and learning. In: Sturmberg, J.P., Martin, C. (Eds.), Handbook of Systems and Complexity in Health Springer. Heidelberg, Germany, pp. 755–766.

Mennin, S., Eoyang, G., Nations, M., 2016. Leadership in Medical Education: Future of the Health Professions Workforce. Human Systems Dynamics Institute, Circle Pines, MN.

Miller, H., 1966. Fifty years after Flexner. Lancet. 288 (7465), 647–654.

Olver, P., 1996. The Management of Educational Change: A Case Study Approach. Arena, Hants, UK.

Quinn, R.E., Faerman, S.R., Thompson, M.P., et al., 1996. Becoming a Master Manager: A Competency Framework. John Wiley, New York.

Schneider, J., 2014. Closing the gap…between university and schoolhouse. Kappan. 96 (1), 30–35.

Walsh, B. 2017, March 31. Re: Creating a culture of innovation vs a transformation [blog comment]. Katie Martin blog. https://katiemartin.com/2015/06/10/creating-a-culture-of-innovation-vs-a-transformation.

Walsh, K., 2014. Cost and value in medical education: The role of discounting. J. Biomed. Res. 28 (5), 337–338.

Wass, V., Southgate, L., 2017. Doctors Without Borders. Acad. Med. 92 (4), 441–443.

Chapter 9

The teacher as a scholar and researcher

Originality is the essence of true scholarship. Creativity is the soul of the true scholar.

Nnamdi Azikiwe

The demonstration of scholarship highlights the contribution made by the teacher to education.

- Every teacher can be a scholar
- Why a teacher-scholar?
- Demonstration of scholarship
- The reflective teacher
- Making evidence-informed decisions
  - Rational thinking and the use of evidence and judgement in teaching
  - What evidence-informed teaching means in practice
  - Finding evidence relating to your practice
  - Reviewing the evidence available
- The teacher as an innovator
  - The role of the teacher
  - The innovation ladder
- The teacher as a researcher
  - Action research
  - Scholarship principles and research
  - Advantages of the teacher as a researcher
  - Potential limitations of the teacher as a researcher
- The teacher as a communicator about their work
  - Sharing your work as a teacher
  - Communication options
  - Writing for publication
- Confronting broader issues in medical education
- Scholarship – a contested concept
- The teacher-scholar, the expert teacher-scholar and the master teacher-scholar
- Take-home messages
- Consider
- Explore further

Every teacher can be a scholar

A teacher is not simply a technician with the skills necessary to deliver a lecture, facilitate a small group or plan an examination. We have described in earlier chapters your role as an information provider, facilitator, curriculum planner, assessor, role model, manager and leader. The teacher, however, is also a scholar, and you can demonstrate scholarship as a teacher in all these roles (Fig. 9.1). Scholarship is sometimes equated with research, with this demonstrated in terms of papers published in peer-reviewed journals. A report from the Canadian Association for Medical Education (CAME) (Van Melle et al., 2012) has broadened the definition of scholarship to include innovation:

> *Education Scholarship is an umbrella term which can encompass both research and innovation in health professions education. Quality in education scholarship is attained through work that is peer-reviewed, publicly disseminated and provides a platform that others can build on. (p. iv)*

The distinction was made in the CAME report between the "teacher" and the "scholarly teacher." We argue that this is not a binary divide, and that you cannot divorce scholarship from the practice of teaching. All teachers have a responsibility to embed and integrate an element of scholarship into their work as a teacher. Your level of engagement and participation in your scholarly role will vary, as does your engagement with other roles. The degree to which you are able to do so will vary with the time

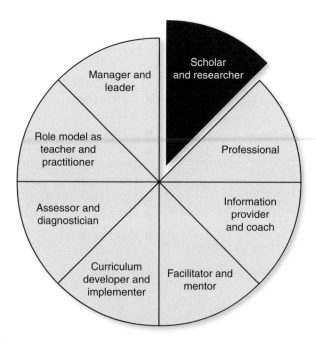

Figure 9.1 The role of the teacher as a scholar

you have available and your expertise. Depending on your interests and activities, you may demonstrate scholarship in different ways. As we define later, not all teachers will be expert or master scholars, but all teachers can be scholars. We describe in this chapter the activities that can contribute to your scholarly role.

Scholarship is not the prerogative of small elite bands of teachers who are education specialists and who have committed most of their time to teaching. Scholarship is not "an esoteric appendix"; rather, scholarship is at the very heart of teaching (Boyer, 1990). Every teacher can be a scholar, as described by Catriona Bell, an experienced clinical teacher and veterinary education researcher (Box 9.1) and from a different perspective, Brian Bailey, an experienced teacher (Box 9.2).

The existence of a scholarship of teaching was highlighted 3 decades ago by Boyer (1990). He argued that there has been too narrow a definition of scholarship in universities around basic research-based activities and publications and advocated the need for a broader definition of scholarship. He went on to describe scholarship in a way that referred to the work of the faculty as four separate yet overlapping functions:

- The scholarship of discovery – the advancement of knowledge through research, including educational research.
- The scholarship of integration – making connections across the disciplines and bringing new insight to bear on original research.

Box 9.1 Becoming a scholar[a]

My role as a teacher has evolved greatly as my career has developed from being a 'vet in mixed practice' who supervised student placements, to a Lecturer in Farm Animal Medicine, and then to my current role as a Senior Lecturer in Veterinary Education. A key aspect of my early roles included designing and delivering practical skills teaching for veterinary students. This was often delivered in challenging teaching spaces and required careful supervision to maintain the safety of the students, the client and the potentially dangerous patient (e.g. examining a lame bull with a group of eight students in a freezing cold barn). However, witnessing a 'lightbulb moment' on a student's face (e.g. when finally identifying a cow's ovary during a rectal palpation examination!) is still one of the most rewarding aspects of my job.

In recent years my role as a teacher has adapted to become a collaborator, curriculum designer, coordinator, scholar, negotiator and mentor in order to lead our school's Faculty Development Programme. Our small team aims to inspire and support colleagues to optimize their teaching and assessment practices through 'engagement with' and 'reflection on' educational Continuing Professional Development and literature, and we are proud of the enthusiastic Community of Practice that has developed.

[a]Catriona Bell, Reader in Veterinary Education, Royal (Dick) School of Veterinary Studies, University of Edinburgh, Edinburgh, UK.

Box 9.2 Reflecting on teaching[a]

Over the years, as a teacher and researcher, my abiding passions have been music and problem-based learning. Reflecting on the reasons for this, looking back, two events were seminal: the famous Live Aid concert for famine relief in 1985 and an international PBL training workshop at McMaster University in 1994. Now each event in its own way clearly moved, clearly affected people, myself included, and, over time, I began to search the respective literatures for the meaning(s) of what happened. To my great surprise – especially regarding music research - most accounts were of a structuralist, cognitive orientation, devoid of substantive, emotional content. I presented a paper to this effect, entitled Does PBL work? Does music?! at the AMEE 2002 conference (a great thrill).

Well that was then. Now, thanks to advances in neuroscience, we know that emotions are at the very core of who we are and what we do – including the doing of thinking and learning – and we have to design our curricula accordingly. Music, as metaphor, offers an ideal model; both expressing and eliciting the ineffable best of the human condition. The instrument that is PBL can play most challenging and enjoyable renditions of that music.

[a]*Brian Bailey, Teacher and lecturer (retired), Edinburgh Napier University, Edinburgh, UK.*

- The scholarship of application – the application of knowledge to problems and practice, with new intellectual understandings arising out the very art of application.
- The scholarship of teaching – a dynamic activity, building bridges between the teacher's understanding and the student's learning.

It is wrong, as is sometimes done, to separate or disaggregate these four elements, as Boshier (2009) described, "stripping them apart." Rather, we consider, as does Boshier, that discovery, integration and application are all interacting elements in the scholarship of teaching.

Why a teacher-scholar?

There are a number of reasons why you should consider yourself as a teacher-scholar:

- Scholarship in teaching is evidence of professionalism. As a teacher, you are not simply a technician but a professional, as we describe in Chapter 10.
- As a teacher-scholar, you gain more job satisfaction from your work as a teacher.
- Working as a teacher-scholar helps you think about and keep abreast with developments in teaching.
- Scholarship is often a major factor influencing decisions about appointments and career progression.
- Your scholarship can help you gain recognition more generally for your work through awards and publications.

- As a teacher-scholar, you are part of a community of teachers with similar interests with whom you can communicate at conferences or by email.
- You can obtain grants to support your education activities.
- You can serve as a mentor and guide other staff.
- Finally, and importantly, as a teacher-scholar you can contribute to improving and bringing about change where necessary in the education process locally, nationally or internationally.

Demonstration of scholarship

You can demonstrate your scholarship as a teacher in a number of ways relating to all four of the scholarships described by Boyer (1990) and relating to the other seven roles of the teacher described in this text. As a teacher-scholar (Fig. 9.2), you should:

- **Reflect** on your own teaching. You are not simply a technician approaching your work as a teacher without thought or consideration in the absence of any understanding of the basic principles as to what works and what does not work in your context (*the scholarship of teaching*).
- **Make evidence-informed decisions** with regard to curriculum, teaching and learning methods, the assessment approach and other aspects of the education process, while at the same time bringing new insights to bear on an appreciation of the available evidence (*the scholarship of integration*).
- **Innovate** and introduce new approaches to aspects of your work as a teacher based on educational principles that are aimed at making student learning more effective and efficient. This may include a new curriculum, new learning approaches or a new assessment method (*the scholarship of application*).

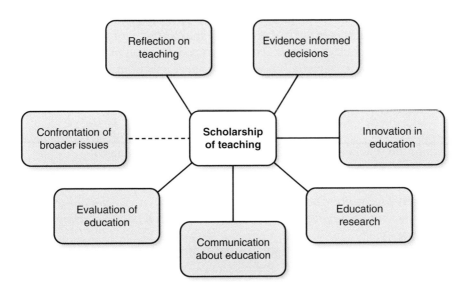

Figure 9.2 Seven features of the scholarly teacher

- **Undertake research,** perhaps in the form of action research related to your own teaching. You may also be part of a research programme examining an issue in medical education (*the scholarship of discovery*).
- **Communicate** about your experiences and lessons learned to other teachers. Your work and experience should be made public (*the scholarship of teaching*).
- **Evaluate** your teaching through student and peer review and other methods, as described in Chapter 10. This is a key feature of your professionalism (*the scholarship of teaching*).
- **Confront** broader issues in medical education, such as the impact of the education programme on improving the health of the community. Later in this chapter we discuss this less well-recognised perspective on scholarship (*the scholarship of application*).

These features represent different elements and perspectives of the scholarship of teaching. As we suggested, too often the definition of the scholarship of teaching is unnecessarily narrow and is equated with research in education, with the other elements not recognised. This may be particularly evident when faculty promotion is under consideration, as noted by Fincher et al. (2000):

Faculty who are essential to the core educational mission of their medical schools often are not promoted because they do not engage in accepted forms of scholarship. Yet, the same faculty may conceptualize, design, implement, or evaluate new curricula, interdisciplinary courses, assessment instruments, web-based learning materials, and high-quality course syllabi. Others may excel as course directors, teachers, and/or highly respected role models. These educational activities may extend beyond the privacy of the classroom to the public domain, where the products of faculty educational efforts may be reviewed by peers and adopted by faculty at other schools. Some educators may be invited to share their expertise with faculty in their department or at other schools, and through presentations at regional or national meetings. Nevertheless, despite the peer review and dissemination inherent in these activities, they may not meet the current promotion criteria for scholarship. (p. 887–8)

In an issue of the journal *Australian Higher Education Research and Development*, devoted to the scholarship of teaching, Chalmers (2011) has noted:

…while there has been significant progress made to date, the ultimate symbols of recognition and reward – promotion and tenure – are proving to be elusive but not unattainable for those who focus on the Scholarship of Teaching. (p. 25)

Fortunately, things are changing, and research is not now considered as the only indication of scholarship. Promotion committees usually look for something beyond simply the intensity of teaching undertaken and its evaluation by the students, and many schools have a teaching promotion track that recognises the broader definition of scholarship, as we describe in this chapter.

A teacher's educational activities can be viewed along a progression, with increasing evidence of scholarship over time. Hafler et al. (2005) have described the progression of a clerkship director's educational scholarly activities at appointment, within 1 year of appointment and later. Initially, the clerkship director knows the literature in the area and assumes a role of investigator in his or her own clerkship, answering questions such as "How do grades vary by month or by year?" With time, the emphasis is on advancing knowledge in medical education more widely beyond the clerkship.

The reflective teacher

Sometimes, like other teachers, you act in relation to your teaching without thinking, by routine and habit. You deliver the same lecture as the previous year, you suggest to your students the same learning resources, you offer learning experiences similar to those offered previously and you continue with the same expected learning outcomes and the assessment of these. For at least part of your time, however, you should critically review your teaching and reflect on what you are doing as a teacher. Are there any changes required in the curriculum and what is expected of the students that should be reflected in your teaching? Based on your previous experience, are there ways whereby you could make the students' learning more effective and efficient? Have you considered and responded to the problems identified in the students' feedback? John Sandars, an experienced teacher, describes in Box 9.3 how he reflects on his teaching and critically questions what he is doing. As described by Squires (1999, p. 16) "Practitioners have to disengage temporarily from the immediacy of practice to think about what they are doing and about what they are thinking."

Box 9.3 A reflective approach[a]

My different roles in teaching are underpinned by a personal and educational philosophy that values the learner. Valuing the learner means to me that I appreciate that each learner is a unique individual, with different life experiences, interests, expectations, aspirations and preferences for learning. My teaching has to recognise that "no one size fits," requiring me to use a variety of content and teaching styles. An essential aspect of valuing the learner is to actively involve the learner as a co-creator of their learning experience, contributing their ideas and knowledge to mutually enrich both the teaching and learning. I also believe that it is essential to offer a more holistic education and not merely provide training, with teaching focussed on simply passing examinations. For me, education is a process of personal and professional growth that is deeply rooted in the complexity of real world challenges. This requires a constant reflective approach that critically questions what we are doing, why we are doing it that way, and how we can do it differently. These questions are essential for the learner to consider but also they are equally applicable for my scholarship as a medical teacher.

---

[a]*John Sandars, Professor of Medical Education, Edge Hill University, Ormskirk, UK.*

The teacher as a scholar reflects on her or his teaching, incorporating other peoples' ideas but without blindly adopting them in their situation. As argued by Hammersley (1993):

> *...the teacher is (or ought to be) a skilled practitioner, continually reflecting on her or his practice in terms of ideals and knowledge of local situations, and modifying practice in light of these reflections; rather than a technician merely applying scientifically produced curriculum programmes. (p. 426)*

In the AMEE Guide on "The use of reflection in medical education," Sandars (2009) has suggested:

> *a process of constant reflection-on-action is an essential requirement for professional expertise and is typical of the 'enquiring mind' that explores and tries to obtain multiple perspectives to enrich their view of the world. (p. 691)*

Reflection is valuable not only for the medical practitioner but also for the teacher. Service expectations and demands on your time may make it difficult for you to find time to reflect on your teaching, but this should not preclude it. Reflection on your teaching is a mark of a scholar, and almost certainly you spend at least some time doing so.

We describe later in this chapter the move to evidence-informed teaching. Do not expect, however, to find the answers to all the day-to-day problems from available evidence about what works. Even if evidence is available, you need to reflect on the issues to be addressed in your own context and on the most appropriate action because each situation is different, and the same rules do not always apply. A basic understanding of educational principles can support your reflection. We described the FAIR principles for effective learning in Chapter 4. As a teacher, you need to reflect on how you can apply these to your teaching – providing feedback to the learner, engaging the learner through active learning, individualising and tailoring the learning to each student and making the learning relevant. Many aspects of the education programme are determined centrally but almost certainly there are aspects of your teaching where you have a measure of autonomy and the ability to implement your own solution to a perceived problem. You may be scheduled to deliver a lecture on a specific topic, but you should reflect on your approach to the task and what sort of lecture the students will receive.

Making evidence-informed decisions

Rational thinking and the use of evidence and judgement in teaching

In the past, it was unusual for teachers, even those with a background in research in their discipline, to apply a research-based approach to address such questions. Ruth Beard (1967) wrote that "it is striking to find that university graduates, with sometimes years of research experience, were unable to apply to teaching the same methods of scientific enquiry they would have presumably used in their own discipline." (p. 1)

Teachers make decisions using a PHOG approach based on their **p**rejudices, **h**unches, **o**pinions or **g**uesses. More recently, van der Vleuten (1995) noted that although medical teachers are trained to make medical decisions based on available evidence, when they put on their teacher's hat, they seem to abandon their critical thinking about what works and does not.

Many medical teachers pay little attention to or ignore evidence about what works and what doesn't in medical education or why it works, although these positions are changing. We can recognise at least four types of teachers who are not engaged with the concept of evidence-informed teaching:

- *"Dr No"* is sceptical about research in medical education. He believes that teaching is a craft and not a science and, in any case, is more committed to his research than his teaching (Fig. 9.3).
- *"Dr As Before"* believes that new methods proposed are simply fads that will go away. Traditional methods have stood the test of time and have contributed to the successful training of cohorts of doctors (Fig. 9.4).
- *"Dr By Chance"* is a keen teacher but has not had time to think seriously about the approaches he adopts and chooses whatever method is available at the time (Fig. 9.5).
- *"Dr Keen"* also is an enthusiastic teacher and has been using technology to support his teaching. However, he has not kept up to date with new developments, including computers and what is now available (Fig. 9.6).

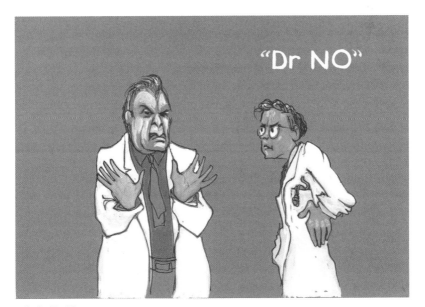

Figure 9.3 Dr No

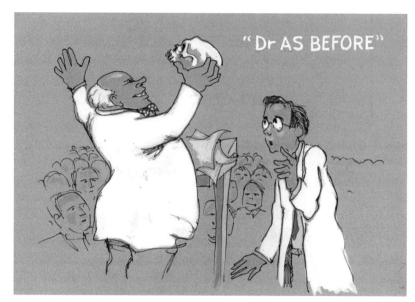

Figure 9.4 Dr As Before

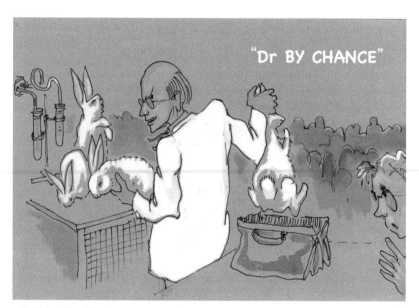

Figure 9.5 Dr By Chance

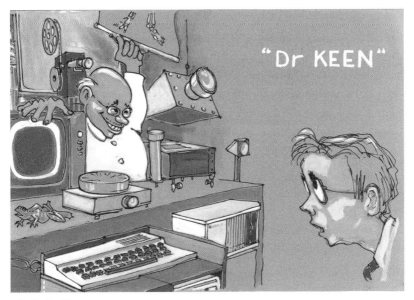

Figure 9.6 Dr Keen

In clinical practice, attention has focused on evidence-based medicine. Decisions about the management of a patient based on the clinical judgement of the doctor are influenced by available evidence about the most appropriate management approach for the patient. Although this approach to evidence-based decisions has legitimacy in medicine, the situation in education has been less certain. It has been argued that compared with research in medicine, research in education is more complex, confounding factors may be more apparent, content may be more implicit and controlled trials may be difficult. Moreover, the impact of education on patient care and the health of the community is less direct than with medical interventions, such as a new drug or a surgical procedure. Many disagree with this negative view of research in medical education, and Davies P. (1999) has argued that when compared with medicine, education faces very similar, if not identical, problems of complexity, context specificity, measurement and causation. Many of the problems relating to the complexity of education interventions and their evaluation also apply to health care. Studies of agents for treating hypertension, for example, have frequently been based on the measurement of the reduction in blood pressure and have ignored issues such as patient satisfaction, quality of life and time absent from work.

An AMEE Conference held in Linkoping in August 1999 concluded that medical teachers should endorse the principle of best evidence medical education (BEME). This was defined as the implementation, by teachers in their practice, of methods and approaches to education based on the best evidence available.

The medical teacher is faced with the following and similar questions in his or her teaching practice. BEME reviews provide answers:

- Are there benefits of introducing students to clinical medicine in the early years of the course?
- What aspects of simulation lead to more effective learning?
- Is team-based learning more effective than traditional approaches?
- Are work-based assessment approaches reliable and valid as a tool for summative assessment?

Since it was established in 1999, the BEME Collaboration has demonstrated that evidence is available in a number of areas and this can be used by the teacher to inform day-to-day decisions in their teaching practice (www.bemecollaboration .org). There is no doubt that at least to some extent, you can move as a teacher from an opinion-based approach to teaching to an evidence-informed approach.

What evidence-informed teaching means in practice

As a teacher-scholar, you should adopt an evidence-informed approach to your teaching. You should:

- Reflect on your teaching practice, as described above.
- Identify from the evidence available what is best practice relating to your teaching. In the case of simulation, for example, do you take into account the ten principles shown to lead to effective learning, as described in the BEME guide by Issenberg and colleagues (2005)?
- Modify your teaching, as appropriate, in light of the evidence.
- Evaluate the results of any changes made and share and communicate the lessons learned.

Although a move to evidence-informed teaching is to be commended, the unpredictability and complexity of what is expected requires you as a teacher to make professional judgements as to the most appropriate action or decision. Atkinson and Claxton (2000) have described the teacher as an "intuitive practitioner" – "(intuition) allows the teacher to read the context at a glance and to adapt the preconceived plan in the light of the changing context."

Decisions on what to do as a teacher should be based both on your professional judgement and on the best evidence available.

Finding evidence relating to your practice

Evidence as to how you might make your teaching practice more effective is available from a number of sources, such as:

- Systematic reviews of the topic. A number of BEME reviews are available covering a range of topics in medical education (www.bemecollaboration.org).

- A personal literature search. The number of potential sources relevant to a search in medical education is vast and confusing. There is, however, a core of databases that should be consulted (Haig and Dozier, 2003). These include Medline, Embase, ERIC (the Education Resource Information Centre), the British Education Index and Google Scholar. Google Scholar is being increasingly used as the first choice for a search.
- AMEE's MedEdWorld.
- Medical education journals, such as *Medical Teacher, AMEE MedEdPublish, Medical Education, Academic Medicine* and *Teaching and Learning in Medicine*.
- Medical education conferences, such as the AMEE Annual Conference, where more than 1,500 papers and posters are presented on a wide range of topics of current interest in medical education.
- Books on medical education, such as *International Handbook of Research in Medical Education* (Norman et al., 2002) and *A Practical Guide for Medical Teachers* (Dent et al., 2017) or books on specific topics, such as *The Definitive Guide to the OSCE* (Harden et al., 2016).
- Consulting experts with experience in the topic.

Reviewing the evidence available

Having found evidence or information as a result of your enquiry, the next step is to evaluate its applicability to your own situation. The QUESTS criteria can be used for this purpose (Harden et al., 1999; Fig. 9.7):

- *Q*uality: How good is the evidence?
- *U*tility: To what extent can what is described be transferred and adopted in your context without modification.
- *E*xtent: What is the extent of the evidence?
- *S*trength: How strong is the evidence?

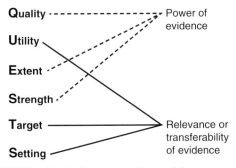

Figure 9.7 The QUESTS criteria for evaluating evidence

- *T*arget: What is the target? What is being measured? How valid is the evidence?
- *S*etting: How close does the context or setting approximate to yours? How relevant is the evidence?

Quality of Evidence

It has been suggested that only evidence from randomised controlled trials (RCTs) should be considered where, for example, method A is compared with method B. Even in medicine, however, RCTs do not necessarily represent the gold standard. What one should aim to establish is not simply whether method A is better than method B, but what aspects of method A lead to more effective learning. Qualitative research methods that illuminate this may be of more value than quantitative methods.

What is perceived as the robustness of the evidence will vary and, as advocated by the BEME Collaboration, you should adopt the best evidence available. In decreasing order of robustness (Fig. 9.8), these are:

- BEME Guides – evidence from meta-analyses of studies researching the topic.
- AMEE Guides – authors' recommendations based on a personal review of the literature and their experience.
- Medical Teacher Twelve Tips articles – authors' recommendations based on their personal experience.

Case studies, professional experience and professional judgement should not be excluded as useful sources of evidence. Knowledge that an approach has been successfully adopted for several years in another school and has been accepted by students and staff, while another approach was rejected after a year's experience, may be useful in helping you to come to a decision in relation to your own situation.

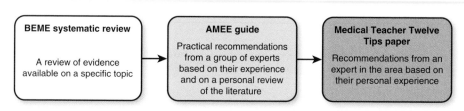

Figure 9.8 Decreasing levels of robustness of evidence

The Utility of the evidence

The utility of the evidence is the extent to which the method or intervention, as reported in the original research report, can be transplanted to another situation without adaptation. You find in a published report on problem-based learning (PBL) that groups of eight students were used but, for logistical reasons, you can arrange only groups of twelve students. Does it matter, and should the group work be arranged differently to take account of this? To what extent does it matter if teachers with experience of the PBL approach, as described in the original report, are not available? Can teachers be given appropriate training in your institution?

Changes can also be made to the approach described in the original research report with the aim of improving what has been described. There may be the expectation but not the certainty that this will lead to improved results.

Extent of the evidence

Evidence may be based on a single study at one site or a multi-centre study, or it may be based on a number of studies conducted over time by different groups. Although the results of a single study have to be interpreted with caution, they can be helpful. An example is a study by Worley in Australia, where eight students were based for 1 year in a rural community (Worley and Lines, 1999). Only a small number of students was studied, but the experience described encouraged others to pursue educating students in rural communities for at least part of the time.

The Strength of the evidence

When we first described the criteria for evaluating evidence, Geoff Norman pointed out that we had left out the concept of the strength of the evidence. Sometimes, conclusions are drawn about the educational significance of the difference between two groups or two approaches studied, when the results have only marginal statistical significance. Such differences should be interpreted with caution.

The Target of the evidence

The target or aim of the study should be considered. Was it the students' attitudes or views on an intervention, their response in a knowledge-based written examination or their clinical performance in practice? The outcomes of interest to you may be different from what was looked at by the authors of the study.

The Setting or context of the evidence

How similar is the setting reported similar to your own? If you are interested in the design of an online learning programme, and in particular in the features likely to lead to the successful delivery of a continuing professional development programme for family physicians in the UK, you may be less interested in the results and conclusions based on an online programme developed for children in Singapore.

The value of the QUESTS criteria

Three of the QUESTS criteria relate to the power of the evidence available – the quality, extent and strength of the evidence. The other three criteria relate to the relevance or transferability of the evidence to your practice – the utility (the extent to which you have to adapt the approach described to suit your own teaching practice), the target (the extent to which the outcomes expected by you and the author are similar) and the setting (the cultural, professional and other differences between you and the author).

The QUESTS criteria can help you as a teacher evaluate published reports and arrive at the best approximation of the applicability to your own teaching practice.

The teacher as an innovator

The role of the teacher

Not every teacher has the opportunity, the time or the motivation to be responsible for a major innovation in medical education, such as the introduction of the objective structured clinical examination (OSCE), the use of programme-focused assessment or the concept of the assessment pyramid, as described by Miller (1990). Every teacher can, however, innovate in some way with regard to the education programme in her or his institution. You may introduce an innovation following reflection on an existing teaching problem when you identify aspects for which changes would be advantageous. Minor innovations may develop into major innovations. This was the case with the OSCE (Harden et al., 1975).

Teachers have an important role in bringing about change in a school. This was noted in the Malaysia Education Blueprint (Ministry of Education, Malaysia, 2013), which set out plans for the further development of education in Malaysia: "Teachers have been identified as the key role players, the catalysts and the motivators to bring about the visionary school outcomes."

As a teacher-scholar, you can have an important role to play by supporting, contributing to or initiating innovations in your school. This was discussed in Chapter 8. Innovations may be at different levels.

At an institution level, examples might be:

- The introduction of a new course in the curriculum.
- The planning of the education programme and allocation of time for a core curriculum and for options or student-selected components.
- Regulations as to the requirements of the students, such as attendance at lectures.

At a course level, examples might be:

- The use of a flipped classroom to replace lectures.
- The introduction of elements of interprofessional education, with medical students learning alongside student nurses or other healthcare professionals for part of the course.
- The design of a new form of assessment for the course.

At an individual level, examples might include:

- A new approach to a lecture for which you are responsible.
- The development of a virtual patient to support the students' studies.
- The introduction of a new approach to student feedback for the part of the course for which you are responsible.

Writing in the foreword to the *OECD Handbook for Innovative Learning Environments*, Schleicher (OECD, 2017) noted:

> *If there has been one lesson learned about innovating education, it is that teachers, schools and local administrators should not just be innovative in the implementation of education change but they should have a central role in its design. (p. 104)*

The innovation ladder

An innovation may be at different levels, as shown on the innovation ladder (Table 9.1), from no change at the bottom of the ladder to a transformation of the education programme or an aspect of it at the top.

Table 9.1 Stages on the innovation ladder

Level	Features
1	"No change", "just a fad", "will go away" – the ostrich approach
2	"Window dressing" – continuing as before but with some token change, such as preparation of a list of learning outcomes but no impact of these on the teaching and learning programme
3	"Renovating" – doing better what one is already doing, such as some improvements in lectures and learning resources
4	"Reformation" – addition of new elements to the existing educational programme, such as the introduction of a clinical skills centre or a flipped classroom
5	"Transformation" – implementation of something completely different, such as an adaptive curriculum, with learning personalised and tailored to the needs of the individual student

The innovation may be a development of and in line with existing practice in the school. Examples are changes in the method for selecting students to the school, the introduction of a new standard setting procedure to be adopted for the student assessment, and the introduction of a new programme or course on pain management. The innovation may represent a move in a new direction and may be considered a fundamentally different approach from current practice. This is a "disruptive innovation." A disruptive innovation is one that makes existing approaches obsolete. The automobile was an early example, disrupting the market for horse-drawn vehicles. An example of what might be considered as a disruptive innovation is the introduction of outcome-based education across the curriculum, where the duration of the course is not fixed but varies, depending on the time taken by the student to achieve the learning outcomes. Another example is a commitment across the curriculum to refocus a traditional education programme with a new emphasis on community-based education or on interprofessional education.

Although an innovation may be transformative, the conservatism of the medical profession in terms of education and training programmes is a powerful inhibitor of change. Suggestions about the introduction of interprofessional education, with medical students taught alongside other healthcare students, the shortening of the education programme from its current length of 4 to 3 years or 5 to 4 years or moving from a time-based to a standard-based programme initially attracted negative responses. Progress, however, has been made on all three fronts. As Mandela said, "It always seems impossible until it's done."

The innovation with which you are associated may be specific and of relevance only to the education programme in your own institution, or it may be a concept that could be adopted in other schools in your region or internationally.

The teacher as a researcher

Action research

As a teacher, you are also a researcher. An unhelpful view of research in medical education is one where the teaching is seen as being done by the teacher, while the education research is done by an educationist or another teacher with training and qualifications in educational research (Fig. 9.9). Teachers should be seen not just as consumers of research but as providers of research. Research should be not just "for" teachers but "by" teachers (Fig. 9.10). Writing on scholarship in education, McGaghie (2009) has argued:

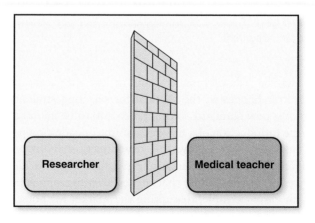

Figure 9.9 An unhelpful view of research in medical education

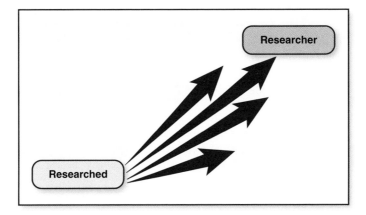

Figure 9.10 Research in medical education is not just *for* teachers but *by* teachers

> *Health professions education is enriched when its scientists and scholars*
> *take time alone and with others to look beyond today's agenda items*
> *toward a longer horizon. (p. 590)*

As a teacher, you are in the best position to appreciate and understand the education programme, its problems and how it can be improved. Research is not simply about what works and what does not work. It is about understanding and illuminating why it works and the educational circumstances in which it works. In what ways, for example, is the flipped classroom better than the traditional lecture, and how can it most effectively be included in the education programme? As a teacher, you have an important role in extending our understanding by contributing answers to these and other problems.

As a teacher, you can engage in what has been described as action research, studying your own practice as a teacher and solving problems. You can do this on your own or in collaboration with colleagues or educational researchers. I (RMH) developed the OSCE after I found in a small study that the traditional clinical examination was unreliable (Wilson et al , 1969). A description of action research on the topic of education climate is given in Box 9.4.

Cohen and Manion (1980) have provided a useful description of action research:

> *Small scale intervention in the function of the real world and a close*
> *examination of the effects of such intervention. Action research is*
> *situational – it is concerned with diagnosing a problem in a specific context;*
> *it is usually (though not inevitably) collaborative – teams of researchers and*
> *practitioners work together on a project; it is participatory – team members*
> *themselves take part directly or indirectly by implementing the research*
> *and it is self-evaluative – modifications are continuously evaluated within*
> *the ongoing situation, the ultimate objective being to improve practice in*
> *some way or another. (p. 186)*

Box 9.4 The teacher as an action researcher[a]

In a paper with Jack Genn as lead author we suggested that studies of the medical education environment could serve as an example of an area on which the teacher as an action researcher could focus (Genn and Harden, 1986). We cited the work of DeYoung (1977) as a model for the practising teacher. DeYoung established the actual climate in his social science classroom and at the same time ascertained what his students would desire as the ideal climate of the class. He introduced changes in his teaching programme the following year to tackle the differences he found between the actual and the ideal climate. The result was greater student satisfaction, increased class attendance and higher examination scores. Many teachers across the globe have now undertaken similar action research related to the education environment.

[a]*Ronald M Harden, General Secretary, AMEE, Professor of Medical Education (Emeritus), University of Dundee, Dundee, Scotland, UK.*

As noted by Winter (1996), action research can be described as follows:

Ways of investigating professional experience which link practice and the analysis of practice into a single productive and continuously developing sequence...Practitioner action research is thus part of the general ideal of professionalism, an extension of professional work, not an addition to it. (p. 9–10)

Action research puts the teacher at the centre of educational development. Goodnough (2010) has described the benefits derived when teachers in schools engaged in action research. One teacher commented:

Action research has benefits for teachers, students, other educators, and policy-makers. Teachers can improve their own teaching repertoires and therefore improve their classroom practice. Other educators can learn from our studies and use this information to improve their own teaching. In addition, policy-makers can use this research to guide policy. It provides considerable insight into current educational issues. (p. 176)

As a senior lecturer in the Department of Medicine at the University of Glasgow, I (RMH) had responsibility for the endocrinology course for third-year medical students. I was unhappy that the course was predominantly lecture based. There was a reluctance, however, to replace lectures with independent learning resources (at that time, tape or slide programmes) because it was thought that students would only learn the subject if they attended lectures. The value of independent learning was accepted, however, after I demonstrated that a small group of students who learned endocrinology using tape and slide programmes instead of attending lectures did as well as, or better than, students who attended lectures (Harden et al., 1969). This is an example of research that can be carried out by teachers as part of their teaching responsibilities. Another example is a more recent study by Khogali, a cardiologist, and other teachers in Dundee.

They implemented a blended learning programme in cardiology and demonstrated that online programmes can be integrated with lectures, PBL, and experiences in the clinical skills centre (Khogali et al., 2011). The teachers found that the students used the resources in different ways – some preferring to work individually, others in pairs or small groups, some preferring an audio commentary, others a visual text and some preferring to assess their competence using a self-assessment component early in the programme rather than doing so only at the end.

A further example where I (RMH) integrated research into the work of a teacher was a study of the scoring of student answers in multiple true/false questions. The question was raised at a meeting of the assessment committee as to whether a point should be deducted for incorrect answers. To tackle the question, a study was undertaken in which students first answered the multiple-choice questions (MCQs), knowing that a point would be deducted for incorrect answers, and then answered questions not previously answered. For some students, this made no difference, but for others it significantly improved their score (Harden et al., 1976).

Action research is at the heart of medical education, and all teachers should inquire into their own practice and modify their future behaviour on the basis of the findings.

Scholarship principles and research

Crites et al. (2014) have suggested that research as it relates to scholarship in teaching can be guided by Glassick's six core principles of excellence for scholarship (Glassick, 2000):

- Setting clear goals – decisions about appropriate questions to be asked.
- Adequate preparation – preparation of a research plan.
- Use of appropriate methods.
- Achievement of significant results.
- Effective communication of the results.
- Reflective critique of the work.

A useful introduction to research in education has been given in the AMEE Guide by Ringsted et al. (2011). A more detailed account is available in *Researching Medical Education* (Clcland and Durning, 2015).

Advantages of the teacher as a researcher

Establishing a culture whereby research by teachers is considered as the norm and where teachers have education research, as well as their own teaching responsibilities, is challenging (Hill and Haigh, 2012). However, when undertaken by teachers, research relating to their teaching responsibilities has a number of advantages.

- The work tackles practical rather than theoretical issues and is more likely to have implications for teaching and learning. Small-scale action research can have a positive impact on the teaching and learning experience offered to students (Dexter and Seden, 2012). The development of the OSCE is an example.

- It helps identify the teacher as a stakeholder in change, empowering the teacher and providing the teacher with greater interest and insight in their work. Lawrence Stenhouse (1975) has reflected on this: "it is teachers who in the end will change the world of the school by understanding it." Johnson (1993) has noted that "the concept of teacher-as-researcher is included in recent literature on educational reform, which encourages teachers to be collaborators in revising curriculum, improving their work environment, professionalizing teaching, and developing policy." Woods (2011) has argued for "...the co-creation of new ideas, opportunities and conditions that connect and interact with other initiatives and help build momentum for transformative change."
- Research undertaken contributes to recognition and reward of teaching. The number of papers published as a result of research is a commonly used metric for assessing faculty performance. We are not arguing that teachers' excellence should be assessed for promotions, tenure and other purposes solely in terms of the number and quality of publications. It does, however, provide useful additional evidence of contributions made to teaching.

Undertaking research can contribute to the development of the individual and can be a powerful faculty development activity. "Action research provides the necessary link between self-evaluation and professional development" (Winter, 1996). This was certainly my experience (RMH) working with education colleagues.

Potential limitations of the teacher as a researcher

There are questions to be asked, however, in relation to the role of the teacher as a researcher.

Is a teacher's understanding of the findings of research and possible improvements shaped by their own personal self-interests and prejudices?

You can guard against this by working as part of a community of research practice in which you are assisted by more experienced researchers (Hill and Haigh, 2012). I (RMH) had the benefit of working in Glasgow as a novice with Willie Dunn, an experienced researcher, who brought to education both theoretical insight and pragmatism. In addition to his wide experience in education, he had served with the armed forces in Malaysia as chief instructor in jungle warfare. This undoubtedly shaped his vision of problems and their solutions.

Can such small-scale investigations by a teacher lead to genuine new insights into the curriculum?

Are they too minimal to be valued? This is not the case. My own work on the OSCE has demonstrated that the initiatives and research of a teacher can lead to work that has a broad impact (Harden et al., 1975).

Does a teacher have the necessary training and skills to be a teacher-researcher?

Such training can now be readily acquired, and courses such as AMEE's Research Essential Skills in Medical Education (RESME) are available for new researchers. Some teachers acquire more in-depth insights and skills through Masters in Medical Education courses. You may find the AMEE Guides series on research (www.amee.org) and texts such as *Researching Medical Education* by Cleland and Durning (2015) of value. An understanding of research can also be acquired through working with an education expert. As a medical teacher, you may be more familiar with quantitative rather than qualitative research. Qualitative research is important in education; Cleland (2017) has provided a short introduction about how it enables a deeper understanding of what is being studied.

The teacher as a communicator about their work

Sharing your work as a teacher

As a teacher-scholar, you have a responsibility to share your thoughts, wisdom, expertise and experiences in medical education with teachers, researchers, decision makers and other stakeholders. Making public your work has been widely accepted as a distinguishing but not essential feature of scholarship. Shulman (2000) has advocated:

> *we develop a scholarship of teaching when our work as teachers becomes public, peer-reviewed and critiqued, and exchanged with members of our professional communities so they, in turn, can build on our work. (p. 50)*

Communication options

You can share your work in a number of ways.

- Publishing papers on a medical education topic either in a medical, medical education or education journal. Key medical education journals for the practising medical teacher include *Medical Teacher, Academic Medicine, Medical Education, Teaching and Learning in Medicine* and the recently introduced *AMEE MedEdPublish*. A range of other, more specialised journals also exists. Suggestions about writing for publication are given below.
- Reviewing papers submitted for publication. In addition to contributions as an author, you can also share your experience and expertise by reviewing papers. This may be by invitation, but all readers of *AMEE MedEdPublish* can review papers, add their personal star rating and collect credits for doing so.
- Contributing to medical education conferences and meetings. These may be local, national, regional or international meetings. The annual AMEE

Conference, for example, offers opportunities for the presentation of workshops, short communications, research papers or posters to an international audience.

- Contributing to faculty development programmes. The faculty development programme may be a local one for staff in your institution or may be a national or international programme. The programme may be face-to-face or online. Your contribution may address the general theme of medical education or target a specific topic, such as team-based learning or the OSCE.
- Serving as a mentor for one or more colleagues. This is an important role for the teacher, as discussed in Chapter 4.
- More generally, engaging with the wider community of teacher-scholars, particularly those with similar interests in medical education.

As pointed out by Simpson et al. (2007), the breadth and scope of this scholarly engagement may be local, national or international and may vary with faculty rank and institution. Networking and sharing experiences can be facilitated by membership of medical education associations such as AMEE and/or local or regional associations. You may participate in education committees, working groups or discussion forums.

Writing for publication

Publication of a paper in a recognised journal is a key activity for the teacher-scholar. Indeed, as we have mentioned, appointment or promotion decisions may be heavily influenced by the number of publications in leading journals in the field. Publishing, however, is not easy (Fig. 9.11). Journals such as *Medical Teacher* are able to publish fewer than 10% of papers submitted.

Barriers to writing for publication

There may be barriers to writing for publication that stop the teacher. These include:

- Lack of time. Teachers have many demands on their time, and sufficient priority may not be given to the task. Some authors overcome this by binge writing, when they allocate several days to work exclusively on writing a paper. Others prefer to schedule a regular series of 1-hour time allocations. One author we know sets aside 1 hour before going to work in the morning. There is no correct answer. You need to do what works best for you.
- Lack of the requisite skills. You may not have received formal training in writing for publication and depend only on learning what is expected by studying examples of papers published. In this case, you may find the brief overview in this chapter helpful. It summarises recommendations

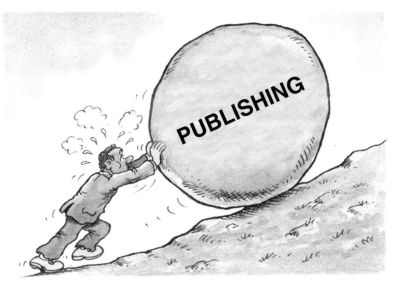

Figure 9.11 Publishing is not easy

from more detailed accounts in books on the topic, including *Guide to Publishing a Scientific Paper* (Korner, 2008), *How to Write a Paper* (Hall, 2012) and *How to Write and Publish a Research Paper* (Wankhade, 2012). The AMEE guides, *Writing for journal publication* (Parsell and Bligh, 1998) and *Writing for academia: Getting your research into print* (Coverdale et al., 2013) also provide useful information and suggestions about publishing.

- Difficulty in getting started. You may procrastinate and find getting started on writing the paper a problem. One suggestion is to make time to write simply the first paragraph. Alternatively, start writing a section of the paper that is easiest for you. This may be the methods or the results sections or even what you see as the "take-home" messages from the paper.

- Perfectionism. A high standard of writing is required if the paper is to be published. Papers should only be submitted if they meet the minimum standards described below. Some authors, however, striving for perfectionism, continue to try to modify, update or in some way improve their paper. In a chapter, "The Reluctant Writers," in her book, *The Forgotten Tribe: Scientists as writers*, Lisa Emerson (2016) has recorded a senior scientist's concerns perfectly:

> *I'm a very good writer. I hate it. I hate it. Well, really, I'm a very good editor and a lousy writer. I have this terrible problem with the tyranny of the blank page. You know, I sit down and look blankly*

at it. I find it difficult to get started. Which is why I'm a much better editor. Somebody else has started it. There's something there to work on. It's the getting started that I find difficult. I think the reason I don't like it and prefer somebody else to get started is that because I like it to be right – I'm a bit of a perfectionist. If I'm writing from scratch myself, I waste a lot of time getting it word perfect; just getting it down and going back and editing it. I'm a slow primary writer. I edit my own work as I'm writing. (p. 75)

A question that may concern potential authors is "When is the paper good enough?" If you are in doubt, it may be helpful to show your draft to a colleague and ask for her or his opinion.

Manuscript features that create interest

When writing your paper, think of the paper not as the one you want to write but that others will want to read. McGaghie (2009) has suggested the following features that will attract the reader and serve as a useful checklist for the author:

- Importance of the question – "Who cares?"
- Timeliness – of current interest
- Originality, with fresh data or ideas
- Grounded in current knowledge
- Relevance to journal readers
- Quality presentation

Sections of a paper

A paper has a number of sections.

The title – The title is a key part of the paper. It may attract or discourage potential readers and reviewers and may be informative, confusing or, even worse, misleading. Time spent on the title is time well spent. Give careful thought to the title as it provides the first impression of the paper. Here are some suggestions:

- Keep the title relatively brief. We find that papers with long titles are less likely to be accepted for publication in *Medical Teacher*.
- Use the title to arouse interest, and avoid boring or uninformative titles.
- Include keywords that are identifiable to search strategies.
- Avoid acronyms or abbreviations.
- Use short declarative sentences.
- Avoid cryptic titles that do not reflect the paper's content.

Here are two possible titles for a paper on task-based learning:

"Task-based learning supports integrated and problem-based learning in the clinical years"

"A study over 2 years of TBL as an educational strategy in the later years of a medical school in Europe with an integrated problem-based and student centred curriculum where student engagement is emphasised"

The first is preferable.

The abstract – The abstract is also a key element of the paper. Reviewers and readers may look only at the abstract. When a group of teachers was asked how they decided whether or not to read an article, the most common approach described was a quick scan of the abstract. The abstract may be structured or narrative. Here are some suggestions relating to the abstract:

- The abstract should stand alone. The reader should be able to understand it without reading the paper.
- Describe in the abstract:
  - Why the study
  - What was done
  - What was found
  - What does it mean
- Do not include references.
- Do not use abbreviations.

The introduction – Every paper should have an introduction section. The length should relate to the length of the paper and should probably be no more than 10% of the paper. The total length of the paper itself should be in line with papers published in the selected journal and for many journals, but not all, will range from 3,000 to 5,000 words. The introduction should address:

- What question is the paper addressing?
- Why is this important?
- What is already known – include a few references.
- How does this paper advance the field?

The methods section – The methods section should describe what was done in sufficient detail for the reader to repeat the study. Unfortunately, because of pressure for space, this is not always the case in published papers. Include the following in the methods section:

- The study population and how it was selected.
- The setting and context for the study.
- What was done.
- How data were collected and analysed.

The results section – The results section is likely to include tables and figures:

- Present the information clearly and in a logical order.
- Avoid unnecessary repetition of data in the text and in figures and tables.
- The legends for tables and figures should be concise and should summarise the content.

The discussion – After reading the abstract many readers next turn to the discussion. In the discussion:

- Do not repeat the results, but summarise the major findings and provide an understanding of them in the context of what is already known about the subject.
- Discuss possible limitations of the study, such as context specificity, response rate, number of students studied or length of study.
- Explore the implications of the study and the take-home messages. This is very important, but do not speculate too much or overestimate the significance of the study.

Submission of the manuscript

It is essential to follow the journal's instructions for authors when submitting your paper. It is surprising how often authors fail to do so, and this may result in an immediate rejection of the paper. The paper should be accompanied by a supporting letter and what is required may vary from journal to journal.

It is unlikely that your paper will be accepted for publication without some modifications suggested by peer reviewers:

- Study comments from the editor and referees carefully.
- Respond in detail to every comment in turn, positively and non-defensively.
- Conform with most but not necessarily all suggestions with thoughtful, well-argued and reasoned responses.
- Return the revised manuscript with a detailed response in relation to the comments received.

Rejection of a manuscript

Unfortunately, you may find that your manuscript is not accepted for publication. This does not necessarily mean, however, that there are serious flaws with the paper. The number of papers that a journal can publish is limited, and even "good" papers may be rejected as not a top priority for publication. In our experience, the most common reasons for papers being rejected by *Medical Teacher* are noted below:

- The topic of the paper and the question addressed are not appropriate.
  - The main theme is not education (e.g. the topic relates to healthcare delivery rather than education).
  - The target audience is too specialised (e.g. it addresses a detailed analysis of psychometrics).
  - The conclusions are not generalizable (e.g. they are likely to be restricted to and relevant to a specific group of students in a specific context). As noted by Ringsted et al (2011):

    The challenge to the researcher is to place a concrete idea, interest, or problem within a general context of learning, teaching, and education. ... One aspect of generalizability is how the study contributes general new knowledge about learning, teaching and education. (p. 696)

- The paper does not significantly add to our understanding of the topic and is unlikely to have an impact.
  - There is no clear take-home message noted in the abstract.
  - The introduction does not indicate why the study is important.
  - The practical significance and conclusion are not highlighted in the discussion.
  - The conclusions go beyond the data presented.
- There are methodology flaws, including:
  - Inappropriate research design
  - Small sample size
  - Poor response rate
  - Too preliminary
  - "Salami slicing" – with unnecessary fragmentation and the same study reported over several papers
  - Old data
- There are problems with the presentation of the paper, including:
  - The manuscript does not correspond to the style of the journal.
  - The English and grammar are poor.
  - The methods and results are not clearly presented.
  - The discussion is poor.
  - The paper is too long.

What are your options if the paper is rejected?

If your paper is rejected, do not be too pessimistic. Show it to a colleague, and ask for advice. Your options include:

- Revise your paper, taking into account any comments from the editor or referees and submit to another journal.

- Carry out further work and prepare a new paper.
- Abandon the paper.

As noted by Coverdale et al. (2005), the key to successful writing is patience and perseverance. At the same time, enjoy the process and have fun.

Three final tips

We were once asked what would be our three important tips on writing a paper. Here they are:

- Write a paper that readers other than yourself will want to read.
- Spend time perfecting the title and abstract. The paper may be judged by them. Check them with a colleague who is not an author of the paper.
- Be certain that the paper is in the required format for the journal to which it is to be submitted.

Confronting broader issues in medical education

Kreber (2013) has suggested that scholarship of teaching should take on a broader meaning than what we have discussed in this chapter to date. She noted that scholarship should also include the intention to create a better world in which to learn, teach and live. In the medical context, this would include addressing issues such as whether the doctors trained reflect the diversity of the population they will serve. Will the doctors choose to work in the community in rural areas after graduation? Do changes in our curriculum result in changes in medical practice that lead to improvements in the health of the community? These questions relate to the overall validity of the education programme. To engage with such issues as part of scholarship may be beyond what is expected of the teacher. Nonetheless, it is worthwhile taking them into consideration as part of a broader view of scholarship. This identifies scholarship as more than researching and innovating in medical education. It means engaging publicly with broader issues, as noted by Kreber (2013), "so that different perspectives can be heard and debated."

Although studies of "what works" are important, the scholarship of teaching is enhanced, Kreber suggests, by a consideration of the desirability of our practices and the extent to which we address these broader issues, as described earlier. This perspective of the scholarship of teaching is challenging, is not usually included in descriptions of the scholarship of teaching and may be beyond what is seen as your remit as a teacher. For this reason, "confrontation of broader issues" has been included in Fig. 9.2 with a dotted line. We argue, however, that the scholarship of teaching is not just about the processes of education but about its purpose, which ultimately includes the improvement of health care in the patients we serve as healthcare professionals locally and more globally. Walpole and colleagues (2017) have studied curriculum development for medical schools addressing the theme of environmental and sustainable healthcare delivery. There has been some discussion, for example, about whether a socially responsible medical school and, by implication the teachers in the school, should have climate change as part of their remit. Kreber (2013) has noted that:

> Moreover, my intent here is to argue for a broader vision of the scholarship of teaching, one where endeavours aimed at improving learning, and creating a better world within which to learn and teach, are nested within the larger concern for creating a better world. Enquiries into "what works," "what is to be done" and "why do it" hold the greatest promise to empower the scholarship of teaching and to address issues of justice and equality in and through higher education. (p. 866)

Today, there remains a need to look at the broader issues in medical education. Consistent with this is the move to outcome or competency-based education and the concept of an authentic curriculum, as described in Chapter 5.

Scholarship – a contested concept

The definition of the scholarship of teaching remains a contested concept. Some believe that the scholarship of teaching is different from what is conceived as "real" scholarship, as demonstrated through research in the basic or clinical sciences. Some schools still have difficulty recognising the scholarship of teaching as a case for promotion. This is particularly true in research-intensive universities. We hope that our description of scholarship in this chapter will help the teacher-scholar be recognised.

As argued by Boshier (2009), the scholarship of the teacher may be a hard sell. One difficulty relates to confusion between scholarship of teaching and exemplary or good teaching, as defined by excellence in the technical skills, described in the inner circle in our diagram of the excellent teacher (see Fig. 1.3). Good teaching, as defined simply by the technical skills and a strong commitment to teaching, is usually insufficient to convince a committee when promotion is under consideration. The premise we have taken in this book is that all teachers are scholars, and this involves more than technical skills. Teachers can demonstrate scholarship as described in this chapter by reflecting on their teaching, making evidence-based decisions, innovating and researching in medical education and communicating about their work as a teacher and sharing their experiences.

The teacher-scholar, the expert teacher-scholar and the master teacher-scholar

The teacher-scholar

The teacher as a scholar reflects on their own teaching and how it might be improved. They communicate their experience to other teachers. They may also engage in research into their own teaching and introduce innovations based on this.

The expert teacher-scholar

Expert teacher-scholars, in addition to reflecting on their own teaching, are recognised for their research relating to it and on the impact it has had. They communicate their experiences through publications and conferences.

The master teacher-scholar

The master teacher-scholar is recognised nationally and internationally for contributions to medical education through innovations and research in the field. They contribute to the advancement of the subject through their reflective publications and communications.

Take-home messages

1. Every teacher can be a scholar if they reflect on their teaching and make informed decisions relating to it.
2. The teacher-scholar innovates in his or her teaching.
3. Teacher-led research (action research) has an important contribution to make to medical education.
4. The scholarly teacher shares his or her experiences with other teachers.

Consider

- Consider how you can demonstrate scholarship in your teaching through the aspects of scholarship, as highlighted in Fig. 9.2.
- Are there lessons to be learned from your experience that would benefit others and that might be shared at meetings on medical education or in journals?
- Are there new approaches or traditional approaches relating to your teaching that could be evaluated to illuminate what works and why?

Explore further

Atkinson, T., Claxton, G., 2000. Intuitive Practitioner: On the Value of Not Always Knowing What One is Doing. Open University Press, London.

Beard, R., 1967. Research into Teaching Methods in Higher Education. Society for Research into Higher Education, London.

Boshier, R., 2009. Why is the scholarship of teaching and learning such a hard sell? High. Educ. Res. Dev. 28 (1), 1–15.

Boyer, E.L., 1990. Scholarship Reconsidered: Priorities of the Professoriate. Jossey-Bass, San Francisco.

Chalmers, D., 2011. Progress and challenges to the recognition and reward of the Scholarship of Teaching in higher education. High. Educ. Res. Dev. 30 (1), 25–38.

Cleland, J.A., 2017. The qualitative orientation in medical education research. Korean J. Med. Educ. 29 (2), 61–71.

Cleland, J.A., Durning, S.J., 2015. Researching Medical Education. http://onlinelibrary.wiley.com/book/10.1002/9781118838983.

Cohen, L., Manion, L., 1980. Research Methods in Education. Croom Helm, London.

Corey, S., 1953. Action Research to Improve School Practice. Teachers College, Columbia University, New York.

Coverdale, J., Louie, A., Roberts, L.W., 2005. Getting started in educational research. Acad. Psychiatry. 29 (1), 14–18.

Coverdale, J.H., Roberts, L.W., Balon, R., et al., 2013. Writing for academia: Getting your research into print: AMEE Guide No 74. Med. Teach. 35 (2), e926–e934.

Crites, G.E., Gaines, J.K., Cottrell, S., et al., 2014. Medical education scholarship: an introductory guide: AMEE Guide No 89. Med. Teach. 36 (8), 657–674.

Davies, A., 1999. Educational assessment: A critique of current policy. Impact. 1 (1), vii–49.

Davies, P., 1999. What is evidence-based education? Br. J. Educ. Stud. 47 (2), 108–121.

DeYoung, A.J., 1977. Classroom climate and class success: A case study at the university level. J. Educ. Res. 70 (5), 252–257.

Dent, J.A., Harden, R.M., Hunt, D., 2017. A Practical Guide for Medical Teachers, fifth ed. Elsevier, London.

Dexter, B., Seden, R., 2012. "It's really making a difference": How small-scale research projects can enhance teaching and learning. Innov. Educ. Teach. Int. 49 (1), 83–93.

Emerson, L., 2016. The Forgotten Tribe: Scientists as Writers. University Press of Colorado, Perspectives on Writing. Boulder, CO.

Fincher, R.E., Simpson, D.E., Mennin, S.P., et al., 2000. Scholarship in teaching: An imperative for the 21st century. Acad. Med. 75 (9), 887–894.

Genn, J.M., Harden, R.M., 1986. What is medical education here really like? Suggestions for action research studies of climates of medical education environments. Med. Teach. 8 (2), 111–124.

Glassick, C.E., 2000. Boyers's expanded definitions of scholarship, the standards for assessing scholarship, and the elusiveness of the scholarship of teaching. Acad. Med. 75 (9), 877–880.

Goodnough, K., 2010. The role of action research in transforming teaching identity: Modes of belonging and ecological perspectives. Educ. Act. Res. 18, 167–182.

Hafler, J.P., Blanco, M.A., Fincher, R.M., et al., 2005. Educational scholarship. In: Fincher, R.M. (Ed.), Guidebook for Clerkship Directors, third ed. Alliance for Clinical Education, Omaha, NE. (Chapter 14).

Haig, A., Dozier, M., 2003. BEME Guide no 3: systematic searching for evidence in medical education—Part 1: Sources of information. Med. Teach. 25 (4), 352–363.

Hall, G.M., 2012. How to Write a Paper, fifth ed. Wiley-Blackwell, Hoboken, NJ.

Hammersley, J., 1988. Changing the world of the classroom by understanding it: A review of some aspects of the work of Lawrence Stenhouse. J. Curr. Sup. 4 (1), 30–42.

Hammersley, M., 1993. On the Teacher as Researcher. Educ. Act. Res. 1 (3), 425–445.

Harden, R.M., Brown, R.A., Biran, L.A., et al., 1976. Multiple choice questions: To guess or not to guess. Med. Educ. 10 (1), 27–32.

Harden, R.M., Grant, J., Buckley, G., et al., 1999. BEME Guide No 1: Best Evidence Medical Education. Med. Teach. 21 (6), 553–562.

Harden, R.M., Lever, R., Dunn, W.R., et al., 1969. An experiment involving substitution of tape/slide programmes for lectures. Lancet 1 (7601), 933–935.

Harden, R.M., Lilley, P., Patricio, M., 2016. The Definitive Guide to the OSCE. Elsevier, London.

Harden, R.M., Stevenson, M., Downie, W.W., et al., 1975. Assessment of clinical competence using an Objective Structured Clinical Examination. BMJ. 1 (5955), 447–451.

Hill, M.F., Haigh, M.A., 2012. Creating a culture of research in teacher education: Learning research within communities. Stud. High. Educ. 37 (8), 971–988.

Issenberg, B.S., McGaghie, W.C., Petrusa, E.R., et al., 2005. Features and uses of high-fidelity medical simulations that lead to effective learning: A BEME systematic review. Med. Teach. 27 (1), 10–28.

Johnson, B., 1993. Teacher-as-researcher. https://www.ericdigests.org/1993/researcher.htm.

Khogali, S.E.O., Davies, D.A., Donnan, P.T., et al., 2011. Integration of e-learning resources into a medical school curriculum. Med. Teach. 33 (4), 311–318.

Korner, A.M., 2008. Guide to Publishing a Scientific Paper. Routledge, London.

Kreber, C., 2013. Empowering the scholarship of teaching: An Arendtian and critical perspective. Stud. High. Educ. 38 (6), 857–869.

McGaghie, W.C., 2009. Scholarship, publication, and career advancement in health professions education: AMEE Guide No 43. Med. Teach. 31 (7), 574–590.

Miller, G.E., 1990. The assessment of clinical skills/competence/performance. Acad. Med. 65 (9 Suppl.), S63–S67.

Ministry of Education, Malaysia, 2013. Malaysia Education Blueprint 2013-2025. Kementerian Pendidikan Putrajaya, Malaysia.

Norman, G.R., van der Vleuten, C.P.M., Newble, D.I., 2002. International Handbook of Research in Medical Education. Kluwer Academic Publishers, London.

OECD, 2017. The OECD Handbook for Innovative Learning Environments. OECD Publishing, Paris. http://dx.doi.org/10.1787/9789264277274-en.

Parsell, G., Bligh, J., 1998. AMEE Guide No 17: Writing for journal publication. Med. Teach. 21 (5), 457–468.

Ringsted, C., Hodges, B., Scherpbier, A., 2011. The research compass": An introduction to research in medical education: AMEE Guide No 56. Med. Teach. 33 (9), 695–709.

Sandars, J., 2009. The use of reflection in medical education: AMEE Guide No.44. Med. Teach. 31 (8), 685–695.

Shulman, L.S., 2000. From Minsk to Pinsk: Why a scholarship of teaching and learning? J. Schol. Teach. Learn. 1 (1), 48–53.

Simpson, D., Fincher, R.E., Hafler, J.P., et al., 2007. Advancing educators and education by defining the components and evidence associated with educational scholarship. Med. Educ. 41 (10), 1002–10009.

Squires, G., 1999. Teaching as a Professional Discipline. Falmer Press, London.

Stenhouse, L., 1975. An Introduction to Curriculum Research and Development. Heinemann Educational Books, Newcastle, UK.

van der Vleuten, C., 1995. Evidence-based education. Adv. Phys. Educ. 14 (1), S3.

van Melle, E., Curran, V., Goldszmidt, M., et al., 2012. Toward a common understanding: advancing education scholarship for clinical faculty in Canadian medical schools. Canadian Association for Medical Education, Ottawa, Canada.

Walpole, S.C., Vyas, A., Maxwell, J., et al., 2017. Building an environmentally accountable medical curriculum through international collaboration. Med. Teach. 39 (10), 1040–1050.

Wankhade, L., 2012. How to Write and Publish a Research Paper: A Complete Guide to Writing and Publishing a Research Paper. CreateSpace Independent Publishing Platform.

Wilson, G.M., Lever, R., Harden, R.M., et al., 1969. Examination of clinical examiners. Lancet 293 (7584), 37–40.

Winter, R., 1996. New Directions in Action Research. Routledge, New York.

Woods, P.A., 2011. Transforming Education Policy: Shaping a Democratic Future. The Policy Press, Oregon, USA.

Worley, P., Lines, D., 1999. Can specialist disciplines be learned by undergraduates in a rural general practice setting? Preliminary results of an Australian pilot study. Med. Teach. 21 (5), 482–484.

Chapter **10**

The teacher as a professional

Professionalism is not a label you give yourself – it's a description you hope others will apply to you.

David Maister, True Professionalism

As a teacher, you are a professional and not simply a technician. Understanding your professional responsibilities will help shape your life as a teacher.

- Knowledge, autonomy and responsibility
- Embedding professionalism in your roles as a teacher
- A standard of behaviour and responsibilities
- Teaching skills and keeping up to date
- Evaluating your competence as a teacher
  - Student ratings of teaching

- Your well-being as a teacher
  - The problem of stress and burnout
  - Promoting well-being
  - "Civic" professionalism
- The professional teacher, an expert professional, a master professional
- Take-home messages
- Consider
- Explore further

Knowledge, autonomy and responsibility

Every teacher is a professional with responsibilities as described in this chapter (Fig. 10.1). Like scholarship, however, professionalism is a contested area. Three issues are often the focus of attention when professionalism is considered – knowledge, autonomy and responsibility (Furlong et al., 2000; Hoyle and John, 1995).

Knowledge

The teacher like the doctor (and the lawyer) has a specialised body of knowledge and skills, which has been identified as important for their practice as a teacher. It includes both content and pedagogical knowledge. As noted by Hoyle and John (1995):

> *Professionals, through specialist and usually long periods of training, are taught to understand this research validated knowledge and to apply it*

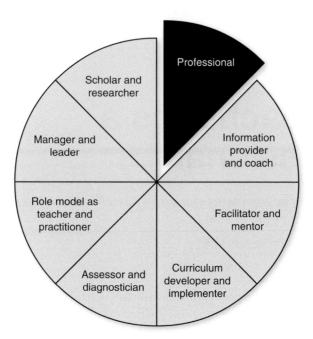

Figure 10.1 The teacher as a professional

*constructively and intelligently according to the technical rules governing
the conduct of the profession. (p. 46)*

Teachers who have this knowledge of teaching are more effective than those who do
not.

Autonomy

Professionals require an element of autonomy as they work in complex and unpredictable situations, as noted by Hoyle and John (1995):

*As professionals work in uncertain situations in which judgement is more
important than routine, it is essential to effective practice that they should
be sufficiently free from bureaucratic and political constraint to act on
judgements made in the best interests (as they see them) of the clients. (p. 77)*

We see to some extent a loss of autonomy of teachers in medical schools, as illustrated
in Box 10.1. This loss of autonomy may even contribute to stress, as described later
in the chapter.

Responsibility to their "clients"

This is manifest in a set of principles and the realisation of these through daily
professional activities (Furlong et al., 2000):

It is because professionals face complex and unpredictable situations that they need a specialized body of knowledge: if they are to apply that knowledge, it is argued that they need the autonomy to make their own judgements. Given that they have that autonomy, it is essential that they act with responsibility – collectively they need to develop appropriate professional values. (p. 5)

Box 10.1 Loss of autonomy

The decision was taken by a university IT department to change to a new learning management system in the medical school. There was no consultation with academic staff. It was decreed that the transfer from the old to the new system would be done only by members of the IT staff. Academic staff were banned from adjusting the resources themselves, and any changes required had to be notified by email to the IT department. Although these arrangements may have been appropriate for inexperienced staff, they made no sense to staff who had expertise in both the old and the new systems. The reduction in the teachers' autonomy had a negative effect on the morale of the enthusiastic teachers whom the school should have been encouraging.

There has been a move, highlighted by Solbrekke and Englund (2011), for professional responsibility to be ignored in the face of an increasing emphasis on professional accountability. This may be associated with a push for high standards, often with centralised control, and with greater accountability of the teacher for the content and quality of training. In the UK, for example, where teachers in medical schools previously had control over the students' final examination and decisions as to whether a student merited a medical degree, there has been a move by the General Medical Council to follow the US model, where the responsibility lies with a national examination board. Countries such as Indonesia and Russia now have national objective structured clinical examinations (OSCEs) at the point of graduation, and teachers are held accountable for their students' performance in the examination. Schools are accredited by national accreditation bodies, which are in turn recognised internationally by the World Federation for Medical Education. Schools are also held to account through published university rankings, which, although discredited as an indication of teaching quality, have a powerful influence on policy decisions in a university.

As discussed by Solbrekke and Englund (2011, p. 853): "Contesting claims on professionals will always create a tension between what is evaluated as good and efficient in terms of "(ac)countable" and "economic" priorities and what is good and "efficient" in terms of morally responsible actions."

Contrasting responsibility and accountability, they noted that key synonyms for "responsibility" are trustworthiness, capacity, judgement and choice. In contrast, key definitions of "accountability" include answerability, blame, liability and obligation. Solbrekke and Englund (2011 p. 854) have summarised the differences as: "'Accountability' emphasises the duty to account for one's actions and concerns what is rendered to another, while 'responsibility' is a moral obligation assumed by oneself or bestowed upon a person to be used, as for example in nursing, to be and act for another."

In medical education, when thinking about the role of the teacher, have we moved too far from responsibility to accountability? At the Association for Medical Education in Europe (AMEE) 2017 Conference in Helsinki, Pasi Sahlberg, a leading educationalist in Finland, suggested that one reason why Finland's schools ranked first internationally on a number of dimensions was that the teachers were trusted. Teaching has changed fundamentally in different ways, and this has altered what we expect professionally of a teacher.

Embedding professionalism in your role as a teacher

As a teacher you are a professional (see Fig. 10.1). Birden et al., as reported by Wass and Barnard (2017) in *A Practical Guide for Medical Teachers*, have defined professionalism as:

> ....*a concept associated with the education, training, attitudes and ethical practices of a group of workers or practitioners. It includes a regulated educational and training system that has specific standards that are monitored and maintained. It has an ethical framework, concerned with good working practices between practitioners and their clients. Professionalism is characterized by a variety of reflective practices that practitioners engage in to maintain their skills. (p. 290)*

Although this was written to describe professionalism in a doctor, it is applicable also to a teacher. As a teacher, you should see yourself as a professional with certain responsibilities and not simply as a technician. This is highlighted in the three-circle outcome model, as shown in Fig. 1.3 (Chapter 1). In the inner circle are the technical competencies expected of a teacher, such as the ability to deliver a lecture, facilitate a small group or write multiple choice questions – doing the right thing. In the middle circle is how you should approach your work as a teacher – with an understanding of educational principles, the appropriate attitude and ethics, an evidence-based approach to decision-making and the necessary teamwork skills – doing the thing right. The outer circle represents your professionalism as a teacher – the right person doing it. This professionalism (Fig. 10.2) requires you to:

- Follow the standard of behaviour expected of a teacher, and accept the associated responsibilities and teaching roles.
- Acquire the necessary teaching competencies, and keep yourself up to date not only in your own discipline but also in approaches to education.
- Enquire into and evaluate your own competence and performance as a teacher.
- Take responsibility for your own well-being, and avoid unnecessary stress and burnout.
- Consider your "civic" responsibility.

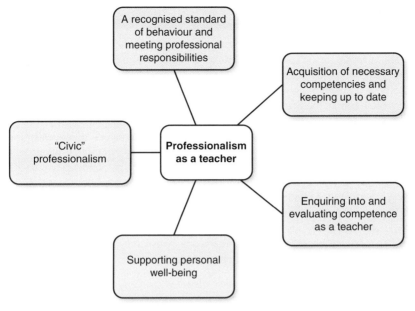

Figure 10.2 Five manifestations of professionalism in a teacher

Professionalism should be embedded in each of the other seven roles described in this text:

- As an information provider, ensuring that students have and know how to find it the necessary information
- As a facilitator, taking responsibility for your students' learning and for their achievement of the learning outcomes
- As a role model, providing an example of the expected professional behaviour
- As a curriculum developer and implementer, understanding the curriculum and how it is delivered in your institution
- As an assessor, assessing students in a fair, reliable and valid way and providing students with the necessary feedback to support their future learning
- As a manager, leader and change agent, engaging with the decision making process, managing elements of the curriculum and leading and supporting change
- As a scholar and a researcher, identifying what works and what does not work, applying the evidence to practice and sharing your experience with others

Anita Laidlaw highlights how, for her, the roles of facilitator, scholar, researcher, professional and role model are all integrated (Box 10.2).

Box 10.2 The teacher as a professional[a]

I view three of the roles of a medical teacher as particularly important and also complementary. These are: a facilitator of learning, a scholar, researcher and professional who enquires into their own competence as a teacher, and a role model. The core skills and attributes of researcher and professional closely overlap (Laidlaw et al., 2009) suggesting that an excellent professional medical teacher should embody these attributes to be a good role model. These roles can be encapsulated in the habit of being a reflective practitioner (Ruona and Gilley, 2009; Schon, 1984). When a learning experience occurs, an excellent medical teacher should be able to identify the opportunity, reflect on it and try to evaluate what the learner gained from it. Such practice ensures that should such an opportunity present itself again, maximum benefit could be gained. This process can be explicit to learners, thereby providing a platform for role modelling such practice. This means that a learner sees how reflecting on an experience to enquire what they themselves have gained from it in terms of skills, knowledge or attitude is a shift towards lifelong learning (Kolb, 1984). This reflection taken a step further by either teacher or learner leads to research, so the reflective practitioner becomes a scholar practitioner (Dunning and Laidlaw, 2015).

[a]Anita Laidlaw, Head of the Division of Education, School of Medicine, University of St. Andrews, St. Andrews, Scotland, UK.

A standard of behaviour and responsibilities

Doctors accept an established standard of behaviour as set out, for example, by the Hippocratic Oath or a modified version of it. This describes the behaviour expected of a doctor and the responsibilities for patients under their care. As teachers, we should also follow a code of conduct that sets out how we should relate to the students for whom we are responsible. You have a responsibility not only to the students, but also to all the stakeholders, including the colleagues with whom you work, the other healthcare professionals, the public and the government. An example of a code of conduct for a teacher is given in Table 10.1. This addresses the relationship between the teacher and the student and the responsibilities of the teacher in terms of their approach to teaching.

Teaching skills and keeping up to date

Professional teachers have the necessary teaching skills and keep themselves up to date. For many years, it was believed that the doctor, on qualifying and without further training, had the necessary skills to teach students. It became obvious, as argued in Chapter 1, that this is certainly not true today. If teachers are to fulfil their roles as a teacher, they need to acquire a range of competencies and an understanding of the educational process. Many medical schools now expect teachers to have training in education.

As a teacher, you should have a basic understanding of the roles of a teacher as a provider of information, a facilitator of learning, a curriculum developer, an assessor of students' competence, a manager and leader and a scholar. You should also be

Table 10.1 A Medical Teacher's Charter (AMEE)

1. Medical teachers believe in the power of medical education across the continuum, from undergraduate through postgraduate to continuing education, to make a difference to the practice of medicine and to the health care of communities throughout the world.

2. As teachers, we are committed to give our students and trainees the best education possible for them to lead fulfilling, purposeful and productive lives as healthcare professionals.

3. Medical teachers set high standards for every learner and respond to individual needs. We challenge students to be all that they can be as doctors, to set demanding goals for themselves and to work as effective members of the healthcare team.

4. We have expertise in teaching and learning and provide opportunities that engage each student's capacity to learn. We help our students achieve the learning outcomes expected of them.

5. We provide a stimulating and supportive learning environment. We help create medical school and postgraduate education settings that welcome students and trainees and foster the achievement of the prescribed learning outcomes, including appropriate attitudes and professionalism.

6. We inspire learners to discover the joy of learning, drawing them into a world of knowledge, skills, ideas and creativity. Our ambition for all is a lifelong engagement with learning.

7. Our practice as a teacher reflects the essential balance between conserving and renewing the best of current teaching practice and anticipating and developing new approaches. In achieving this, we work in partnership with colleagues and other professions.

8. We act and make decisions in relation to our teaching based on our judgement and on the evidence relating to good practice in the area.

9. We take responsibility for advancing the professionalism and scholarship of medical education.

10. The medical teaching profession sets itself demanding standards. We act with judgement, integrity and respect to build the trust and confidence of all the stakeholders including the public, the government, the healthcare professions and the learners.

Modified from the Australian Curriculum Studies Association. Charter for Teachers. (www.acsa.edu.au)

aware of your importance as a role model. Further expertise, and training where necessary, is likely to be required with regard to roles for which you have a specific responsibility. This may relate to an approach to teaching such as team-based learning, to curriculum design such as the development of an outcome-based approach, to assessment such as organising an OSCE or to the selection of students for admission to the medical school.

Development of the teacher's competence is important, as highlighted by Irby et al. (2015 p. 705), not just for the individual teacher in terms of competence and job satisfaction, but also for the institution: "The goal of faculty development is to empower faculty members to excel in their varying academic roles, and to create organizations characterized by vitality."

In the UK, the professional development of medical teachers and trainers is now a requirement of the General Medical Council. This aims to ensure that all teachers have the necessary competencies to promote the quality of undergraduate and postgraduate education.

McLean et al. (2008) have suggested that minimum requirements for professionalising teaching practice are:

- Faculty development as an integral mission of every medical school. This includes orienting new staff members into the culture of the school, and enabling the development of generic teaching competencies and the development in staff of more specific skills relating to their role as a teacher.
- An institutional culture that recognises and rewards teaching excellence and scholarship equally with research and clinical service.

Faculty development programmes are now widely available and should be tailored to the needs of the individual teacher and the roles expected of them. Features that contribute to how effective a faculty development programme will be for you, as identified in a systematic review of faculty development programmes (Steinert et al., 2016), include:

- The relevance of the training programme to your teaching responsibilities.
- The provision of opportunities for application of the ideas in practice, either during the programme or in the workplace.
- The design of the educational programme based on educational principles, including the provision of feedback.
- Opportunities for reflection on your practice in the light of ideas addressed in the programme.
- Your participation in educational projects that allow you to apply the principles in the workplace.
- Collaboration and networking with other teachers, including peer evaluation of your teaching and the availability of role models.
- A supportive learning environment and institutional support, including financial support and release of time for the teacher.

Appropriate faculty development can improve your effectiveness as a teacher and, at the same time, increase your confidence and job satisfaction.

We have moved away from the concept of faculty development as simply attendance at a course or education training programme to an appreciation that faculty development is a continuing process. John Cotton Dana, on being asked to supply a Latin quotation for inscription on a new building at Newark State College in New Jersey, was unable to find a suitable quotation and, instead, offered one of his own making – "Who dares to teach must never cease to learn." As a teacher and a professional, you have the responsibility not only to acquire the necessary teaching skills but also to keep yourself up to date both with developments in your own discipline and with changes in educational practice. In medicine, the idea of mastery of a subject has given way to the recognition of lifelong learning. The same is true in medical education. Effective teachers are also good learners and keep themselves up to date. Here are some examples of changing practice relating to the different roles of the teacher:

- As an information provider, you have to continually reassess what information and skills should be acquired by the students. You should recognise that the approach to information, as we describe in Chapter 3, is changing, and that doctors now practise in an age in which information is ubiquitous and widely available (Friedman et al., 2016).
- As a facilitator of learning, you should appreciate the increasing understanding of how students learn and the changes in approaches to learning, such as the use of team-based learning, the move from the traditional lecture to a "flipped" classroom, the use of simulation and the concept of longitudinal, integrated clinical clerkships.
- As an assessor, you should understand the assessment process in your school and where your school sits on the seven continua relating to trends in assessment practice, as described in the PROFILE model in Chapter 6.
- As a role model, you should be aware of what is expected of you in the light of changes in healthcare delivery and public expectations.
- As a manager or leader, you have to keep abreast of your management and leadership responsibilities, taking into account the increasing complexity of teaching practice and the increasing need for collaboration.
- Innovating and responding to change is key for the teacher as a scholar and researcher.

At a time of rapid developments in the field of education, keeping up to date with current best practice is a formidable challenge. This can be facilitated both at an institutional and personal level through:

- Local, national or international medical education courses. The AMEE Essential Skills in Medical Education courses provide one example and are available both face-to-face and online, addressing general or more specialised topics.
- Medical education conferences. There are many international conferences where examples of current best practice in education can be explored. Examples are the AMEE annual conference, the Asia-Pacific Medical Education Conference, the International Medical Education Conference, the International Conference on Medical Education, the Ottawa Conference on the Assessment of Competence in the Health Care Professions and the International Association of Medical Science Educators annual meeting.
- Reading print and online journals that cover the subject of medical education. Examples are: *Medical Teacher, Medical Education,*

Academic Medicine, Teaching and Learning in Medicine and *AMEE MedEdPublish*.

- Joining webinars with a medical education theme.
- Reading published textbooks on the subject. A number of references are presented in this book in the "Explore further" section at the conclusion of each chapter. A more detailed account of some issues addressed in this book can be found in *A Practical Guide for Medical Teachers* (Dent et al., 2017) and *Essential Skills for a Medical Teacher* (Harden and Laidlaw, 2017).
- Being part of a community of practice and participating in online updating services such as MedEdWorld and MedEdPORTAL. Alexis Wiggins, a school teacher with 15 years' experience, described in her blog an interesting approach to her own continuing education, as reported in the *Washington Post* (Strauss, 2014): "I waited 14 years to do something I should have done my first year of teaching." She was referring to shadowing a student for a day, doing everything the student was supposed to do. She was amazed at what she learned and wished that she could go back to every class of students she had taught and change a minimum of ten things in her own teaching. We do not know personally anyone who has done this in a medical school but it could be a useful exercise and a day well spent.

Evaluating your competence as a teacher

A professional teacher will have acquired the appropriate teaching competencies. They will also assess their own performance as a teacher. A professional has been defined as someone who is an enquirer into his or her own competence. For each of the roles described in this book, we have suggested that you consider your own position and what is expected of you as a teacher, as an "expert" and as a "master" teacher. Have you the necessary skills and competence to fulfil your role as a teacher? Assessing your own competence and performance as a teacher is part of your professional responsibilities. If you present lectures, for example, you may find viewing a video recording of your lecture helpful. Self-assessment and reflection on your roles as a teacher is important but it is not enough. Other ways you can evaluate your performance as a teacher include:

- Evaluation by students. Student assessments of lectures or other teaching contributions and of the course for which you are responsible can give you valuable feedback, but does have limitations as highlighted in the Dr Fox effect, described in Chapter 5.
- Peer assessment by a colleague. This can involve peer observation of a teaching session, such as a lecture or peer review of course materials. It is helpful if the colleague is someone whose opinion you value.
- Assessment by a student assigned a specific role as assessor. A student can be appointed who is formally trained as an assessor both with regard to what to look for and how to provide feedback to the teacher.

- Performance of students in the final examination. This too should be interpreted with caution. In one study, it was found that students had higher marks in the questions relating to the subject covered by what was recognised as the poorest lecturer – the lectures were so bad that students had no option but to explore the subject themselves and read the relevant textbooks.
- More formal assessments, such as the objective structured teaching exercises (OSTEs) (Lu et al., 2014). Alice Fornari highlights the role of the OSTE in assisting teachers to evaluate their own performance (Box 10.3).

Much has been written about the merits of these and other sources of evidence (Berk, 2006). Each source can supply unique information but is fallible, and the results from different sources should be triangulated to form a judgement of teaching effectiveness. Talking about teacher assessment Shulman (1988, p. xxiii) has suggested that we create "'A union of insufficiencies' in which various methods of assessment are combined in such a way that the strengths of one offset the limitations of the other."

Box 10.3 Self-assessment of teaching[a]

I have been a teacher in higher education full time since 1983 with a transition to medical school education in 2003. This transition has opened me up to the world of medical school faculty across the continuum of undergraduate, graduate and continuing medical education. The most eye-opening observation for me as a medical educator, and important to my own professional development, is the need to connect medical faculty interested in clinical teaching education to form a "community of practice" specific to their education roles. Faculties are connected clinically and this education role is not always natural, even with expressed interest. My intent supports a "community of practice" created over time by a shared pursuit, educating learners within the clinical environments that patient care is delivered.

One strategy I value to engage faculty and help them become more confident in their teaching skills is the objective structured teaching encounter (OSTE). OSTEs support experiential practice and assessment of clinical teaching skills. This approach to clinician educator training assures professional development of new roles goes beyond traditional "one-off" seminars and workshops. Clinician educators build confidence while enhancing their teaching skills. Through self-assessment and debriefs, they engage in dialogues on the true challenges of teaching that is common to all clinical settings. This experiential approach, anchored in self and peer formative assessment, supports more engaged educators who will then approach clinical teaching with more skill, confidence and enthusiasm. For me as a medical educator, this approach is a "win-win" for all involved in embracing the role of the clinical teacher.

---

[a]Alice Fornari, Assistant Vice President of Faculty Development, Associate Dean of Education Skills Development, Professor of Science Education, Population Health and Family Medicine, Hofstra Northwell School of Medicine, USA.

You can keep a portfolio of your teaching experiences, and this can be used to support promotion submissions. It can include:

- Your teaching commitments
- Reflections on your teaching and changes you have made
- Membership in committees and working groups
- Further study or courses undertaken
- Publications and communications at conferences
- Teaching awards or scholarships received locally or nationally

Student ratings of teaching

Student ratings are the most widely used approach to evaluate teaching and have been the primary measure of teaching effectiveness. Although they are of value, student ratings may be biased, and their limitations should be recognised (Berk, 2013). They are a necessary but not sufficient source of evidence to assess teaching effectiveness comprehensively. An example of a rating sheet for the evaluation of a lecture is given in Fig. 10.3.

Ratings may be perceived by the teacher as unfair, resulting in a feeling of resentment, and interviews with students or groups of students may be helpful. Traditionally, student evaluations were paper and pencil based but there has been a move to online rating, which offers ease of administration, low cost and rapid turnaround of the results. The results of the two approaches have been found to be the same with the exception of unstructured or open-ended items, for which longer and more thoughtful comments are often provided online.

Consideration should be given to the number of evaluations students are expected to complete because too many result in response fatigue and a low response rate. A strategy to improve the response rate for an end-of-course assessment is to require the evaluation form to be completed before students are given their grades or marks.

In the UK, increasing importance has been attached to the annual National Student Survey of the quality of teaching in UK universities. The production of a league table based on the results has been a driver for institutions to take the need to enhance the students' learning experience seriously (van der Velden, 2012). Indeed, in one medical school, a poor performance proved to be a stimulus for setting up a department of medical education. The results of the student survey have also been used as a significant element in the UK Teaching Excellence Framework assessment of teaching quality in UK universities.

Your well-being as a teacher

Increasing attention is being paid to the importance of your well-being as a teacher. An emphasis on well-being is a recognised feature of contemporary life and, as a

	Definitely yes	Probably yes	Uncertain	Probably no	Definitely no
1. The content of the lecture addressed the course learning outcomes	☐	☐	☐	☐	☐
2. The delivery of the lecture was clear and paced correctly	☐	☐	☐	☐	☐
3. Visual aids were used effectively	☐	☐	☐	☐	☐
4. I found the lecture stimulating	☐	☐	☐	☐	☐
5. The lecturer actively engaged students during the lecture	☐	☐	☐	☐	☐
6. Opportunities were provided to ask questions	☐	☐	☐	☐	☐
7. Useful handouts were provided	☐	☐	☐	☐	☐
8. The learning experience was valuable	☐	☐	☐	☐	☐
9. The lecture was pitched at the right level	☐	☐	☐	☐	☐
10. The lecturer kept to the time allocated	☐	☐	☐	☐	☐
11. The lecture was well prepared	☐	☐	☐	☐	☐

Name of lecturer: _____

Date: _____

12. What did you most like about the lecture

13. What did you like least about the lecture

14. Any other comments

Figure 10.3 Evaluation of a lecture

professional, you have a responsibility, not just for your students' well-being but also for your own. It is likely that at times as a teacher you will feel stressed, overworked and not appreciated. This does not mean that you are a less good teacher. It means that you are human.

The problem of stress and burnout

There have been alarming pronouncements about the growing prevalence of stress and burnout in teachers and the adverse effect this has had, not only on the teacher but also on the education programme. Three aspects of burnout have been described (Pierce and Molloy, 1990):

The first is the development of increased feelings of emotional exhaustion and fatigue. Second is the tendency for teachers to develop negative, cynical attitudes towards their students. The third aspect of burnout is the tendency to evaluate oneself negatively, resulting in feelings of lack of personal accomplishment.

A number of factors contribute to job stress for the teacher (Harden, 1999). These relate to:

- An increased workload and the day-to-day demands on the teacher. The number of students admitted to medical school has increased, often without a matching increase in funding.
- The many changes taking place in education. These include curriculum developments, new approaches to teaching such as blended learning, with face-to-face and online instruction integrated, changes in assessment with the move to more authentic assessment and improved approaches to the selection of students.
- A reduction in the freedom, autonomy and discretion the teacher has in relation to his or her work as a teacher. Teachers now have less control of their work, as discussed earlier in this chapter, and this sense of powerlessness can contribute to stress.

No longer are teachers left to deliver the teaching in their own subject independently. This must be done in collaboration with their colleagues as part of an integrated curriculum and with colleagues in other professions if interprofessional education is to feature as part of the educational programme. A possible loss of autonomy has been suggested as a criticism of outcome-based or competency-based education. It can be argued, however, that a level of conformity and standards for medical training, as set out for specified learning outcomes, is required. Once the learning outcomes are agreed, however, the teacher has a greater measure of freedom about how she or he can facilitate the student to achieve the expected outcomes.

The greatest degree of stress is found in jobs that are characterised by high demands and a low decision latitude, and stress may be seen in this circumstance as a function of the job and not the person.

- They have more continuous teaching throughout the year, without a break. This may be due to an increase in the length of the working year or the engagement of the teacher with a number of modules throughout the course. The clinician, for example, may be required to teach in the early years of the course as well as in the later years. Such continuous pressure with no time to recover can be a significant cause of stress.
- Patients may be less readily available for teaching, with changes in healthcare delivery. This places an additional burden on the teacher, with the need for the teacher to arrange experiences for students with patients

and at the same time become familiar with new approaches such as simulation.

- The teacher may be required to assume new roles in the teaching programme. Stress may result from a mismatch between the requirements and demands of the job and the person's role or perceived ability to meet these demands. Some roles expected of the teacher may be unfamiliar and require further training and experience. An example might be designing an assessment procedure and implementing a standard setting approach.
- Conflicting demands on the teacher as a result of their teaching, research, clinical and administrative functions may result in role stress. The teacher may be confronted by a range of demands and expectations from a number of sources that cannot all be met at the same time.
- There may be insufficient recognition, rewards, salary incentives or promotion prospects for teachers relating to their teaching responsibilities. Unfortunately in many universities, research continues to be rated and valued more highly than teaching.
- Finally, there may be a lack of support or resources to assist teachers in meeting their commitments.

Some stress may be inevitable but, for a teacher, it can represent a potentially serious problem. The stress facing a teacher can be represented in this formula:

$$S = (WL + DA + IR + LP)/(RR + RC + JS + PS)$$

where stress (S) is a function of increased workload (WL), decreased autonomy (DA), an inappropriate teaching role (IR) and lack of preparation for the teaching responsibilities (LP) and where stress is reduced by rewards and recognition (RR), respect and civility at work (RC), job support (JS) and personal support (PS).

In considering burnout and stress, the emphasis has been switching from the problem of the individual to the problem in the work environment. Improving the quality of social encounters and greater civility and respect in the workplace can result in a reduction in burnout among staff (Maslach and Leiter, 2016).

Healthcare professionals who are personally engaged in their work in patient care and teaching with dedication and absorption are more resilient, experience less burnout and are healthier (van den Berg et al., 2017).

Promoting well-being

Stress and well-being of teachers in medicine need to be recognised and strategies developed at individual and institutional levels to alleviate stress and promote well-being. Action required includes:

- Improving job satisfaction for the teacher and rewarding commitment and excellence in teaching

- Specifying and clarifying the prescribed roles expected of the teacher and ensuring that teachers are given roles in which they can operate most effectively
- Ensuring that the workload is spread appropriately and individual teachers are not overloaded
- Providing teachers with educational, administrative and personal support
- Involving teachers in planning the teaching programme and decentralising it as far as possible to reduce feelings of a lack of autonomy
- Ensuring participation by staff in staff development programmes, including programmes on mindfulness.

Programmes developing mindfulness have been shown to be of value. The role of mindfulness programmes is now established and can have a long-term beneficial effect on perceived stress (van Vliet et al., 2017). Mindfulness involves:

- Paying close attention to emotions and raising the level of introspective awareness
- Creating emotional space and the ability to see a problem without feeling part of it
- Self-compassion and being kinder to oneself and realistic in expectations of success.

A mind-body medicine course, developed at Georgetown University, takes into account the connectedness between mind and body. It consists of a programme that encompasses experiential sessions of specific mind-body techniques such as meditation, relaxation and guided imagery (Karpowicz et al., 2009).

However, the issue of your personal well-being does raise problems. For example, there may be confusion in terms of your professionalism as to whether you owe it to your students to work long hours teaching and preparing for your teaching or whether you owe it to yourself to keep stricter divides between home and work. It may be a struggle to resolve such dilemmas. As suggested by Craig and Fieschi (2007):

> All caring professions may seem to present fuzzy boundaries. Indeed
> professions are, in part, held to be so because of a particular relationship
> with the "client" (be it a patient, a pupil or a lost soul) defined by the
> professional's willingness to offer both expertise and individual advice and
> attention. This meant, always, a level of closeness and commitment that
> went hand in hand with high levels of trust. (p. 10)

Maladaptive behaviour in the teacher may also affect the student, as highlighted by Lemaire and Wallace (2017) in their editorial: "Burnout is one consequence of the "hidden curriculum" in medical education, where learners witness and adopt their teachers' maladaptive behaviours, which are often reinforced throughout their careers."

"Civic" professionalism

Your professional responsibilities reflect both moral and social aspects of being a teacher and extend beyond your responsibilities to the individual student. They encompass the broader perspective of scholarship, as discussed in Chapter 9. You are responsible not just for the students you teach, but for the patients they will treat as medical practitioners and for wider issues, such as globalisation and climate change. This has been described by Sullivan (2005) as your "civic professionalism."

In medicine, there has been vigorous debate about the scope of a physician's responsibility for issues such as health inequalities and the need for system change. This relates to the boundaries of a physician's professional obligations and responsibilities (Hubinette et al., 2017). In the same way, we argue that the teacher has a responsibility to consider these wider issues. Writing about the new academic professionalism, Nixon (2001) has argued that professionalism is not just doing what the teacher does and how he or she does it, but about asking why it is done and how it will affect the community:

> *Such values prefigure a professional reorientation which requires of its practitioners a willingness to reconceive and radically readjust the relation between their own "small world" of professional interests and the wider public interests of the world "out there". (p. 179)*

The professional teacher, an expert professional and a master professional

The professional teacher

As a professional teacher, you accept your responsibilities in relation to your behaviour, your competence, the evaluation of your performance and your personal well-being.

An expert professional

In addition to accepting these professional responsibilities, you develop particular expertise in one or more of the areas and take a leadership role in relation to it.

A master professional

You undertake research and development work in one or more of the areas and are recognised nationally or internationally for your expertise in respect of this

Take-home messages

As a professional, you have a responsibility to:
1. Meet the standards of behaviour expected of a teacher
2. Acquire and keep up to date your competencies as a teacher
3. Evaluate your performance as a teacher
4. Look after your personal well-being.

Consider

With regard to your professionalism as a teacher, consider whether you:

- Meet the expected standards of behaviour, as set out in the teacher's charter in Table 10.1
- Have acquired the necessary understanding and skills required for your role as a teacher
- Evaluate your performance as a teacher, adjusting your approach as necessary
- Consider and respect your personal well-being.

Explore further

Berk, R., 2006. Thirteen Strategies to Measure College Teaching: A Consumer's Guide to Rating Scale Construction, Assessment, and Decision Making for Faculty, Administrators, and Clinicians. Stylus Publishing, Terling, VA.

Berk, R.A., 2013. Top five flashpoints in the assessment of teaching effectiveness. Med. Teach. 35 (1), 15–26.

Birden, H., Glass, N., Wilson, I., et al., 2014. Defining professionalism in medical education: A systematic review. Med. Teach. 36 (1), 47–61.

Craig, J., Fieschi, C., 2007. DIY Professionalism: Futures for Teaching. Demos, Glasgow.

Dent, J.A., Harden, R.M., Hunt, D., 2017. A Practical Guide for Medical Teachers, fifth ed. Elsevier, London.

Dunning, R., Laidlaw, A., 2015. The application of the Practitioners in Applied Practice Model during breaking bad news communication training for medical students: A case study. Scottish Med. J. 60 (4), 170–175.

Friedman, C.P., Donaldson, K.M., Vantsevich, A.V., 2016. Educating medical students in the era of ubiquitous information. Med. Teach. 38 (5), 504–509.

Furlong, J., Barton, L., Miles, S., et al., 2000. Teacher Education in Transition: Re-Forming Professionalism? Open University Press, Philadelphia.

Harden, R.M., 1999. Stress, pressure and burnout in teachers: Is the swan exhausted? Med. Teach. 21 (3), 245–247.

Harden, R.M., Laidlaw, J.M., 2017. Essential Skills for a Medical Teacher. Elsevier, London.

Hoyle, E., John, P.D., 1995. Professional Knowledge and Professional Practice. Cassell, London.

Hubinette, M., Dobson, S., Scott, I., et al., 2017. Health advocacy. Med. Teach. 39 (2), 128–135.

Irby, D.M., O'Sullivan, P.S., Steinert, Y., 2015. Is it time to recognize excellence in faculty development programs? Med. Teach. 37 (8), 705–706.

Karpowicz, S., Harazduk, N., Haramati, A., 2009. Using mind-body medicine for self-awareness and self-care in medical school. J. Hol. Health. 6 (2), 19–22.

Kolb, D., 1984. Experiential Learning: Experience as the Source of Learning and Development. Prentice Hall, Upper Saddle River, NJ.

Laidlaw, A., Guild, S., Struthers, J., 2009. Graduate attributes in the disciplines of Medicine, Dentistry and Veterinary Medicine: A survey of expert opinions. BMC Med. Educ. 9, 28.

Lemaire, J.B., Wallace, J.E., 2017. Burnout damages more than just individuals. BMJ 358, 183.

Lu, W.H., Mylona, E., Lane, S., et al., 2014. Faculty development on professionalism and medical ethics: The design, development and implementation of Objective Structured Teaching Exercises (OSTEs). Med. Teach. 36 (10), 876–882.

Maister, D., 1997. True Professionalism. Simon and Schuster, New York.

Maslach, C., Leiter, M.P., 2016. Understanding the burnout experience: Recent research and its implications for psychiatry. World Psychiatry. 15 (2), 103–111.

McLean, M., Cilliers, F., van Wyk, J.M., 2008. Faculty development: Yesterday, today and tomorrow. Med. Teach. 86 (4), 421–428.

Nixon, J., 2001. 'Not without dust and heat': The moral bases of the 'new' academic professionalism. Br. J. Educ. Stud. 49 (2), 173–186.

Pierce, C.M.B., Molloy, G.N., 1990. Psychological and biographical differences between secondary school teachers experiencing high and low levels of burnout. Educ. Psych. 60 (1), 37–51.

Ruona, W., Gilley, J., 2009. Practitioners in applied professions: A model applied to Human Resource Development. Adv. Dev. Hum. Resources. 11 (4), 438–453.

Schon, D., 1984. The Reflective Practitioner: How Professionals Think in Action. Perseus Books, New York.

Shulman, L., 1988. A union of insufficiencies: Strategies for teacher assessment in a period of reform. Educ. Leadership. 46, 36–41.

Solbrekke, T.D., Englund, T., 2011. Bringing professional responsibility back in. Stud. High Educ. 36 (7), 847–861.

Steinert, Y., Mann, K., Anderson, B., et al., 2016. A systematic review of faculty development initiatives designed to enhance teaching effectiveness: A 10-year update: BEME Guide No 40. Med. Teach. 38 (8), 769–786.

Strauss, V., 2014. Teacher spends two days as a student and is shocked at what she learns. https://www.washingtonpost.com/news/answer-sheet/wp/2014/10/24/teacher-spends-two-days-as-a-student-and-is-shocked-at-what-she-learned/?utm_term=.f414162f28c0.

Sullivan, W.C., 2005. Work and Integrity: The Crisis and Promise of Professionalism in America. Jossey-Bass, San Francisco.

van den Berg, J.W., Mastenbroek, N.J.J.M., Scheepers, R.A., et al., 2017. Work engagement in health professions education. Med. Teach. 39 (11), 1110–1118.

van der Velden, G., 2012. Institutional level student engagement and organisational cultures. High Educ. Q. 66 (3), 227–247.

van Vliet, M., Jong, M., Jong, M.C., 2017. Long-term benefits by a mind-body medicine skills course on perceived stress and empathy among medical and nursing students. Med. Teach. 39 (7), 710–719.

Wass, V.J., Barnard, A., 2017. In: Dent, J.A., Harden, R.M., Hunt, D. (Eds.), A Practical Guide for Medical Teachers, fifth ed. Elsevier, Edinburgh.

THE TEACHER AS A PROFESSIONAL

Chapter 11

The roles of the teacher today and in the future

Teaching is impossible. If we simply add together all that is expected of a typical teacher...the sum makes greater demands than any individual can possibly fulfil.

Lee Shulman

A consideration of the roles of a teacher is important both for the teacher and for the institution. These roles will change with time.

The eight roles of the teacher

We have described in this book eight roles for the teacher (Fig. 11.1):

The teacher as an information provider

We have argued in Chapter 3 that the role of the teacher as an information provider is changing from a conductor of information to a curator of information where the

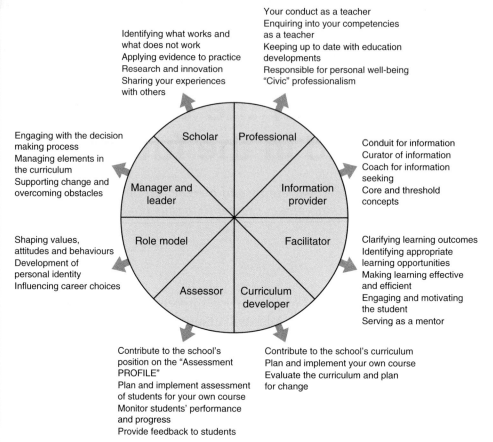

Identifying what works and what does not work
Applying evidence to practice
Research and innovation
Sharing your experiences with others

Your conduct as a teacher
Enquiring into your competencies as a teacher
Keeping up to date with education developments
Responsible for personal well-being
"Civic" professionalism

Engaging with the decision making process
Managing elements in the curriculum
Supporting change and overcoming obstacles

Conduit for information
Curator of information
Coach for information seeking
Core and threshold concepts

Shaping values, attitudes and behaviours
Development of personal identity
Influencing career choices

Clarifying learning outcomes
Identifying appropriate learning opportunities
Making learning effective and efficient
Engaging and motivating the student
Serving as a mentor

Contribute to the school's position on the "Assessment PROFILE"
Plan and implement assessment of students for your own course
Monitor students' performance and progress
Provide feedback to students

Contribute to the school's curriculum
Plan and implement your own course
Evaluate the curriculum and plan for change

Scholar · *Professional* · *Manager and leader* · *Information provider* · *Role model* · *Facilitator* · *Assessor* · *Curriculum developer*

Figure 11.1 The eight roles of the teacher

objective is to make information available to students when they want it and need it. The teacher acts as a human filter drawing attention to what might be important and useful for the student. This makes the learning more efficient and saves the student time. The teacher acting as a coach also encourages the student to search for and evaluate information they need.

The teacher as a facilitator

Rethinking your role as a facilitator as highlighted in Chapter 4, is a challenge with the move from information provider, where the emphasis is on transmitting or transferring knowledge to one of facilitation of the students' learning. This has been referred to as a move from "sage on the stage" to "guide on the side." If the student is to achieve the specified learning outcomes, it is your responsibility as a teacher to help them do so by ensuring that they understand the required learning outcomes and that they engage in appropriate learning activities that will enable them to achieve the learning outcomes. You may also have a role as mentor.

The teacher as a curriculum planner and developer

The teacher has a responsibility for developing and implementing an authentic curriculum in their school, which prepares students for their career as healthcare professionals. This includes, as described in Chapter 5, identifying the expected learning outcomes, adopting appropriate educational strategies, designing learning opportunities or experiences, developing a suitable learning environment and organising an assessment process to check if the student is achieving the required standards.

The teacher as an assessor

The role of the teacher as an assessor has changed from an activity solely designed to certify that the student has reached the required standard (assessment-*of*-learning) to one which also supports the student's learning (assessment-*for*-learning), as described in Chapter 6. The assessment of the student should represent not an assessment at one point in time, but should be an evaluation of the student's performance across the course.

The teacher as a role model

The importance of the teacher as a role model is often neglected or ignored in staff development programmes. It is, however, one of the most important roles. Students model themselves on the behaviour they see in practice and not on what they are told to do in the lecture. We described in Chapter 7, how as a role model the teacher shapes the student's values, attitudes and behaviours and can influence their career choice.

The teacher as manager and leader

The teacher is a member of a team, at times taking a management or leadership role. Every teacher, to a greater or lesser extent, has management and leadership responsibilities, as described in Chapter 8. The teacher may have an important role to play in the management of change.

The teacher as a scholar and researcher

Every teacher should be a scholar, reflecting on their own teaching, trying to improve on it in light of what is known about different education approaches and undertaking action research in relation to their own teaching. This is discussed in Chapter 9.

The teacher as a professional

Teachers are not technicians but professionals who have a code of conduct, ensure that they have the skills required as a teacher and keep themselves up to date, are responsible for evaluating their own competence and are concerned about their own health and well-being. We have extended this to include "civic" professionalism.

As you will have seen, we have taken a broader perspective of each of these roles than may be customary – for example, the information provider, who not only provides the student with information but educates the student to find information, the scholar who is more than a researcher and the professional who takes a broader view of her or his responsibilities as a teacher.

Factors affecting the roles expected of a teacher

A number of factors may affect the roles expected of a teacher.

The phase or stage of education

The expected role of the teacher will change as the student passes through the training programme, with students expected to take more responsibility for their own learning in the later stages of undergraduate education and in postgraduate education (Dron, 2007). This represents a shift from a role of information provider to one of facilitator.

The cultural background

Different cultures vary in their expectations of the teacher. The teacher's responsibilities as an information provider and lecturer are emphasised more in some cultures than others. The expectations of the teacher as a manager or leader also vary in different cultures.

The size of the team

In some situations, the teacher may work as part of a large team, in which responsibilities can be shared between a number of teachers. One teacher may be responsible for assessment and serve as chair of an assessment committee, another may be responsible for curriculum development and another may be responsible for aspects of the teaching and learning programme, including a clinical skills unit. In other contexts, where there are fewer teachers, the teacher may be expected to take a wider range of teaching roles.

Educational support available

The extent to which educational assistance is available to support the teacher may vary. An educationalist or psychometrician, for example, may be responsible for standard setting as part of the assessment process and for testing the reliability of the examinations. In other settings, these may be the responsibility of the teacher. Education support may or may not be available in the form of an educational technologist to support technology developments.

The context of teaching

The relative importance of the different roles may vary with the context of the teaching. In the clinical situation, the teacher assumes greater importance as a role model.

The educational strategies adopted in the curriculum

The education strategy adopted in the school may dictate the roles expected of the teacher. The teacher's role as facilitator, for example, is important in problem-based learning.

The public's expectation

We have seen situations in which parents attempt to exert an influence on the role adopted by the teacher. They may express the view that they are paying for their son or daughter to be taught and raise objections when there is a move away from formal lectures, and students are given more responsibility for their own learning.

Multiple roles for a teacher

Consideration of your role as a teacher is important. As a teacher, you should:

- Recognise the different roles a teacher has in supporting students to achieve their objectives. We have described eight roles.
- Be familiar with the roles to allow you to have a better understanding of the education process and to assist you to carry out your day-to-day work as a teacher most effectively and with job satisfaction. We describe below, for example, how you can gain a new insight into the task of lecturing by considering the different roles you can play in relation to a lecture.
- Appreciate that you have a responsibility for all of the roles, but you may have a greater responsibility with regard to some roles.

As described by Joyce et al. (2009), thinking about the different roles expected of you is not easy:

> *Thinking about the roles that make up teaching can make you dizzy. Just for starters, these roles include helping students grow in understanding, knowledge, self-awareness, moral development and the ability to relate to others. Simultaneously we are managers of learning, curriculum designers, facilitators, counsellors, evaluators and, reluctantly, disciplinarians. To the best of our ability, we modulate across roles accordingly to individual and group needs as we select and create learning experiences for all our students. (p. 118)*

Sören Huwendiek, an experienced medical educator with a broad interest in clinical teaching and assessment, medical education research and change management describes in Box 11.1 how the teacher can focus on several but not all roles.

Box 11.1 The different roles of the teacher[a]

I myself enjoy most of the roles described in the book. The book nicely shows the many different roles we (might) have. This diversity and the possibilities to support change make my professional life as a medical educator a varied and fulfilling experience. However, I think medical educators can also have a focus on just some of the roles and do not need to fulfil every single role to the fullest.

Most of the roles described in this book were also found in a study exploring the self-definitions of the members of the Association for Medical Education in Europe (AMEE) (Nikendei et al., 2016). In this study, one self-definition was the "Enthusiast". Indeed, I feel that there are so many enthusiasts among medical educators, which makes being part of this community a great privilege.

[a]*Sören Huwendiek, Head of Department of Assessment and Evaluation, Institute of Medical Education, University of Bern, Bern, Switzerland.*

Teaching can be viewed as a complex system involving all eight roles, with the different roles co-existing. Indeed, the teacher with different roles at the same time can be described as "the new normal." Tan Li Hoon, a clinical teacher in Singapore, and Eliana Amaral, a senior teacher in Brazil, describe their multiple roles as a teacher in Boxes 11.2 and 11.3.

Box 11.2 Multiple roles[a]

I am a core faculty member in the institute of the Sing Health Anaesthesiology Residency Programme, and in charge of the teaching programme. As an information provider, I introduce the module, provide the teaching schedule and discuss the learning outcomes and assessment plans. I edit and compile the reading material provided for the learners, using chapters contributed by the teaching faculty. This is done on a 3-4 year basis, with a new edition in preparation.

In addition to a being a role model in my clinical and professional practice, I demonstrate a personal commitment to continuous professional development, a willingness to learn and an openness to feedback. I facilitate the implementation of the programme and curriculum by carefully planning the module, identifying learning outcomes, selecting teaching methods and organising the logistics. In consultation with other teachers, I decide on the assessment methods and blueprint the questions to the curriculum. I also organise an end of month assessment. In addition, I also collect from the learners an evaluation of the teaching programme.

[a]*Tan Li Hoon, Consultant, SingHealth Anaesthesiology Residency Programme, Singapore.*

We can take the lecture, one of the most common tasks facing a teacher, as an example of the multiple roles assumed by a teacher:

- The teacher is seen traditionally in this context as predominantly an information provider.

Box 11.3 A spectrum of roles[a]

According to local bylaws, a faculty member must integrate teaching, research, and extension of the discipline knowledge to the community. As such, and being a full-time professor, tenured at a public research-oriented university in Brazil, trained and practising as an obstetrician, I had the opportunity to experience a spectrum of roles during my professional trajectory. This included being a clinical care provider, health service administrator and advisor, as well as facilitator of learning, curriculum planner, developer and evaluator, educational and academic manager, scholar, researcher and change agent. I also served as a role model for undergraduate and graduate students, residents, and faculty members. Becoming a teacher-of-teachers, a faculty developer for my own department, institution, as well as national level, new skills and specific knowledge were required.

The mix and relevance of each role varied along my career from the role of healthcare manager to a senior academic position which amalgamated clinical and educational roles. Each experience was a platform for the one that followed, and offered lessons for me to learn from and share. Helping to improve services, produce new knowledge, while training new and better professionals is energising, and keeps eyes sparkling – intense and exciting, stressful and chaotic on occasions. Anyway, the balance is positive – no doubt a perfect professional choice.

[a]*Eliana Amaral. Professor of Obstetrics, Head of Faculty Affairs, State University of Campinas (UNICAMP), Sao Paulo, Brazil, and FAIMER Institute Fellow.*

- The teacher can also facilitate learning with the use of breakout discussions during the lecture or the use of a "flipped classroom."
- The use of an audience response system during the lecture, or providing students with the opportunity to assess their own knowledge after the lecture, illustrates the role of assessor.
- The lecturer also serves as a role model and his or her comments, attitude and behaviour may influence the student. We have commented earlier in this text, for example, on the negative effects on the student of the lecturer who consistently arrives late for the lecture and the hospital-based lecturer who makes disparaging comments about the value of the student's community attachments.
- As a curriculum planner, the lecturer looks at how the lecture contributes to the overall education programme and the students' achievement of the expected learning outcomes. The lecturer is also concerned with how the lecture relates to the other learning experiences offered to the students.
- As a scholar and a researcher, the lecturer evaluates what they are doing and shares innovative ways of delivering a lecture with others.

Although we have considered each of the eight roles of the teacher in separate chapters, they should not be treated in isolation. This example of the lecture illustrates how the different roles interact with and affect each other. How the eight roles relate to the common tasks facing a teacher is illustrated in Table 11.1. All tasks require multiple roles of the teacher, and all roles are reflected in different tasks.

Table 11.1 The eight roles of a teacher: How they apply in different degrees to the activities expected of a teacher

Education activity	Teacher role							
	Information provider	Facilitator of learning	Curriculum planner and implementer	Assessor	Role model	Manager and leader	Scholar and researcher	Professional
Lecture	+++	++	+	+	+	+	+	+
Small group	+	+++	+	++	++	+	+	+
Development of learning resources	+++	++	+	++	+	+	+	+
Clinical teaching	++	++	+	+	+++	+	+	+
Examination	+	+	++	+++	+	+	+	+
Feedback to student	++	++	+	++	+	+	+	+
Curriculum planning	+	++	+++	+	+	+	+	+

Cutting across all the other roles is the need for teachers to be a professional – evaluating their own practice whether as a lecturer, a clinical teacher, a curriculum planner or an examiner and taking steps to keep themselves up to date with respect to their work as a teacher. As scholars, they should reflect on their experiences and communicate lessons learned to others.

Nor are the boundaries between the different roles rigid. By identifying as an information provider the necessary core information to be learned, the teacher is also facilitating learning. The teacher is also facilitating learning if he or she provides feedback to the student following an examination. The roles are mutually interactive through complex interdependent relationships, and trade-offs and compromises may have to be made between the different roles.

There may be an element of conflict between the different roles: for example, the teacher as information provider and facilitator (when should the student be given the information or be expected to find it for themselves?); the teacher as a facilitator and assessor (can the same person act as teacher and assessor?); the teacher as a role model and information provider (does the behaviour of the doctor in practice differ from what is described in the lectures relating to ethics?).

The multiple roles of the teacher are important in the clinical situation. The good clinical teacher needs to fulfil a range of teaching roles (McAllister et al., 1997). The multiple roles needed in a single clinical teaching experience were referred to by White and Ewan (1991), and Irby (1994) has described how clinical teachers need to provide information, facilitate learning and assess learners' knowledge. As teaching opportunities arise, a good teacher will move instinctively between different roles.

Changing roles

Your roles as a teacher are likely to vary with changes in your career. The roles may alter when you are promoted to more senior appointments, with management and leadership roles assuming increased importance. Your relative responsibilities and priorities relating to teaching, research, clinical work and administration may also change over time, and this too may influence the role(s) you fulfil as a teacher. Although some roles may become more prominent with time, all will remain relevant. Even if a new assessment unit is established, with trained psychometricians and assessment experts, your understanding and input to the assessment process will still be important. If an integrated curriculum is introduced, and your subject no longer features prominently, you still have to take responsibility for how your subject is embedded in the programme. The creation of a new central management structure will not absolve you from the management of aspects of your own teaching programme. As we discussed earlier, financial constraints should not inhibit your role as scholar and change agent but should stimulate further efforts to examine and adapt current education practices critically.

As a teacher gains more experience, it is recognised that not only will their roles change, but their views on teaching are also likely to change. This may include a shift from an emphasis on teaching to an emphasis on learning (Kugel, 1993).

Your personal role as a teacher

Your role as a teacher in your institution should ideally match the roles for which you are best suited. If this is not the case, it may be because your potential contribution to the curriculum has not been fully appreciated or because there is a mismatch between what is required in a curriculum and the expertise or experience of the available staff in the institution. This may be the situation, for example, when a new school is established or when a fundamentally different approach to the curriculum is adopted in a traditional school approach to teaching.

We discussed in the earlier chapters your involvement in all eight roles and highlighted what is expected of you as a teacher in relation to each role. We also suggested how you can demonstrate particular expertise in a role.

Case studies of the roles of a teacher in practice

The different contributions teachers can make to the curriculum are illustrated in the eight case studies in Box 11.4. Each teacher made a significant contribution to the education programme but this varied, depending on their background, other commitments and interest in teaching. The behavioural science teacher; the anatomist; the surgeon; the ear, nose and throat (ENT) surgeon and the obstetrician all contributed to the teaching of their subjects and to the overall specified learning outcomes as information providers. They also all served as role models. They facilitated the students' learning in different ways. The general practitioner promoted a more community-oriented approach to the curriculum, and the obstetrician introduced an interprofessional education programme. The behavioural scientist and the ENT doctor had a major impact on assessment. Many demonstrated evidence of scholarship, and the cardiologist was promoted to a professorial position on the basis of this. The basic scientist offered students experience in research, served as a role model of a research worker and provided students with a glimpse of the future of medicine. Some had particular responsibilities as chair or member of a committee, but all had a significant impact on the curriculum.

The institution's responsibilities

The importance of the teacher

No medical school can truly succeed without great teachers. The teachers are as, if not more important than the curriculum, the physical building and the learning resources available. I (RMH) remember working with a new medical school where for the first year after the launch of the school, only temporary buildings and limited resources were available, and the curriculum had some areas that needed refinement. The staff and students were enthusiastic, however, and committed to working together

Box 11.4 Case studies of teachers and their roles

The committed behavioural science teacher

J.S. is actively engaged in research in the behavioural sciences but takes seriously her responsibility for teaching the subject to medical students. She restructured the behavioural science course to make it more relevant and appealing to the students, while at the same time bringing it in line with the nationally specified behavioural science core learning outcomes to which she had an input. She collaborates with general practitioners and other clinicians in implementing the programme. Students are encouraged to assess their progress, and they receive personal feedback. Students, most of whom come from a biomedical model background, admire her passion and enthusiasm about the relevance and importance of the behaviour sciences to medical practice and begin to appreciate the value of the subject.

The innovative anatomist

P.M., an anatomist with a medical background, engages with the students with new approaches including body painting to teach surface anatomy. To help students understand the relevant anatomy, he prepares specimens using a 3D printer. He is not on the curriculum committee but is familiar with learning outcomes expected of the students and demonstrates how his course contributes not only to the students' knowledge of anatomy, but also to their mastery of generic competencies such as communication skills and team working. He also offers an elective for students who wish to study anatomy in more detail. Although the time allocated to teaching anatomy has decreased, the clinicians now feel the students have a better grasp of anatomy and are more able to apply their knowledge to clinical problems.

The busy surgeon

R.P. is a busy surgeon. He contributes to teaching in the gastrointestinal block and is in charge of its organisation. He is also responsible for students during their surgery clerkships in his surgical unit and, despite his heavy clinical workload, takes his teaching responsibilities and commitments seriously. The students' portfolios demonstrate the rich and comprehensive experience they receive during the clerkship. Some students report that studying with R.P. has inspired them to take up surgery as their career choice.

The inspirational ENT surgeon

M.G. is responsible for the ENT teaching in the medical school. Students had previously not taken the subject seriously, at least in part because their competence in the field was not assessed in the final examination. M.G. negotiated with those responsible in the school for the final OSCE to include one ENT station, with an ENT surgeon as an examiner. He worked closely with the students and helped them to take more responsibility for their own learning in ENT, including peer learning and peer assessment as a formal part of the programme. Under his guidance, some students developed learning resources covering the topic. The students involved became interested in medical education and presented papers on the subject at medical education conferences. Students now value the course highly.

The enthusiastic cardiologist

T.L. was responsible for the cardiovascular system course in the curriculum. She also served on the school's curriculum committee. In collaboration with colleagues, she identified

Continued on next page

Box 11.4 Case studies of teachers and their roles—cont'd

the core knowledge and skills expected of the students in relation to the cardiovascular system along with twelve threshold concepts relating to the system, which were key for the students' understanding of the subject. She presented a paper on her work on threshold concepts at an international medical education conference. She also contributed to the local staff development course for new teachers and designed an objective structured teaching evaluation to assess teaching competencies. She was promoted in the school to a professorial position on the basis of her teaching contributions and scholarship.

The research-oriented molecular biologist

B.H. was an internationally recognised researcher in molecular biology. He had little time to spend on teaching but, when he did contribute to the course, he attempted to make his lecture inspirational and relevant to the future of medical practice. He offered students work in his laboratory as a student-selected component or option in the curriculum. This provided valuable research experience for the students and was highly rated by them.

The dedicated general practitioner

H.M. was a general practitioner with an appointment in the University Department of General Practice. She provided a much valued perspective of general practice in different courses throughout the curriculum and also was responsible for arranging community-based experiences for students in the first and later years of the curriculum. Students admired her as a role model, and a number indicated that she was the sort of doctor they would want to look after themselves and their family.

The imaginative obstetrician

R.S. was professor of obstetrics. He served on the school's curriculum committee and chaired the phase 3 and the reproductive system block committees. He was dedicated to teaching obstetrics and gynaecology but was also a powerful proponent of the contribution his subject made to the overall curriculum and the school's learning outcomes. Students' participation in prenatal clinics contributed to the health promotion learning outcome, and the audit of deliveries and maternal outcomes contributed to their understanding of patient safety, quality control and prevention of errors. He also had a vision of the importance of the doctor as a member of the healthcare team and introduced interprofessional education in the problem-based sessions in the reproductive system block, where the medical students learned alongside midwifery students. He carefully constructed the problems so that the more theoretical knowledge of the medical students and the more practical experience of the midwifery students were both required to tackle a problem.

The popular orthopaedic surgeon

R.T., an orthopaedic surgeon, received the student Best Teacher Award. Students found his lectures and his clinical teaching inspirational. He was appointed as director of a newly created clinical skills centre and went on to develop an interest in simulation and new approaches to clinical teaching including the use of ambulatory care clinics. He studied for and was awarded a Master's degree in Medical Education and, at his graduation, students as a group stood and applauded the conferment of the degree on him.

ENT, Ear, nose and throat; *OSCE,* objective structured clinical examination.

to make the programme a success. Years later, after everything had been completed, a general feeling was that the students' experience during this first year had matched or even surpassed their experience in later years, confirming the importance of the teachers (and the students) rather than the curriculum or the physical environment. Too often in a medical school, we focus on the curriculum and the physical resources rather than on the teachers who, working with the students, are the key ingredient in the education programme.

In his TED Talk, "How to Escape Education's Death Valley," which attracted over one million views, Ken Robinson highlighted the importance of teachers. He argued that investing in teachers is not just a cost but an investment, and that no education system is better than the teachers in the system (Robinson, 2013). In the classic text on the curriculum, Kelly (2004) stressed the importance of the teacher: "…the teacher as the central figure and his/her competence as the crucial factor in the quality of the educational experiences provided."

Matching the roles and teachers

The dean or those responsible in an institution need to ensure that all the eight roles described are represented by the teachers in the school. An individual teacher does not need to make a major contribution to all the roles but, for the success of the programmes, one or more teachers should be assigned to each of the roles as a major responsibility.

A teacher's level of commitment and expertise relating to a role may vary from a basic understanding and engagement with the role to a greater expertise and involve-ment. For each role, we have suggested both the expectation for every teacher in relation to the role and also the higher level of commitment expected of an expert or master teacher, who represents excellence and outstanding performance relating to the role. A teacher is not expected to be an expert in all eight roles. The challenge for school teachers in this respect has been described in a 2016 blog by Sir Michael Barber, formerly Chief Education Advisor to Pearson:

> For most of the past century we have bundled a very complex set of
> disparate skills into a single role we call the "classroom teacher." Teachers
> must have deep content knowledge to understand the scope and sequence
> of a curriculum, and pedagogical expertise to plan effective lessons and
> evaluate student comprehension and mastery. We also ask them to be
> charismatic presenters, a coach/mentor to provide student support and
> motivation for students to persevere, and project managers able to keep
> track of each student's academic process. It is incredibly difficult, and
> perhaps unrealistic, to expect to find such a diverse skill-set in a single
> individual. As a result the past few years has seen various attempts to
> "unbundle" the teacher.

Different roles require different skills and abilities of the teacher, and teachers may have a preference about the roles where they want to have the greater impact.

This should be taken into consideration when roles are assigned. We recall one teacher who was rated badly as a lecturer and who felt uncomfortable giving lectures. When reassigned to supporting students and facilitating their learning in the learning resource area, she performed magnificently and was highly rated by the students. She also had greater job satisfaction. Sending her on a faculty development programme to improve her lecturing skills would, almost certainly, have been less productive.

It is a useful exercise to ask teachers to compare their current role in the school with what would be their preferred role. When this exercise was carried out at the medical school in Dundee, there was a good match between actual and preferred roles (Harden and Crosby, 2000). Some differences were found, however. One surgeon who had not had a significant part to play in the development of the curriculum indicated his wish to do so and was appointed as a member of the curriculum committee, with excellent results. Another member of staff indicated a wish to be more involved in the assessment programme and was given responsibility as coordinator of an objective structured clinical examination (OSCE). An example of a questionnaire that can be used to determine teachers' views on their roles is given in Table 11.2.

Mismatch between a school's requirements and the available teaching skills

Deficiencies or gaps between what is required and what is provided by existing staff may arise, particularly with regard to specialist expertise in areas such as assessment, the development of a curriculum map, the implementation of a blended learning programme or even the use of a flipped classroom or team-based learning. In these circumstances, there are a number of options (Harden and Crosby, 2000):

- Ignore the deficiencies. This is usually a recipe for disaster, with frustration developing on the part of both staff and students. An adverse effect on the quality of teaching is almost inevitable.
- Change the curriculum to accommodate the available teaching roles. If, for example, a school is populated by good lecturers who lack expertise in group facilitation, one can design the curriculum to place a greater emphasis on lectures rather than on problem-based learning, where there is a need for tutor-facilitated small group work. The compromises that such an approach entails may or may not be acceptable, and an institution has to make this judgement. The decision is not an easy one and it could be argued that a lecture-based curriculum with excellent lectures is preferable to a problem-based curriculum with poor problem-based facilitation.
- Retrain staff in the institution to fulfil the required roles. This is possible but requires a commitment from the staff and administration and an energetic and focussed staff development programme.

Table 11.2 Questionnaire to assess a teacher's perception of his or her current personal commitment and preferred future commitment to each of the eight roles

Teacher's role	Current personal commitment					Preferred personal future commitment				
	None	Little	Some	Consid-erable	Great	None	Little	Some	Consid-erable	Great
	1	2	3	4	5	1	2	3	4	5
Information provider and coach										
Facilitator and mentor										
Assessor and diagnostician										
Curriculum developer and implementer										
Role model as teacher and practitioner										
Manager and leader										
Scholar and researcher										
Professional										

THE ROLES OF THE TEACHER TODAY AND IN THE FUTURE

- Recruit new staff who have the appropriate expertise to fill the roles. This is easier in a new school but may also be implemented in an established school when staff leave or when new appointments are created.
- Make special arrangements to meet the need by appointing temporary staff or consultants. This option should be considered if the other options are not available or are less attractive.

Teacher evaluation

Consideration of a teacher's roles in the curriculum should be a part of the teacher evaluation system. A teacher rated by students and peers as a poor lecturer, may perform well, as we have described, with small groups of students or, alternatively, as a developer of resource materials. Students may express different levels of satisfaction with the same teacher, even in the same course, according to the model of teaching being assessed (Husbands, 1996). We discussed different approaches to teacher evaluation in Chapter 10.

The time commitment of staff to teaching can be assessed in terms of not just contact hours in face-to-face teaching in lectures or clinics, but also in the fuller range of activities expected of the teacher, as defined in the roles. The involvement of staff across widely varying teaching roles, including time spent on curriculum planning and production of resource materials, can be incorporated into measures of teacher activity (Bardes and Hayes, 1995).

A school's responsibilities for the teachers employed

The medical school has responsibilities to the teachers employed. We have called these responsibilities "the five Rs," and they are directly or indirectly related to the roles of a teacher (Fig. 11.2).

Recruitment of teachers

The roles required in a school should be taken into consideration when a teacher is appointed. What is needed in a medical school is a balanced team of staff responsible for delivering all aspects of the curriculum. This may be reflected in job specifications and in staff contracts. A school may not need five staff with special expertise in assessment, but it certainly needs one.

Each staff member can bring something special and different to the school, as described by John Sexton, President Emeritus, New York University (Sexton, 2004):

> ...for it to be rational for people of great talent to choose to be university teachers, stereotypes of status must be broken. All faculty must come to think differently about their colleagues. Everybody will have a role and respect, but that does mean that everybody will have the same rights and responsibilities, just as appreciating a percussionist and a violinist in a symphony orchestra does not mean that they are the same. The university

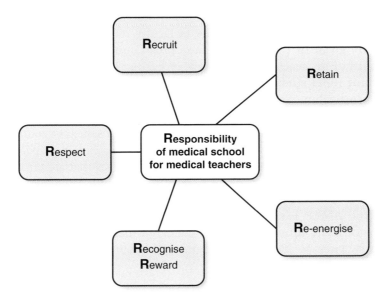

Figure 11.2 Five responsibilities of a medical school for its teachers

I envision will not be one that devalues roles, but one that genuinely values different kinds of faculty.

Other factors may be important in the recruitment of teachers, including content knowledge, clinical expertise, research ability and revenue earning potential.

Retain the teacher

Efforts should be made by an institution to retain teachers appointed. The annual turnover in the departments of medicine and surgery at the University of Arizona was reported by Schloss et al. (2009) to be between 4.9% and 8.3%, at an overall annual cost to the university of more than $400,000. It was argued that the magnitude of the costs warranted substantial efforts to foster faculty success in retention. We argue in this book that explaining to staff the different roles expected of them and matching, as far as possible, their preferences with the roles assigned leads to greater job satisfaction and, as a result, greater retention of staff. Teachers should be helped to own the process by working with them in identifying their optimum role. The school also has a responsibility, if they wish to retain a teacher, to provide the necessary infrastructure to support the teacher in whatever role is assigned and also to give him or her sufficient time to meet the demands of the role.

Re-energise the teacher

It is important to keep the teacher enthusiastic about teaching and also up to date in medical education practice. A medical school has a responsibility to ensure that teachers have relevant staff development opportunities, and a school-wide faculty development programme can contribute to faculty retention (Ries et al., 2009). Examples are given in Chapter 10. Many programmes focus on the technical skills required of the teacher – how to give a lecture, how to manage a problem-based learning (PBL) student group, how to assess students in an OSCE or how to design a curriculum. Some look at the educational or theoretical underpinning of teaching and learning. Often neglected, however, is an understanding of the different roles of a teacher and how these are changing. Introductory courses should explore the different roles and the expectations of a teacher in respect to these roles. Teachers should participate in more advanced courses that are targeted at the roles assigned to them, where the role is examined in more detail, along with the necessary understanding and skills. Face-to-face and online courses are available, including the AMEE Essential Skills in Medical Education (ESME) courses, which provide basic introduction, and courses which examine in more detail roles such as assessor, leader and researcher (https://amee.org/amee-initiatives/esme-courses).

Faculty development programmes are now a feature of the support for teachers in medical schools. If delivered appropriately, they can result in more effective teaching for the student and more job satisfaction for the teacher (McLean et al., 2008; Steinert et al., 2016; Steinert, 2017).

The programme for a teacher should be tailored to meet the needs of the individual teacher; this may succeed where the "one size fits all education" model may fail (Tyree, 1996). The aim of a staff development activity may be to make teachers better at what they are already doing and/or to help them to acquire new skills and fulfil new roles that were previously not within their remit.

Staff development, as discussed in Chapter 10, should be based not only around courses, and staff can be stimulated and encouraged by supporting their participation in conferences and meetings. This provides an opportunity to rekindle their enthusiasm by talking with colleagues with similar interests and problems, and also helps them acquire new ideas and approaches that may be valuable in their own setting.

A lack of funds allocated by a medical school to support such activities is a false economy. Supporting teachers' participation in education courses, face-to-face or online, and their attendance at conferences are good investments for an institution. Financial resources devoted to faculty development programmes can also result in significant financial benefits for the institution (Topor and Roberts, 2016).

Recognise the teacher

Teachers should be recognised for their achievements in the roles with which they are identified. For each of the eight roles, we have described the additional features that can distinguish excellent or outstanding performance. Such achievements should be recognised with promotion or financial incentives. We have come a long way since

Roger (1987) in a text, *Flexner: 75 years later,* expressed concern about the failure to recognise teachers' contributions to the education programme:

> *Let's cut out talking nonsense about how we will reward faculty for teaching and show that we really mean it. I don't need to spell out what this implies in the way of recognition, salaries, promotion, and the like. But if we want faculty to value teaching as an important part of their lives, the changes here must be profound. We've played sanctimonious games here for years. (p. 42)*

More recently, Michael Whitcomb (2003), former editor of *Academic Medicine,* highlighted the need to recognise faculty:

> *...there is widespread agreement that those members of the faculty who are most committed to, and involved in, the education of medical students must be supported and rewarded, both professionally and financially, and that the central administration of the school must play a key role in seeing that this happens. (p. 117)*

Recognising the teachers for their input to the curriculum and the value of their roles and what they offer are important and bring vitality to a school.

Respect the teacher

Finally, it is important for teachers to be shown respect for the difficult job they are doing and for the different roles expected of them. In his leading text on the subject of respect, Sennett (2003) wrote "Lack of respect, though less aggressive than an outright insult, can take an equally wounding form. No insult is offered another person, but neither is recognition extended; he or she is not seen – as a full human being whose presence matters."

In a chapter *Productivity through People* in their classic text *In Search of Excellence,* Peters and Waterman (1986, p. 238) highlighted the importance of respect: "There was hardly a more pervasive theme in the excellent companies than respect for the individual. That basic belief and assumption were omnipresent."

Respect for teachers is important. Lack of respect for general practitioner teachers was identified in the report *By Choice – Not By Chance* (Health Education England and Medical Schools' Council, 2016) as an important factor in students not choosing general practice as a career. Teachers will have a range of roles in a successful curriculum, and all of these should be respected.

An institution's commitment to teaching

The recognition by an institution of the different roles of a teacher and their importance helps make explicit the institution's commitment to teaching. A review of the roles can contribute to an evaluation of the educational programme, and the elements of the roles valued indicate the philosophy underpinning the school's education programme. Consideration of the roles can also facilitate the process of change, with which all schools must engage. This includes identifying traditional as well as new roles for the teacher.

Disjunction between beliefs and practice

There may be a disjunction between a teacher's knowledge, competence and performance. Even if teachers have the knowledge and are competent, they may not perform because they do not believe in the approach being implemented in the school (Fig. 11.3). Problems arise when a teacher agrees to a role in public but, in fact, does not accept the role that is out of tune with their personal beliefs. This disjunction between the teacher's conception of teaching and her or his teaching practice inevitably influences the delivery of the teaching. An example is the teacher who does not believe in a problem-based approach in the curriculum but is required to serve as a facilitator with the PBL discussion groups. In PBL, the teacher has an important role to play, but this is as a facilitator of the students' learning rather than as an information provider. The teacher who has not accepted or understood this role of facilitator falls back on the more comfortable direct teaching or didactic style, and the small group session assumes the form of a tutorial rather than a group exploration of the issue.

Knowledge, competence and performance	Action
The teacher knows what to do, is capable and will perform	Performs
The teacher knows what to do, is capable but does not perform	Competent but logistic problems or a lack of belief prevents performance
The teacher knows what to do, but is not capable and cannot perform	Understands but is not competent and does not perform
The teacher does not know what to do, is not capable and cannot perform	Does not understand, is not competent and does not perform

Figure 11.3 Knowledge, competence and performance of the teacher

Norton et al. (2005) have found that teachers' **intentions** with regard to their teaching practice were more oriented towards knowledge transmission than their **beliefs or conceptions** of teaching, which favoured more facilitation of learning. This may be the result of the constraints of the context in which the teacher operates. It may also at least in part be the result of teachers not having thought about their educational approach sufficiently to operationalise their beliefs in appropriate teaching strategies.

Describing this disjunction, Opfer and Peddler (2011) have suggested:

> *...although individual teachers have their own beliefs and practices about teaching and learning, schools collectively also have beliefs and practices about teaching and learning that constitute what complexity theorists refer to as the 'collective conceptual orientation'. (p. 392)*

We believe that the answer to what is a not uncommon disjunction between beliefs and practice is for the teacher and institution to focus on the teachers' roles and for more time to be spent on understanding the merits and value of the different roles, rather than the teacher being provided with a how-to-do-it type of prescription for his or her job. Constantly redefining with the school your role as a teacher will help align your teaching practice with the curriculum needs and will increase the likelihood that you achieve job satisfaction and your students learn more effectively.

The future roles of the teacher

Changes in medical education

As teachers, we should not be curators of some glorious medical education past. We should look to our roles as part of an exciting future in which we innovate and support and contribute to changes in medical education. These are likely to include:

- More authentic competency-based curricula designed to meet change in the healthcare delivery system and public expectations.
- Shortened duration of training, with a move from a time-based to a competency-based model.
- Breaking down the barriers between the different phases of undergraduate, postgraduate and continuing education, with more attention paid to a continuum of education.
- Greater collaboration between the stakeholders, not only internationally but also locally and in the different healthcare professions.
- Unbundling the curriculum with sharing of the responsibility for a student's learning and with a single medical school not expected to cover all of the elements.
- Increasing emphasis on scholarship and professionalism in medical education and recognition of the broader responsibilities of a teacher, as discussed in Chapters 9 and 10.
- Training in education for all teachers and a requirement to maintain education competence in the context of the changes taking place.
- Increasing student engagement in the education programme, with students as partners in learning rather than consumers.

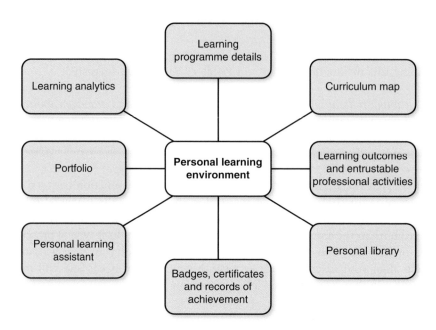

Figure 11.4 The student's personal learning environment

- A greater understanding of how the brain works, with adaptive learning personalised to the needs of the individual students.
- Students having their own personal learning environment that includes the learning resources, or curriculum map showing their planned and experienced progress and evidence of their achievements (Fig. 11.4). Students' interaction with their personal learning environment may be assisted by a personal learning assistant.
- The extensive use of digital maps and analytics to help learners navigate through the education programme and find flexible paths appropriate to their needs.
- Advances in educational technology, including virtual reality and augmented reality.

The future roles of the teacher

It is impossible to predict how these changes will play out in practice, but it is possible to make some educated guesses about how the changes are likely to affect the roles of a teacher. Many of the changes are already with us, and the roles of the teacher are already changing. As William Gibson once said, "The future is already here – it is just not very evenly distributed."

With changes in education and what is expected of the teacher, there may be an element of role inverting or even conflict. The result may be that teachers find themselves in a culture in which their role identity is no longer clear (Colbeck, 1998), and there may be uncertainty about what it means to be a basic scientist or a clinician who is a teacher. Establishing the roles of the teacher is important and, as argued by Stella Lowry (1993): "No proper review of an education system should ignore the role of the teachers."

Here are some suggestions as to how your role as a teacher may change.

Information provider

You will continue to have a role as information provider, but the focus will change. With the continuing expansion of information resulting from advances in medicine and medical practice, the need to identify the required core information and the threshold concepts will become even greater. Learners will acquire the necessary vocabulary and an awareness in medicine of different conditions, investigations and treatments, but not necessarily have detailed information about each.

More emphasis will be placed on your role as a curator of information, in which your role is to filter and make sources of information available for your students. So also will your role in ensuring that students know, when faced with a problem, how to ask the right question, know where to find the answer and know how to evaluate what they find. For the student, learning is not just about knowing the answers to problems; it is about knowing how to ask the right question, find the answers and evaluate them. Your role as an information coach is to ensure that students have these skills.

Facilitator

The move from information provider to facilitator is likely to accelerate, supported by learning analytics and tools such as curriculum maps. With greater student engagement, the relationship between students and the teacher will change. Facilitation of learning will take place not only face to face but at a distance online.

Curriculum developer

The teacher's role in relation to the curriculum will change in line with the developments signalled above. Your understanding of the curriculum and a contribution to its planning will be essential. This will include an appreciation of your role in a blended learning programme that combines face-to-face and online learning.

Assessment

We have discussed trends in assessment in Chapter 6 and the assessment PROFILE for a school. Assessment will no longer be something that happens at the end of a course or module but will be integrated into the teaching programme for which you are responsible. Greater importance will be attached also to your role in helping students develop the motivation and skills to assess their own competence after graduation from the school as part of their preparation for lifelong learning.

Role model

The role of the teacher as a role model will be, if it is not already, a key role for you in the future. This is particularly important in the context of the technical developments in medicine and education.

Manager and leader

This role will also become more important, given the increasing complexity of the education programme that results, for example, in integration and interprofessional education, education at multiple sites and the need to strive for effectiveness and efficiency in the programme. Educational change in medicine will be an imperative in the future, with management and leadership implications. Decisive leadership will be required to address the future challenges.

Scholar and researcher

The concept of the teacher-scholar will be recognised to a greater extent than it is today, with teachers reflecting on their experiences, innovating in relation to their teaching practice and sharing their experiences with others.

Professional

A high standard of professionalism will be expected of teachers, with an appropriate code of conduct and an obligation to evaluate their own competence and to keep up to date in their teaching practice.

Teachers perform more efficiently when motivated, and a major factor in their motivation is that they are able to perform and are comfortable in their assigned roles. As medical education continues to become more complex, identifying and exploring your future personal roles in the teaching programme will become even more important. This text has been written to assist you and to compensate for the emphasis placed to date in medical education on curriculum approaches and teaching, learning and assessment methods, by highlighting and exploring the different roles a teacher performs. Looking to the future, we believe that a better understanding of your role will lead to more effective and efficient teaching and, at the same time, to greater job satisfaction for you as a teacher. The world will continue to need medical teachers. It is just that the roles of the teacher will be different. Richard Sennett (2006), an eminent sociologist, has argued that we are seen as valuable, not for what we have achieved in the past but for what we might do in the future (Craig and Fieschi, 2007).

Take-home messages

1. A consideration of the issues raised in this text with regard to your roles as a teacher will inform your teaching practice, provide you with a better understanding of the process and result in a greater job satisfaction – teaching can be enjoyable and even fun. Your students are also likely to learn more effectively.

2. A description of the roles expected of the teachers in an institution makes explicit the institution's commitment to teaching and the different contributions expected of teachers in the delivery of the education programme.

3. Identifying the roles of teachers that are necessary to allow the school to deliver its education programme will allow an institution to determine better whether staff are available with the competence required to meet the school's needs. This may inform appointment decisions.

4. Consideration of the required roles of the teacher is helpful when curriculum change is planned, particularly when this involves a significant difference in approaches to teaching and learning from those currently embedded in the curriculum.

5. Faculty development programmes should introduce staff to all eight roles of a teacher and provide more advanced training as required for staff to meet specific roles.

6. Consideration of teachers' roles can guide staff evaluation or appraisal, recognising that faculty rated high by students in one role may be rated low in another role.

Consider

- We earlier asked this question: How would the student learn if you were not there as a teacher? It is worth reflecting again on this from your own perspectives of the different roles we have described and your contribution to the curriculum. How would students miss you most if you were not there?
- What are your current roles in the curriculum, and what change in your roles would you wish?
- Looking at your institution, has it accepted the responsibilities for the teacher and his or her roles, as described in this chapter?
- Which of the eight roles should be given more attention or priority?

Explore further

Bardes, C.L., Hayes, J.G., 1995. Are the teachers teaching? Measuring the educational activities of clinical faculty. Acad. Med. 70 (2), 111–114.

Colbeck, C.L., 1998. Merging in a seamless blend: How faculty integrated teaching and researching. J. High Educ. 69 (6), 647–671.

Craig, J., Fieschi, C., 2007. DIY Professionalism: Futures for Teaching. General Teaching Council, London.

Dron, J., 2007. Control and Constraint in e-Learning: Choosing When to Choose. IDEA Group, London.

Harden, R.M., Crosby, J., 2000. AMEE Guide No 20: The good teacher is more than a lecturer – the twelve roles of the teacher. Med. Teach. 22 (4), 334–347.

Health Education England and Medical Schools Council, 2016. By choice—not by chance: Supporting medical students towards future careers in general practice. www.hee.nhs.uk/our-work/hospitals-primary-community-care/primary-community-care/supporting-medical-students-towards-careers-general-practice.

Husbands, C.T., 1996. Variations in students' evaluations of students' lecturing and small-group teaching: A study at the London School of Economics and Political Science. Stud. Higher Educ. 21 (2), 187–206.

Irby, D.M., 1994. What clinical teachers in medicine need to know. Acad. Med. 69 (5), 333–342.

Joyce, B., Calhoun, E., Hopkins, D., 2009. Models of Learning – Tools for Teaching. Open University Press, Buckingham, England.

Kelly, A.V., 2004. The Curriculum: Theory and Practice. SAGE Publications, London.

Kugel, P., 1993. How professors develop as teachers. Stud. Higher Educ. 18 (3), 315–328.

Lowry, S., 1993. Teaching the teachers. BMJ. 306, 127–130.

McAllister, L., Lincoln, M., McLeod, S., et al., 1997. Facilitating learning in Clinical Settings. Stanley Thornes, Cheltenham, England.

McLean, M., Cilliers, F., van Wyk, J.M., 2008. Faculty development: Yesterday, today and tomorrow. Med. Teach. 30 (6), 555–584.

Nikendei, C., Ben-David, M.F., Mennin, S., et al., 2016. Medical educators: How they define themselves – results of an international web survey. Med. Teach. 38 (7), 715–723.

Norton, L., Richardson, J.T.E., Hartley, J., et al., 2005. Teachers' beliefs and intentions concerning teaching in higher education. High Educ. 50 (4), 537–571.

Opfer, V.D., Peddler, D., 2011. Conceptualizing teacher professional learning. Rev. Educ. Res. 81 (3), 376–407.

Peters, T., Waterman, R.H., 1986. In Search of Excellence. Profile Books, London.

Ries, A., Wingard, D., Morgan, C.V., et al., 2009. Retention of junior faculty in academic medicine at the University of California, San Diego. Acad. Med. 84 (1), 37–341.

Robinson, K., 2013. How to escape education's Death Valley. http://www.ted.com/talks/ken_robinson_how_to_escape_education_s_death_valley.

Roger, D.E., 1987. What we might do to improve the medical education process. In: Vevier, C. (Ed.), Flexner: 75 Years Later: A Current Commentary on Medical Education. University Press of America, New York.

Schloss, E.P., Flanagan, D.M., Culler, C.L., et al., 2009. Some hidden costs of faculty turnover in clinical departments in one academic medical center. Acad. Med. 84 (1), 32–36.

Sennett, R., 2003. Respect: The Formation of Character in an Age Of Inequality. Penguin, London.

Sennett, R., 2006. The Culture of the New Capitalism. Yale University Press, London.

Sexton, J., 2004. The common enterprise university and the teaching mission. https://www.nyu.edu/about/leadership-university-administration/office-of-the-president-emeritus/communications/the-common-enterprise-university-and-the-teaching-mission.html.

Steinert, Y., 2017. Staff development. In: Dent, J.A., Harden, R.M.Hunt, D. (Eds.), A Practical Guide for Medical Teachers, fifth ed. Elsevier, London. (Chapter 40).

Steinert, Y., Mann, K., Anderson, B., et al., 2016. A systematic review of faculty development initiatives designed to enhance teaching effectiveness: A 10-year update: BEME Guide No 40. Med. Teach. 38 (8), 769–786.

Topor, D.R., Roberts, D.H., 2016. Faculty development programming at academic medical centers: Identifying financial benefits and value. Med. Sci. Educ. 26 (3), 417–419.

Tyree, A.K., Jr., 1996. Conceptualizing and measuring commitment to high school teaching. J. Educ. Res. 89 (5), 295–304.

Whitcomb, M.E., 2003. The medical school's faculty is its most important asset. Acad. Med. 78 (2), 117–118.

White, R., Ewan, C., 1991. Clinical Teaching in Nursing. Nelson Thornes, London.

Index

Page numbers followed by "*f*" indicate figures, "*t*" indicate tables, and "*b*" indicate boxes.

Time-based approach, 165*t*
Transfer theory, 25
Transmitter of information
    responsibilities as, 38–39
    role of, 36–38
Transportability, 220
Transprofessional education, 127*f*
Transversal competencies, 115, 115*t*
Travelling theory, 24–25
'Troublesome knowledge', 44*b*

Utility, of evidence, 238–239

Validity, 168
Vertical integration, 125
Vision, of medical school, 110–111

Web-based information resources,
    81–82
Wisdom, in information pyramid,
    45, 45*f*
World Federation for Medical
    Education, 261